Skinny Bitch

....

ULTIMATE EVERYDAY COOKBOOK

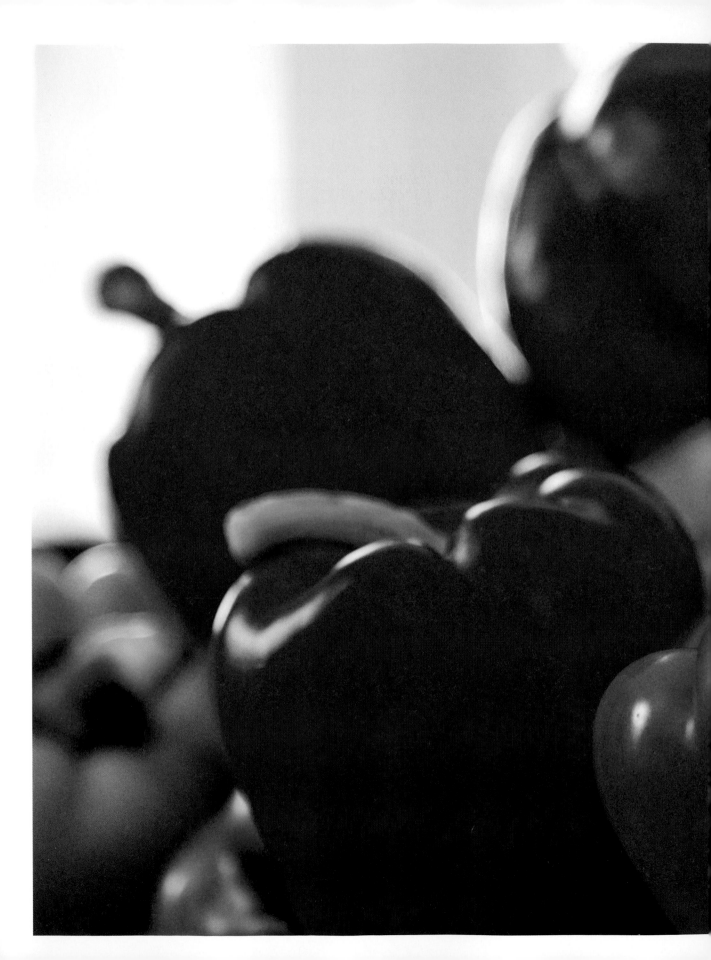

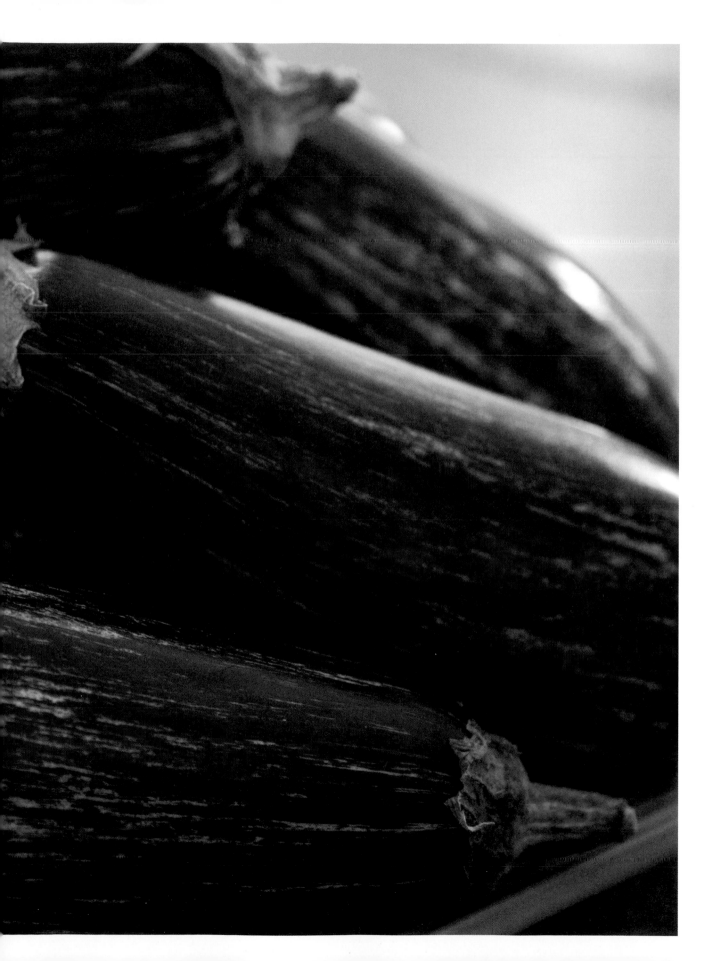

Skinny Bitch

ULTIMATE EVERYDAY COOKBOOK

KIM BARNOUIN

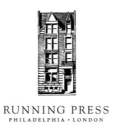

RUNNING PRESS
PHILADELPHIA • LONDON

9   8   7   6   5   4   3   2   1

Digit on the right indicates the number of this printing

Library of Congress Control Number: 2010931148

ISBN 978-0-7624-3937-9

Design by Joshua McDonnell
Photography: Front Cover and pp 2, 3, 8, 11, by Steve Belkowitz
All Other Photography by Matt Armendariz

Edited by Jennifer Kasius

Typography: Archer, Avenir, and Bembo

Running Press Book Publishers
2300 Chestnut Street
Philadelphia, PA 19103-4371

Visit us on the web!
www.runningpresscooks.com

To my son, Jack; Never forget to dream big and to believe in the impossible. And to my husband, Stephane; Thank you for always believing in everything I do.

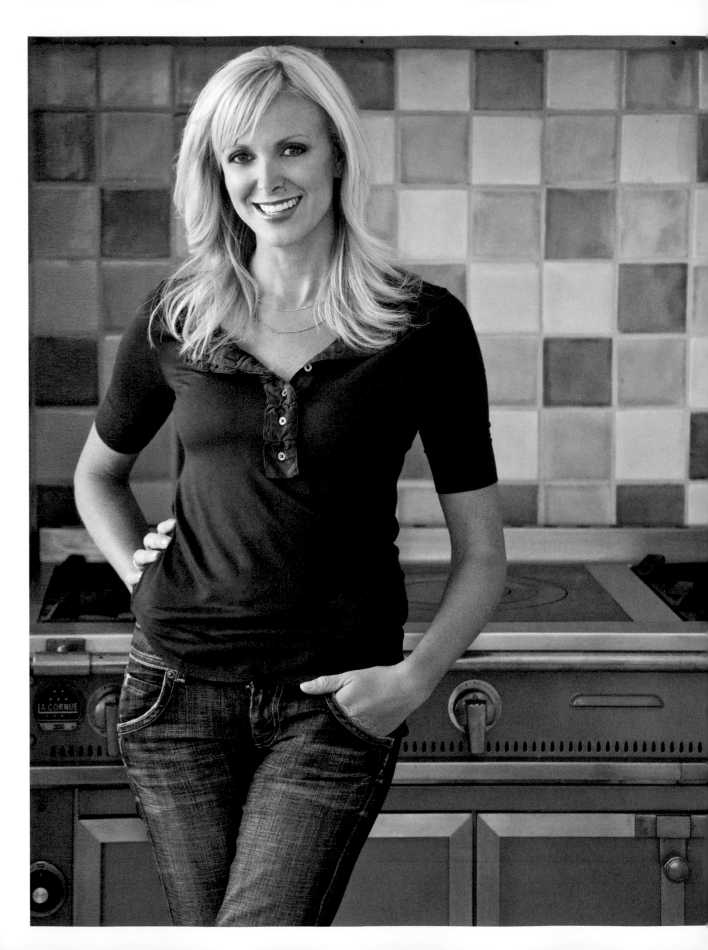

INTRODUCTION

If you had told me ten years ago I'd be writing a cookbook, I would have laughed in your face and squeezed your cheeks. *How cute.* My stove was camouflaged in cobwebs and the only soup I ate came from a can. Cooking just didn't fit into my program; microwaves did. It wasn't until I met my husband, a French chef, that I realized soup was much better made from scratch. What a concept. So, with a bit of fear and an open mind, I slowly started to make my way into the kitchen with baby steps. It took an honest effort, many unsuccessful dates with the Food Network, and a few new ovens. (Sorry, honey!) Eventually, I started to nail it. Cooking started to trigger a release of endorphins. I was on fire. Next task: cooking healthy.

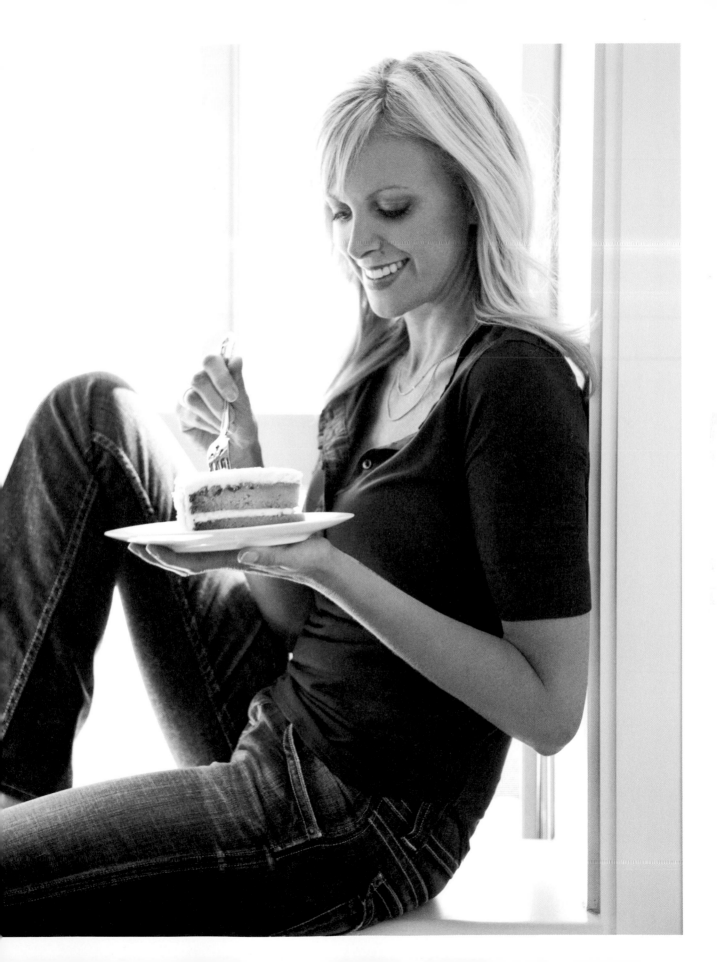

Of course, some of you have always had a reason to put healthy food on the table, and know that eating right is the only way to fuel your body. For others, maybe healthy cooking is new, uncharted territory. You smartened up, had a brief but necessary meltdown, ate the rest of the bon-bons in your freezer, and then gave your diet a complete makeover. I've been there.

Then there are those of you who have been along for the ride since reading *Skinny Bitch*. We meet again, bitches. It seems like only yesterday I was all over your asses for treating your bodies like a garbage disposal. Now, look at us. Our differences are behind us, and our bodies are looking better than ever.

When all is said and done, it doesn't really matter what world brought you into mine. You're here, with this cookbook in hand, for a reason. You know what that reason is, and you should give yourself a pat on the back. Making changes in your life, especially what you put on your plate, is no easy task. It's strenuous, and sometimes compromising. But I found it's also necessary and invigorating.

I should know. In my early twenties, my body was begging for an ultimatum of sorts. You see, I wasn't always the poster girl for women's health. I was consuming more sugar and caffeine than Willy Wonka and liked my pizza hot, cheesy, loaded with toppings—and hand-delivered by a smokin' hot pizza boy. Medical insurance was a luxury I couldn't afford, and I struggled with ongoing panic attacks, anxiety, and depression. I was in a constant "brain fog." I needed to know what the hell was wrong with me.

So, with few resources at my disposal, I turned to the Internet and good old-fashioned books and embarked on a pilgrimage of health and discovery.

It wasn't long before it became clear that what I was eating was indeed, *eating me*.

Every ailment I had pointed straight to food. I would make a small change in my diet, and my body responded immediately. I started to say goodbye to my vices, and everything changed for me—more clarity, happier moods, and the *best* hair days. Then the light blub went on in my head. Food was healing me. How come this wasn't public knowledge? I had a choice. I could go on living life in my little Kim bubble—a pizza addict with an unhealthy tan. Or I could invest in a new lifestyle and tell the world that food has the power to change your health. What would it be, blondie?

I think you know how this story ends.

Though choices are ours to make, I realized I never had much of a choice at all. After doing tons of research and completing a master's degree in holistic nutrition, how could I not open my big mouth? So, I did. I became a "Skinny Bitch." I set out to uncover what was plaguing me and ended up stumbling on what was plaguing a nation. Call it Pandora's box. Call it nonsense, if you will. But for me, and for millions of people who have fallen victim to our immoral food industry, this journey was a revelation. Halle-freakin-lujah.

Since *Skinny Bitch* hit the shelves, a lot has changed. For starters, I have become a wife, a mother, and a pretty damn good chef if I do say so myself. I guess I just grew up. But, deep down, I'm still the same wise-ass with a mouth like a sailor—just more refined. I still drop profanities at my computer screen, forgetting my impressionable four-year-old son is standing right in the doorway. And I'm still the same girl who has a few choice words for my girlfriends who still drink diet soda. What can I say? Some bitches just never change.

But, beyond that, I have realized there is a much bigger picture working for me here. It's not just about a book. My purpose is to guide women in making positive changes in their lives to help themselves and the people they love, like my husband did for me. Once one person makes a change, they have the power to trigger the domino effect throughout their household.

Today, I'm campaigning for yet another change. I am proposing for us to get back in the kitchen.

For some of you, there is no "getting back" in the kitchen. Cooking is an everyday activity, and you enjoy it. Good for you. As you know, it took me a long time to figure this out, so I hope this cookbook gives you some new ideas and tips on getting creative in the kitchen.

But, for the greater majority of us, cooking has become an event reserved for major holidays, graduations, and homecomings. Food is not where we have gone wrong—culture is.

It seems we have taken huge strides *backwards* when it comes to the way we think of food. We've all gotten busier—adopting a "Work Hard, Work Harder" motto—and our meals have suffered as a result. Lack of time and money have certainly played their parts. Trust me, I get it. But there's a bigger cost to all of this.

Without even knowing it, we have devolved into a culture that rushes through life, and quickly gives in to the lure of a cheap, quick meal cour-

tesy of the ubiquitous neighborhood fast-food joints. We continue to put in twelve-hour days, skipping from the office to parent-teacher conferences, dashing to soccer practice and ballet rehearsal, and then opting for a preservative-filled cheeseburger here, a fried chicken finger there. All the while, we exhaust the excuse that we don't have enough time to cook. Somewhere along the way, this has developed into a modern framework of efficiency, the product of a new generation. Long gone are the days when we enjoyed cooking meals with loved ones, followed by hearty family conversation: The jibber-jabber of Dad's promotion, Junior's batting average, Sally's test scores, and Mom's slightly embarrassing obsession with *General Hospital*. Not only have we lost precious family bonding time, we've also lost our health.

For that convenient, cheap thrill in a wrapper, we are doing some serious damage to our bodies. The rise of heart disease, arthritis, osteoporosis, and cancer isn't just a pretty little coincidence. Use your noggin. These diseases are just another by-product of our food industry. Experts even suggest that up to one-third of all cancers are related to diet.[1] Then tag on the calories and refined sugars, and preservatives. As our daily lives grow busier and busier, our waistlines grow thicker and thicker. It's a vicious circle. Every time we forgo a home-cooked meal for the drive-thru, we consume an average of 50 percent more calories, fat, and sodium. Pot bellies and love handles come free with each order! It's no wonder we live in a world with more than one billion overweight adults with a whopping 300 million of them considered obese.[2] We're ordering it right off the Value Menu.

We need to quit using food as a quick fix. Food has a special power. It has a *soul*. It has the ability to bring people together just for the sake of enjoyment. It's time for us to get back to the days when Mom accidentally broiled apple pie and Dad had to reassure the fire department that there was not a problem. The days when roommates bonded over a home-cooked eggplant lasagna and great records. The days when young, independent women chose to cook themselves a good meal rather than sit in their office at 10 p.m. to meet a deadline. I want us to find new ways to enjoy cooking and realize that the kitchen doesn't have to present difficulty. Let's kick the mind-set that quick, savory meals are exclusive to fast food chains and restaurants.

So, what's stopping us?

Without a doubt, most will blame time. Or a lack thereof. I'm not implying that you drop everything and hole up in the kitchen every night of the week. Your pots and pans don't offer the most scintillating social interaction. I hear you. And I wouldn't expect you to give up the restaurant experience. It's fun, and nice to have someone else wait on you every once in a while. What I *am* suggesting is to pick a few days and nights a week when you can enjoy a traditional meal and the timeless beauty of preparing it. Often those days and nights of cooking will lead to leftovers, which save you even more time. Make your kitchen a playground.

Next on the list will be the issue of money. People tend to think that it costs more money to cook homemade meals, but actually, the opposite is true. I cannot dispute that the 99-cent menu is easy on the wallet, but if you shop smart, the ingredients for one dinner can cross over to many. Dinners turn into packed lunches for work or school the next day. Honestly, I couldn't say it better than the highly acclaimed food writer and author Mark Bittman, when he said "You don't need a capital investment for rice and beans, any more than you do for cheeseburgers and fries." Ten dollars can buy you a few key cooking utensils, and in the end, you get enough wholesome calories to live by.[3]

Finally, some of you will be candid and admit that you're just lazy. Or that cooking really isn't your thing. Well, guess what? Though your honesty is refreshing, being an overweight, lazy ass who cries about her cottage cheese thighs isn't really anyone's thing. Challenge yourself. Prepare a healthy dish, ask yourself how you feel and what you liked about it, and make tweaks. Take baby steps. Eating crap has done nothing but make you a statistic. Learn more about how cooking can help turn around your entire life.

To say that I have learned a great deal about cooking is an understatement. Since working on the first cookbook, *Skinny Bitch in the Kitch*, I have learned more about the art of cooking as personal therapy. I have fallen asleep with hundreds of different dog-eared cookbooks sprawled across my chest (each of them wonderful in their own right), formed close relationships with remarkable chefs, and thrown myself into the kitchen head first. As a result, I think I've created something that brings all the ingredients together for one fun, practical, smart-ass cookbook. This is something for everyone. It's about time, dammit.

This book is a reflection of the changes in my life that have led to the way I now look at food. My eating habits have made so much progress. I no longer rely on "fake meats" for every meal, though they were my rock while making the transition from vegetarian to vegan. Don't get me wrong. I still enjoy imitation meats (hence, you will find some in my recipes and need not banish them from your freezer entirely either), but I use them more as a special treat now. My main focus is on fresh, seasonal, flavorful dishes that are quick and easy-to-prepare. I want people to know that it *is* possible to eat well and love every bit of it. It's not difficult. You're a big kid now—spitting out your Brussels sprout in a napkin destined for the bathroom trash bin is not acceptable. Nutritious fare has flourished, devising countless ways to taste delicious. A healthy diet shouldn't be thought of as deprivation but, instead, as bringing you a sense of enjoyment and pleasure that carry the added bonus of helping your body function to the best of its ability.

No matter what your dietary preference, I'm not here to judge. Though all the recipes in this book are technically vegan, this is not a cookbook designed specifically for vegans. The simple dishes in this cookbook were designed to satisfy, and *fool* for that matter, any palate. It's a cookbook meant to reignite the passion for stepping in the kitchen, freeing your mind, making a mess, learning a few things in the process, and setting something on the table that makes you feel empowered.

Remember you don't have to change the way you eat overnight. In fact, I don't recommend it. Make small changes here and there to ease into a new way of eating. Even if it's just eating a few more vegetable dishes a week or cutting back on fried foods, it's a choice and a worthwhile one.

So, my dear friends, it is time for me to wish you the best of luck. Use food to turn your health and life around—it is that powerful. Use food to clear your head. Use food to reunite friends. Use food to bring your family together. Use food to influence change. Use food to get laid, if it helps. *Just use it.* That's what it's there for.

Remember, no matter what led you to this cookbook, this is your opportunity. Invest in yourself, and your body will invest in you. Any positive changes you continue to make in your diet are steps in the right direction, and every choice you make is a new chance to discover just what you're capable of.

Trust me.

Your Friend,
Kim

P.S. For years, I have received e-mails with questions about everything from better nutrition and treating everyday ailments to my favorite food products. While I try to be responsive, I'd be kidding myself to say I have answered every e-mail. So, instead of waiting for you to come to me with questions, I decided I would bring Skinny Bitch to you. My newest baby is a free daily e-mail feed that answers your questions before you even ask. Check it out at www.healthybitchdaily.com.

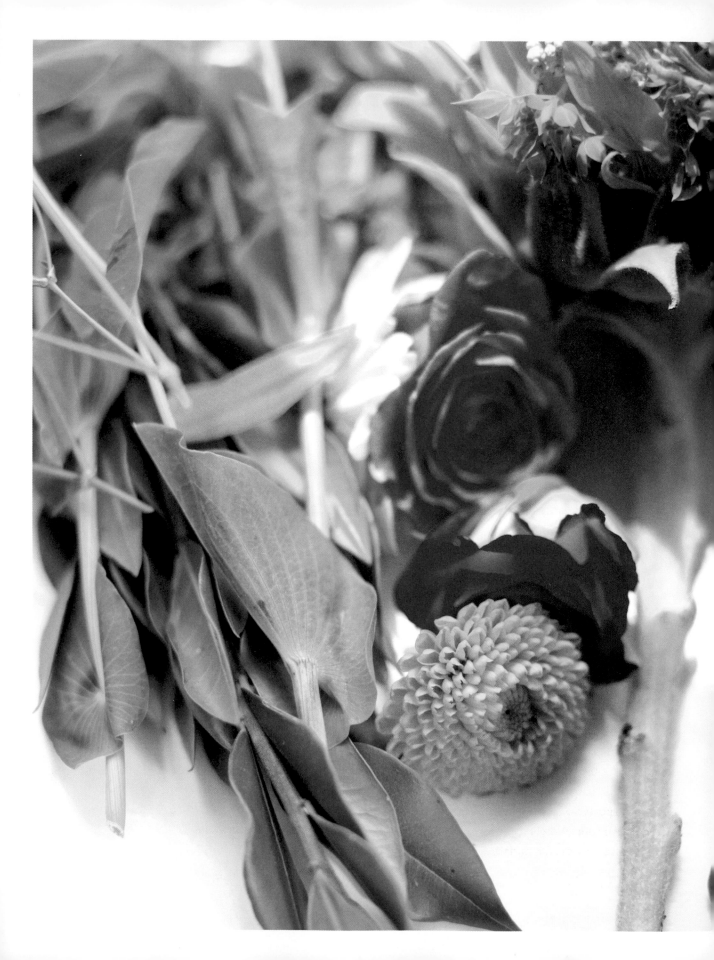

PART ONE

SUSTAINABILITY: A GREENER DIET

Mother Earth has a problem. A problem much bigger than drunk texting or the lack of parking at your local Starbucks. She has a *huge* boo-boo. Not the kind you just stick a bandage on. This one is gonna need some major TLC.

It's called global warming—the very thing that is wiping out our polar bears and giving Death Valley a name to live up to. And, it's not going anywhere. That is, unless we do something about it.

Now, what do our diets have to do with global warming? As it turns out, the planet actually does give a shit whether you have bacon for breakfast or a bowl of cereal.

This is not where I criticize factory farming for its inhumane practices and utter disdain for animal welfare. *Skinny Bitch* already did that. Actually, I've got a whole other bone to pick with the industry: our food system and its immense contributions to greenhouse gas emissions and global warming.

Go figure. The world isn't flat. Everything we do becomes a part of the vicious circle, and what we eat has a lot more to do with this than most think. Animal agriculture makes a 40 percent greater contribution to global warming than all transportation in the world combined; it is the number one cause of climate change.[4]

But, it doesn't end there. According to the United Nations, factory farming is one of the most significant contributors to the most serious environmental problems—land degradation, climate change, air pollution, water shortage, water pollution, and loss of biodiversity—on a local and global scale.[5]

This isn't just a problem. The common cold is a problem. These environmental problems, my friend, are a disease.

So, it's clear, our diets are pissing off the planet. Here are the five major ways our food systems are contributing to our own demise.

1. GREENHOUSE GAS EMISSIONS

Bad news. As much as we would like our foods to be raw, natural, and fresh from healthy soil, they are far from it. On today's consumer farm, our foods are grown with massive amounts of pesticides, herbicides, and chemical fertilizers, all of which are making you, me, and the earth sick.

Raising animals for human consumption is one of the world's leading emitters of carbon dioxide (CO_2), and the number one source of methane and nitrous oxide emissions.[6] Those are just the big guns, but there are more culprits. You can call them ammonia, hydrogen sulfide, carbon monoxide, cyanide, and phosphorus, for starters. As you could have guessed, these greenhouse gases are not something we want spraying into our atmosphere like a fire hose. But they do, trapping heat and depleting the ozone layer, contributing to a third of the globe's total greenhouse gas emissions.[7]

The process by which these manmade gases get from the farm into the air is not exactly what I'd call dinner-table conversation. One way is that farm animals, such as cattle, goats, chickens, sheep, and hogs, emit methane when they exhale to digest their food. Think of it as one disgusting burp. But here is where things get really appetizing. Like humans, animals poop, too. With one major difference: We humans have built waste-management infrastructures like toilets and sewage systems to manage our crap, while animals just do their business and have no choice but to rely on farmers to clean up after them. That's where the problem comes in. There are *billions* of animals pissing and shitting on factory farms. They produce 130 times as much waste as the human population—roughly 87,000 pounds of poop per second. Despite this, there is no safe, reliable system in place for disposing of farmed animal waste. Nobody is hauling it off, nobody is flushing it down the potty, and nobody is regulating it.[8] Instead, we control the problem by storing it in huge, open-air waste lagoons that are the size of football fields. If poop was polite and stayed within the confines of these pleasant lagoons without harming a fly, then maybe, just maybe, it would be a start in the right direction. But this shit is emitting greenhouse gases that, combined, are 324 times more harmful than carbon dioxide.[9] And, we cannot blame the animals. It's the standard diet of more than 756 million tons of grain and corn fed to animals in feedlots per year that causes this unrestricted emission

of methane and nitrous oxide.[10] Remember, by nature's standards, cows are supposed to eat grass and chickens are designed to nibble on wheat, veggies, and grass. But we have decided to play God. Leave it to us.

Now, sometimes farmers recycle manure so they can use it as fertilizer in agricultural fields. This is when nitrogen likes to play a little cloning game and produce even more nitrous oxide. This nitrogen free-for-all is then absorbed by the atmosphere, soil, water, and ocean, further adding to the greenhouse effect.[11] And so goes the circle of life.

Sorry, honey, but I'm not done yet. Indeed, I have saved the best for last. Aside from contaminating our air, water, and dirt, animal's caca also finds a sneaky way to make it into our food, *directly*. More than 40 diseases can be transferred to humans through animal manure in meat. These include *Salmonella, E. coli, Cryptosporidium,* and fecal coliform, which can be 10 to 100 times more concentrated than in human waste.[12] Who's hungry now?

2. WATER SUPPLY AND POLLUTION

We have gotten a little greedy as a culture, and forgotten the concept of give-and-take when it comes to our valuable water resources. A little mistake never hurt anyone, right? Yeah, not so much. Thanks to global warming, we're experiencing record droughts, lakes are shrinking, reservoirs are dropping to all-time lows, and polar ice caps are melting quicker than it takes your nails to dry. At the same time, there is a scarcity of usable water due to water pollution. Yet, human demand is higher than ever. Seems there is a big gap.

Again, livestock production is hard at work here. In fact, it's the largest contributor of water pollutants. Our water is quickly turning into a strange brew, with traces of animal waste, fertilizers, antibiotics, hormones, and pesticides eroding from nearby farm pastures.[13] Let's open the history books for a minute. In 1995, an eight-acre hog waste lagoon in North Carolina ruptured, spilling 25 million gallons of manure into the New River—an incident that until the BP Oil Spill remained the largest environmental disaster of its kind. Actually, twice as big as the MacDaddy of all spills six years earlier, Exxon-Valdez. And we didn't hear a peep. The spill wiped out acres of coastal wetlands and ten to fourteen million fish.[14] The vast body of water that all this shit spilled into is called our ocean, sweetheart. How special.

Aside from polluting our rivers and ground water, what do you think consumes nearly 8 percent of global water? Yup, it goes to hydrating animals and irrigating crops.[15] Suddenly, I feel parched.

3. DEFORESTATION

I've got a new problem for you to put in your pipe, Smokey. It's not a forest fire but, hell, it might as well be. Forget chopping down trees to make paper and pencils. We've gotten so much better at tearing down forest canopies to make room for more factory farms. Each year, we clear more than six million acres of Amazon rainforest to make more space for livestock to burp, crap, and meet their maker.[16] This has led to the second leading cause of climate change—deforestation.[17] Currently, livestock covers 30 percent of the Earth's entire surface, while 260 million acres of forest have been cleared for the meat-based diet.[18,19] Because we can't magically create new land, developers are tapping into our most beautiful natural resources,

yelling " Timber," —and up goes another factory farm. But, it looks like there is some solace for those on a green diet. A low-fat vegetarian diet requires less than half an acre per person to produce that food. Compare that to 2.1 acres per person for the meat eater.[20]

Looks like the grass isn't so green on the other side after all.

4. LACK OF BIODIVERSITY

Moooove over, wildlife. We need to make more room for livestock. Nope, not enough. Still not enough. Why don't we just take over Africa, and call it a day?

As we take down the trees, we are clearing and destroying land that is home to our wild animals for the use of livestock. Our need for *more, more, more,* at a pace of *now, now, now,* is causing serious loss of our natural habitats. Unlike humans, much of the planet's wildlife can only survive in specific regions. So when we chop, flatten, and crush their homes to construct another factory farm, they don't adapt well. They can't find food. They get sick. And they die.

Physical space for livestock is the bulk of the problem. However, we also have to account for land used to grow grain crops to feed the farm animals. Remember, we are talking a huge chunk of land. Today, 80 percent of corn, 95 percent of oats, and 56 percent of all U.S. farmland is dedicated just to beef production. To produce just one kilogram of beef, seven kilograms of grain are required to nurture said cow.[21] (I use the word *nurture* very loosely here.) When you consider that factory farming raises and slaughters more than ten billion land animals each year, that is a lot of space we are clearing for land to grow grain.[22] Let me put this into perspective. C'mon, it will make my day. If the cropland we currently use to produce grain for livestock was redirected for humans, we would be able to feed 800 million people who are starving in third-world countries.[23] That is just on land.

5. FISH DEPLETION

Under the sea, we continue to deplete the ocean of thousands of fish species every day. Unlike our lovely freshwater fish tanks at home, we cannot just refill the ocean with another pretty fishy our kids can affectionately call Nemo. Depletion equals extinction.

The problem is in the way we fish. Forget your idyllic images of fishermen perching on the edge of their boats with a fishing pole in one hand and a soda pop in the other. It's much more complex (and horrifically calculated) than that. Hundreds of thousands of hooks are propelled into the ocean in targeted areas to line and sink the "Catch of the Day." In pursuit of that tasty tuna, they kill plenty of other critters as well. Commercial fishing is quickly wiping out entire populations of mammals (whales, dolphins, polar bears), birds (albatross, penguins), and other beautiful sea creatures (krill, seahorses) as *bycatch*. Bycatch, as in, whatever else has to die in order to get what we're really fishing for.[24]

According to Jaan Suurkula, M.D., and chairman of Physicians and Scientists for Responsible Application of Science and Technology, our evolved way of fishing is a class-act way of telling the fishes to go play on the highway. "A new global study concludes that 90 percent of all large fishes has disappeared from the world's oceans in the past half century, the devastating result of industrial fishing," said Suurkula.[25] Judging by the direc-

tion we're headed, the killer whale will be sitting right next to Tyrannosaurus Rex in the museum, a relic from a lost time.

WHAT CAN WE DO?

The reality is that 99 percent of all land animals eaten, or used to produce milk and eggs in the U.S., are a product of the commercial factory farm system.[26] The very system threatening our ecosystem. There is just no way around it.

You really want to do something? Start kicking meat and dairy to the curb. Toodles. *Adios. Au Revoir.* Screw off.

Studies have found that omnivores contribute seven times the volume of greenhouse gases that vegans do.[27] For those mathematically challenged, that's a lot.

Let me spell it out for you: If every American skipped one meal of chicken per week and substituted veggie foods in its place, the carbon dioxide savings would be the same as taking more than a half-million cars off U.S. roads.[28] You hear that? 500,000 cars. The National Resources Defense Council is quick to throw out bold slogans like "Drive Less" and "Buy Hybrids" to reduce global warming, but they don't have the balls to tell people the number one way they can reduce carbon emissions is by eating vegetarian once a week. Once. That's a small commitment to solve a big problem.

YOUR CARBON FOOTPRINT

We have big feet. *Really* big feet. No matter how cute and dainty they look in those four-inch stilettos, it appears they're leaving a hell of a footprint in their wake. Every year, the average North American produces around twenty tons of CO_2 through their daily activities. To give you an idea of how big that is, Sasquatch, the global average per person is about *four* tons of CO_2 every year.[29] Do the math. We're spewing out sixteen more tons of CO_2 than the rest of the world, every year. And it has nothing to do with our shoe size.

Every day in going about our daily routines—brushing our teeth, driving to work, and eating dinner—we are adding to the scoreboard of greenhouse gas emissions. So, how big of a mark are you making on the planet? What's your carbon footprint? Before you pull out a calculator and start punching in numbers, take a chill pill. It's more complicated than you think. Your carbon footprint is a measure of the impact your actions and activities have on the environment. It considers the amount of energy you use in your home, the number of miles you drive to work, how often you travel, your recycling patterns (or lack thereof), and personal diet, to name a few.[30] But my only job is to help you measure your impact as far as what you put into your mouth. It's time you had your earth and ate it, too.

HOW FAR HAS YOUR FOOD TRAVELED?

Your food is earning more frequent flier miles than a bag of peanuts. And nobody is reaping the rewards. While more than eight hundred million tons of food a year are shipped around the hemisphere, food is traveling 25 percent farther than it did twenty years ago. In fact, it's one of the biggest and fastest growing sources of greenhouse gas emissions. Right behind factory farming.[31] "We are living in the era of the 1,500-mile-meal, where each ingredient typically travels that distance to get to your plate," said Kate Geagan, author of *Go Green, Get Lean.* "Unripe and unready, our food is picked to travel—eating oil and belching emissions. Eating locally is one way to reduce greenhouse gases."

Think long and hard about this: Our food takes an average of seven days just to arrive at the grocery store. It may be another two to five days before you make the mistake of putting it in your cart. What does this say about the freshness of your food? You got it. Diddly-squat.

The best solution is to buy produce locally grown as often as you can. You don't need to be hardcore. Every so often, enjoy foreign foods that aren't grown in your area. I do. You'll even find some ingredients in this cookbook that you cannot always get locally. But work local foods into your diet more often than not. Buying from your neighborhood farmers' market ensures you're not shipping your food in from halfway across the country and you're putting fresh ingredients on the dinner table.

HOW MUCH FOOD ARE YOU BUYING AND WILL YOU EAT IT ALL?

I know, I sound like your freakin' mother. But admit it, she had a point. Before I tell you you're going to bed without any dessert, just ask yourself next time whether you're biting off more than you can chew. If you are only feeding for one, why buy six pounds of carrots—unless you plan on turning into one.

The reason is simple. Nearly half of all the food harvested in the U.S goes to waste each year. Our food system produces about 3,774 calories per person every day, but we only consume about 2,100. The rest gets wasted, either by overeating or by tossing it in the dumpster.[32]

The best solution is to plan out your meals, including snacks, two weeks at a time, and prepare a grocery list that fits the bill. Account for foods that may go bad in those two weeks and possibly plan a bi-weekly trip to your local farmers' market for some fresh produce. (Neighborhood carpool, anyone?)

This isn't me trying to be a hard-ass. All this food that we are aimlessly wasting could help feed the more than eight hundred forty million people that are undernourished, or the twenty-five thousand people that die every day from hunger-related causes.[33]

Stick to the meal plan and you'll scratch the planet on its back.

WHAT KINDS OF FOOD ARE YOU BUYING: PLANT-BASED OR ANIMAL-BASED?

I'll say it again. It takes more than ten times the number of fossil fuels to produce a calorie of beef protein than a calorie of grain protein.[34] It is more energy efficient to grow grain for humans to eat than it is to grow grain, turn it into feed, feed it to animals, and then slaughter the animal—all to end back up in your pretty little mouth. But here's the funny thing: Apart from helping out the earth, eating green is *actually* good for you. The very foods with a high-carbon cost—red meat, pork, dairy products, and processed snacks—are also the foods chock-full of fat and unhealthy calories. When you go meatless, you win. Earth wins. Happy ending for everyone.

If you're having a hard time kicking your bad habit, get creative. When the going gets tough, girls explore their options.

Four Ways to Experiment With a Green Diet:

GET ACQUAINTED WITH YOUR SPICES: Learn how to cook and flavor foods with herbs and spices rather than animal fat. They're packed with health benefits from the Earth's soil, free of preservatives and cholesterol, and they can change up the flavor of a meal in a jiffy. (See pages 58-59.)

GROW A MINI GARDEN IN YOUR BACKYARD OR BUY A GARDEN KIT FOR YOUR PATIO: The distance your food is traveling from food to plate is mere footsteps, and you'll have fresher ingredients, guaranteed.

PENCIL IN MEATLESS MONDAY: If I had it my way, it would be Meatless Monday, Meatless Tuesday, Meatless Wednesday, and so on. But for you non-veggies, mark a set day in the calendar each week when you'll enjoy a meatless meal regardless of whether you're flying solo or cooking for four. It will present a new challenge in the kitchen and lower your carbon footprint. Each week, try to step it up and tag on another day. Before you know it, you'll be celebrating Meatless March!

JOIN A CSA (COMMUNITY SUPPORTED AGRICULTURE): Many traditional farmers are getting savvy and packaging boxes of locally grown produce delivered fresh to your door. It's not traveling far to get to you and you're not gassing up the Benz to pick it up. Most of these services will allow you to check how many times a week you want a new box, and what types of veggies you and your family want. Life made simple.

HOW PROCESSED IS YOUR FOOD?

By now, we are all very aware that processed foods are bad. As in, no good. As in, out to get us. Yet 90 percent of the average American household grocery budget goes toward filling the pantry with processed foods that are teeming with additives and preservatives, with no traceable nutrients.[35]

Whether we're talking about cancer, diabetes, Alzheimer's disease, Parkinson's disease, or coronary heart disease, the rate of food-related disease has been steadily rising. Each year about 550,000 Americans die of cancer, with one-third of these deaths attributed to poor dietary choices.[36] *Why?* Studies are finding a direct correlation with food processing and our health. In today's society, our foods are grown with shitloads of pesticides, herbicides, and chemicals to speed up their growth and preserve their shelf life. The FDA actually estimates that, every year, twenty pounds of pesticides are pumped into each American's food. At least fifty of these pesticides are classified as *carcinogenic*.[37] Just in case you are unfamiliar with the term, let me sound it out for you. Carcinogenic means *to cause or tend to cause cancer*. In layman's terms, our over-processed, pesticide-ridden diets are slowly killing us. And all we have to do is eat.

Need some more evidence? In July 2009, researchers at Rhode Island Hospital published a controversial study in the Journal of Alzheimer's Disease that found a concrete link between death from disease and levels of nitrates, nitrites, and nitrosamines found in processed foods.

According to Suzanne de la Monte, the leader of the Rhode Island Hospital study, we have become a "nitrosamine generation" without even knowing it. "Not only do we consume them in processed foods, but they get into our food supply by leeching from soil and contaminating water supplies used for crop irrigation, food processing, and drinking," said de la Monte.[38]

SMART BITCHES READ LABELS

All that really matters to grocery stores and retailers is that the food appears edible. By any means necessary. Too bad that apple had to be picked unripe, transported a great distance, then gassed to ripen it for sale. That's one way of doing it. The other route is to pump the foods with preservatives and irradiation to keep it stable for transport and sale. What? You're outraged? Well, luckily, these aren't your only options. There are two simple things you can do to guard yourself against this fate:

1. Buy Organic
2. Read Your Labels

CHOOSING ORGANIC: THE GLOBAL FRESCA DIET

Ever since major food companies caught wind of the term "organic" and noticed that it lulls consumers into a buying trance, it has become the hottest word in their vocabulary. They have worked overtime to stamp the organic sticker on everything from peanut butter to baby's diapers. But here's the twist: All we did was hear the word, and we jumped on the bandwagon. Did we know what organic *really* meant? Likely not. But we sure liked the sound of it.

While the term gets used and abused, simply stated, the organic sticker earns produce and ingredients the right to say they have been grown without the use of pesticides, chemicals, synthetic fertilizers, sewage crap, genetically modified organisms, or ionizing radiation.[42]

Eight Tips for Understanding What's in Your Food

You stand there in the frozen-food section, underdressed and unprepared for the polar temperatures that fill the aisle. Shit! Of all times to go braless, you chose today. But you'll be quick. You just need to check the calorie count on the Lean Cuisines and you'll quickly sashay to warmer pastures.

Stop right there! Reading the back of a box purely for its calories will get you nowhere. Low calories may seem like the yellow brick road to getting skinny, but they're not the path to getting healthy. Read your labels. Packaged snack foods, canned goods, frozen dinners, and boxed meal mixes can all promise a slashed calorie count, but they're crawling with preservatives and scary ingredients.

Study these tips and you'll become a pro at judging your foods with care:

1. LESS IS MORE: Check the number of ingredients. As a general rule of thumb, the lower the amount of ingredients, the better. Healthier, minimally processed foods tend to contain the fewest ingredients.

2. THE FINICKY FIVE: If fats, sugars, partially hydrogenated oils, or high-fructose corn syrup are in the first five ingredients, back away. Nobody will get hurt. Except for the company that was stupid enough to put it in your food. Now we're talking.

3. COOL IT ON THE CHOLESTEROL: The daily recommended intake is between two hundred and three hundred milligrams a day. Since your liver makes about 80 percent of it for your body to operate as usual (and is capable of making all of it), you don't need to get it through your diet.[39]

4. MONITOR YOUR SODIUM: Sodium is necessary, but when consumed in large amounts, it can stimulate high blood pressure. Choose foods that contain five hundred milligrams or less, with a healthy daily intake of two thousand milligrams or less.[40]

5. THE GOOD FATS, BAD FATS, AND LOW FATS: In general, you want five grams or less per serving, but invest some time in identifying what types of fats your food contains. Saturated and trans-fatty acids are not your friend. The healthy fats, monounsaturated and polyunsaturated, help to keep your heart healthy and lower overall cholesterol. Keep in mind, if the package preaches "low-fat," it usually means that refined starches and sugars are used as replacements to ensure tasting pleasure.

6. THE SECRET OF SUGAR-FREE: Don't let them trick you. Unless it's from a health food store and it's fruit-juice sweetened (agave nectar), it likely contains artificial sweeteners. Sugars, like high-fructose corn syrup and refined sugars, are the devil in disguise.

7. DON'T BE FOOLED BY ADVERTISING JARGON: The terms "all-natural" "fresh," and "no additives" carry little weight. Since these terms are loosely regulated by the FDA, they are tossed around like dollar bills in a strip club.[41]

8. NAMES THAT REQUIRE AN INTERPRETER: If you cannot pronounce it, it is likely to have spent some good time in a laboratory. Don't throw away your spelling bee ribbon just yet. Words like butylated hydroxyanisole, and propylene glycol are hard enough to pronounce, let alone spell (see page 32, The Skinny: Processed Foods).

Benefits of Buying Organic

When you buy organic, you are:

- Limiting your food's travel from production to plate
- Protecting yourself against nasty chemicals and pollutants that are used to grow many commercial consumer products
- Supporting local farmers who follow sustainable farming methods
- Investing in your local community rather than the factory-farm powerhouses that are screwing up our planet

Organic goods are like music to nature's ears. They are biodegradable, and come straight from the ground without shipping harmful pollutants off into our atmosphere and water supply. Rock on, organic. Rock on.

How Do I Know Produce Is Organic?

Often, buying from your local farmers' market or farming community is a good sign you are purchasing organic produce. However, many major commercial supermarket chains are changing their ways to meet the growing consumer demand. Look closer at the labels.

The USDA abides by three important factors to identify the labeling of organic produce:

- **100-percent organic:** Made with 100 percent organic ingredients
- **Organic:** Made with 95 percent organic ingredients
- **Made with organic ingredients:** Made with a minimum of 70 percent organic ingredients with strict restrictions on the remaining 30 percent, including no GMOs (genetically modified organisms)

Products with less than 70 percent organic ingredients may list those ingredients on the side panel of the nutritional information, but cannot brag they are organic on the front of the packaging.[43] Remember to do your due diligence and read the packaging rather than throwing it into the cart like She-Who-Knows-Her Shit. Keep in mind that it is always in your best interest to buy the most raw, true-to-form produce with 100 percent organic ingredients.

Does Organic Taste Better?

Hello?! Are puppies cute? Are thong bikinis uncomfortable? Yes, organic tastes like heaven! Especially when you consider the good you are doing for your body, your mind, the environment, and your community.

But, do-gooding aside, award-winning chefs across the world have been turning to organic food for years for its superior taste and quality. Let's look at the why: They are not shot up with chemical fertilizers and bloated with water to force the rapid growth factory farmers rely on. These fruits and veggies grow the old-fashioned way on a slow timer. Like soaking in a good marinade, they have the chance to absorb and select all the complex elements and nutrients found in carbon-rich soil, giving them time to develop thicker cell walls and more concentrated flavors. They sunbathe in minerals that make them juicy and enriched. In the end, we get a winner: Natural, plump, zesty, fresh produce that contributes to a nutritious, well-balanced diet. Yes, I did say *nutritious*. Studies are showing that organic produce is packed with more antioxidants, vitamins, and phytochemicals than chemically grown produce.[44] As if you needed another reason.

HOW DO I BUY LOCAL?

Purchasing produce *locally* does not imply finding the supermarket chain closest to your home. Sure, that's local and it does follow the path of least resistance, but still no cigar.

Buying locally refers to where the good was grown and produced. Back in the days when Grandpa walked shoeless in the snow to get to school (uphill both ways), local farms were the only option. As populations grew and a fast-food culture swallowed up the food chain, small-scale, traditional farmers were pushed to the side to make room for the big boys—the farms that would produce three times the amount in one-third the time. In the U.S., just four companies produce most of the nation's animal products—81 percent of beef, 73 percent of lamb, 57 percent of pork, and 50 percent of chicken.[45] But all hope is not lost. The "little guys" have survived, though they have not flourished. As we build global awareness of the problems factory farms pose to our generation, we're seeing a return of sustainable, local farmers who believe in the way business used to get done. They also tend to practice more sustainable methods, such as protecting our air, water, and soil quality; minimizing energy consumption; and recycling or composting their waste. Small farms have even been shown to invest more money back into their local communities.[46]

Locating a Farmers' Market Near You

To find a farmers' market or a certified-organic farmer near you, there are a number of great websites to visit:

LOCAL HARVEST: A kick-ass resource, Local Harvest gives you access to a nationwide community of family farms, small farms, farmers' markets and other local and organic food sources near you. The website features products of the month, farm events, and produce subscriptions to get your fresh fruits and veggies dropped off on your doorstep. www.localharvest.org

FARMERS MARKET: This resource offers a detailed directory of farmers' markets across the country, with a basic blog on socially conscious thinking and products. www.farmersmarket.com

EAT WELL GUIDE: This site gives the conscious consumer the opportunity to find farms, farmers' markets, and restaurants within a one-mile to two-hundred-mile radius, on a global scale! Check out the fun and energetic Green Fork blog, designed to keep you up-to-date on sustainable trends. www.eatwellguide.org

LOCAL FARM MARKETS: This website gives similar access to a nationwide directory of local farmers' markets with cool resources for being a smart consumer. www.localfarmmarkets.org

THE DIRTY DOZEN

To buy, or not to buy, organic. Just another one of life's conundrums. You have a hard enough time finding socks to match, now you have to concern yourself with which produce goods are best purchased with the shiny organic sticker? I know, you need a hug.

Well, I am going to make it really easy for you. Are you familiar with the Dirty Dozen? It's the Environmental Working Group's high-profile list of the fruits and veggies that are the most toxic when grown "conventionally" (non-organically). To give you an idea of just how high the risk is, I have also included a score below each. The score indicates how many samples of each good on a scale of one to one hundred, have been found to be pumped with pesticides. The higher the score, the uglier its chances. No ifs, ands, or buts: these are the ones you need to buy organic.

PEACHES: This plump, delicious fruit is sprayed on a weekly basis, from March until harvest, with an assortment of pesticides and fungicides. It is considered the worst on the Dirty Dozen list, according to the EWG. **Pesticide Rating: 100**

APPLES: Talk about taking a bite out of crime. Around forty pesticides, herbicides, and fungicides are approved for use on apples. **Pesticide Rating: 93**

BELL PEPPERS (Red and Green): Growers add their own concoction of toxic spices from among fifty approved chemicals and insecticides, typically sprayed two to six times on the pepper crops during their growth cycle. **Pesticide Score: 83**

CELERY: The FDA suspects that celery is the most likely candidate for pesticide residue, due to its ability to absorb a number of toxins through the soil and groundwater. And if the FDA suspects it, then you know it's dirty. **Pesticide Score: 82**

NECTARINES: Ouch. Nectarine trees take a beating for several months with various pesticides, fungicides, and petroleum-based horticulture oils. **Pesticide Rating: 81**

STRAWBERRIES: Ms. Shortcake would not be a happy camper. More than sixty-five different pesticides, fungicides, and herbicides are registered for use on these babies. **Pesticide Rating: 80**

CHERRIES: Let's skip the cherry on top. Cherries are naturally attractive to insects and pests, and susceptible to viruses and fungal diseases. Yummy! **Pesticide Rating: 73**

KALE: Newer to the Dirty Dozen list, kale has been found to have ten types of pesticide residue, post-rinse. Yikes. **Pesticide Score: 69**

LETTUCE: Leafy greens are considered to be contaminated with the most potent pesticides used on food—fifty of them to be exact. **Pesticide Score: 67**

GRAPES (Imported): The USDA mandates that all grapes imported from Chile be fumigated with methyl bromide when they arrive at the U.S. ports. What a welcome! **Pesticide Rating: 66**

PEARS: Pear crops bear more than fifty nasty chemicals. **Pesticide Rating: 63**

CARROTS: Sure they build brainpower, but more than forty different pesticides have been detected on carrots. **Pesticide Score: 63**

Visit www.ewg.org for updates or additions to the list of the Dirty Dozen.[48]

THE CLEAN FIFTEEN

If I've done my job, you should be a little weary of the word "clean" at this point. But here, you can let down your guard a bit. The Clean Fifteen refers to foods that are okay to purchase *without* the organic stamp of approval. No, they are not perfect. They just aren't big pest targets or they have thick, protective skins that shield the edible stuff from harmful pesticides.

ASPARAGUS: This veggie faces fewer threats from unwanted pests, thus requiring less pesticide use.

How to Pick a Good One: Choose bright green or purplish bunches with tightly bundled tips that aren't flowering. For even cooking, buy bunches that are fairly uniform in size and thickness.

Storage/Instructions: Store in the refrigerator.

AVOCADOS: The thick shell protects the fruit from pesticide buildup.

How to Pick a Good One: The best avocados are slightly tender but won't dent or cave in to the touch. Look for bumpy, dark green to almost black skins.

Storage/Instructions: Store in the refrigerator. If you can find only unripe avocado, store in a paper bag at room temperature until it ripens.

BROCCOLI: Broccoli crops have less trouble with pest threats, so they call for less pesticide use.

How to Pick a Good One: Choose broccoli that is deep green with a grayish-purple tint on the stems. Feel for firm stalks with no wilted leaves or rubbery consistency.

Storage/Instructions: Store in the refrigerator.

CABBAGE: Like broccoli and asparagus, cabbage doesn't need lots of pesticides.

How to Pick a Good One: You want the outer shell to be tight, crisp, shiny, and heavy. If the leaves are yellowing, leave it for the next guy. As far as varieties, bok choy should have deep green leaves with crisp, white stems; savory cabbage (the exception to the rule) will form a looser head with wrinkled leaves.

Storage/Instructions: Store in the refrigerator.

KIWI: This fruit's fuzzy skin acts as a barrier to harmful pesticides and chemicals.

How to Pick a Good One: Choose kiwi that are plump and can take a gradual squeeze. Refrain from buying ones that are too soft, moist on the skin, or show any signs of bruising.

Storage/Instructions: Store in the refrigerator. If you can find only unripe kiwi fruits, store them in a paper bag on the kitchen counter at room temperature until they feel ripe.

MANGOES: Their thick skin protects them from the outside world, even those pesky pesticides.

How to Pick a Good One: Mangoes should be slightly firm but yield to a gentle squeeze. For those with a sweet tooth, the softer varieties are sweeter, but don't go too soft, as this often indicates a rotten one. Look for mangoes bright in color, whether that is red, yellow, or orange.

Storage/Instructions: Store in the refrigerator. If you can find only unripe mangoes, store them in a paper bag on the kitchen counter at room temperature until they feel ripe.

ONIONS: This tearjerker doesn't attract many pests, which means less pesticide use.

How to Pick a Good One: Look for dry, sheer skins and flesh that is full and firm, primarily at the stem end. Avoid any discoloration or soft spots. Pick fresh onions one by one. Refrain from buying by the bag.

Storage/Instructions: Store at room temperature.

PAPAYA: Pesticide residue will stick to the outer skin, which preserves the flesh inside.

How to Pick a Good One: If you plan to serve papaya in the next day or two, choose one with golden color that is soft to the touch, not bruised or shriveled. If you wish to eat it later in the week, pick one intermediate in color, between green and golden.

Storage/Instructions: Store in the refrigerator. If you can find only unripe papaya, store in a paper bag on the kitchen counter at room temperature until they feel ripe.

PINEAPPLE: Its rough, spiny rind shields the fruit from pests, pesticide residue, and unwanted creatures.

How to Pick a Good One: Pull on the leaves at the top to find out if a pineapple is ripe. If a nice little tug rips out a leaf, then you have a ripe pineapple. The rind is so thick that typically bruising on the outside won't reflect on the inside.

Storage/Instructions: Store in the refrigerator. If you plan to eat it in a few days, countertop storage is fine.

SWEET (SHELLING) PEAS: According to the Environmental Protection Agency (EPA), sweet peas are the least likely vegetable to have pesticide residue.

How to Pick a Good One: Pea pods should be bright green in color with no yellowing; a bit leathery but firm. You should be able to feel the beans through the pod.

Storage/Instructions: Store at cool temperatures. Plan on picking up a pound for every cup of peas you want.

SWEET CORN: Corn may require some fertilizer to grow, but it's not likely to end up on the kernels.

How to Pick a Good One: Look for bright green husks that tightly hug around the ear. Pull back the husk to ensure kernels are small, shiny, and firm.

Storage/Instructions: Store at room temperature and do not refrigerate. Corn is best served a few days within purchase.

WATERMELON: Watermelon is a tough cookie. With a rind like this, not many chemicals can fight their way into its juicy, red flesh. Is it summertime yet?

How to Pick a Good One: Go ahead, give it a firm squeeze. Look for a firm rind with a deeper green, even pigment. Avoid bruising or soft spots.

Storage/Instructions: Store in the refrigerator.

TOMATOES: Tomatoes found themselves on the Dirty Dozen list in 2008, but they're in the clear now. The EPA recently identified the tomato as one of the cleanest vegetables.

How to Pick a Good One: Look for glossy, firm skin without signs of bruising. The brighter the color, the riper the tomato. Look for deep, even color and avoid the pale, scrawny ones.

Storage/Instructions: Store at room temperature.

EGGPLANT: Their thick skins call for less pesticide use.

How to Pick a Good One: Skin should appear medium in color, shiny, and not shriveled or wrinkled. When squeezed, a good eggplant should offer some cushion but not be too firm. Typically, bruising on the outside does not indicate any damage to the actual flesh, but it's always best to choose an eggplant with no baggage.

Storage/Instructions: Store on the kitchen counter and do not refrigerate.

SWEET POTATO: Sweet potatoes are not huge pest targets, and therefore are unlikely to be contaminated with a slew of pesticides.

How to Pick a Good One: Choose a sweet potato without any soft areas and avoid those with sprouts, eyes, slits, or a green pigment. For best results when cooking, buy potatoes that are fairly uniform in size and thickness.

Storage/Instructions: Store at room temperature and do not refrigerate.

Visit www.ewg.org for updates or additions to the list of the Clean Fifteen.[49]

Seven Tips
on Shopping for Organic Produce

Below are some tips and things to consider when buying organic produce. Shop smart and you will feel satisfied with spending a little extra on the safer produce.

1. BUY ITEMS IN SEASON: Depending on where you live, those apples and pears may not have had to make the fifteen hundred-mile trip to your local produce aisle, so even organic food will be cheaper when it is in season. Carry a copy of the seasonal chart (see page 31).

2. MAKE THE SWITCH FOR A FEW FRUITS AND VEGGIES: Take advantage of the Dirty Dozen list. Use it. Sleep with it. Tattoo it on your forehead. You can significantly cut your exposure to harmful pollutants and pesticides simply by making the switch for a few of the most toxic goods, and purchasing from certified-organic growers or sustainable farmers.

3. CHAT UP THE STAFF: Have a heart-to-heart with someone who looks friendly in the produce department. Quiz them on where the produce comes from, if it is in season, and if you may have a sample. A little flirting never hurt. It is your hard-earned cash and your right to make sure you are spending it on something that is well worth it.

4. BUY IN BULK: If you are feeding a large family or live to entertain, buy in bulk. At some specialty grocers, like Whole Foods, shoppers earn a 10-percent discount for bulk purchases.

5. STICK TO THE GROCERY LIST: The caramel apples subconsciously call to us, too. They call to everyone. You're not that special. Put together a comprehensive grocery list before you leave that follows a detailed schedule of meals and snacks. Stick to it and you will save moolah.

6. COMPARE ORGANIC-TO-ORGANIC PRICES: Comparison shot, baby. Some major chains are stepping up to the plate and launching their own organic brands, while others still haven't quite gotten with the program, and offer lame organic choices at spiked prices. If the price per pound jumps out at you more than gas prices, do your due diligence and make some calls or hit your local farmers' market or corner produce stand.

7. CLIP ORGANIC COUPONS: Learn something from your mother's coupon-hoarding days: save, save, save. Open up the Sunday paper and grocery circulars and cut out the coupons. You may feel like a dork but your wallet won't.

Mother Earth's Clock: BUYING SEASONAL

Mama Earth is no dummy. She knows just when her soil is right to grow the most delicious, sweetest, freshest, and highest-quality produce.

One of the key factors of buying local is making an effort to purchase fruits and vegetables when they are in season in your region. True, today's commerce has made it simple to get whatever, whenever you want it. That doesn't mean it's okay. Eating seasonal foods in the regions we live in, and nearby, has a lower carbon count, and acts as a way of following nature's cues to get in touch with our surroundings.

Best of all, seasonal produce gives you an opportunity to have some fun in the kitchen. Cooking should never be boring. Not in a *Skinny Bitch* kitch. Cooking with foods in season allows you to experiment with new foods and recipes and introduce some new flavor and spice to your meals. Many organic, seasonal suppliers take advantage of the season by selling wild and foraged produce along with other basic varieties of fruits and vegetables. Depending on the season, this gives you a chance to get crazy and wild! Who wants to cook with one tomato when you can sauté four different sub-varieties? Swap out the garlic powder for some fresh rocket or wild garlic. The opportunities are endless.

Lastly, there is no denying the difference in taste between a fresh, unprocessed, sun-ripened fruit and one plucked two weeks ago, unripe and tired from jet lag. Please, don't take it from me. Try it for yourself.

Seasonal Foods Chart

Excuse me, but earth doesn't exactly have a hotline. How do I know what fruits and vegetables are in season?

Follow this Seasonal Foods Chart and discover the real pleasure of cooking:

SPRING: artichokes, arugula, asparagus, avocados, beets, broccoli, carrots, cauliflower, chard greens, cherries, fennel, kale, leeks, mint, new potatoes, peas, radishes, rhubarb, strawberries, turnips, yellow squash

SUMMER: apricots, arugula, avocados, basil, beets, blueberries, broccoli, carrots, chard greens, cherries, collard greens, corn, cucumber, eggplant, fennel, figs, grapes, green beans, kale, leeks, melons, mint, nectarines, new potatoes, okra, parsley, peaches, pears, peas, peppers, plums, radishes, raspberries, rhubarb, strawberries, tomatoes, yellow squash, zucchini

FALL: apples, artichokes, arugula, avocados, basil, green beans, beets, bok choy, broccoli, Brussels sprouts, carrots, cabbage, cauliflower, chard greens, chestnuts, collard greens, corn, cucumber, fennel, figs, grapefruit, kale, leeks, lemons, limes, mint, new potatoes, okra, oranges, parsley, parsnips, pears, peas, pecans, peppers, persimmons, pomegranates, pumpkin, quince, radishes, raspberries, rutabagas, sweet potatoes, tangerines, tomatoes, turnips, winter squash, yams

WINTER: avocados, beets, broccoli, carrots, cauliflower, chard greens, collard greens, fennel, grapefruit, jicama, kale, kiwi, leeks, lemons, limes, new potatoes, parsnips, persimmon.

Visit www.sustainabletable.org to find fruits and vegetables that are in season in your area.

PART TWO

THE SECRET TO BEING A SKINNY BITCH

There have been some misconceptions about what it means to be a *Skinny Bitch*. And I think it's time I cleared that up before I find another gray hair.

Over the years, it has become habitual for women, most of whom have never read a single page of the book, to give me their "two cents." If I had a dime for every time a lady at a cocktail party asked me how I could encourage women to be supermodel thin, I'd be a Coinstar. She stands there, a White Russian waving in one hand, teriyaki beef skewer in the other, hypothetically asking: *How could you encourage women to be skinny? If all women were a size 2, we'd live in such a boring place.*

I clear my throat [ahem], and so kindly reply, *Yes that would be very boring.*

So, rather than individually reply to each of these well-rehearsed comments, I thought it better to tell it like it is. *Skinny Bitch* has nothing to do with being *skinny*. And it has nothing to do with being a *bitch,* either. Though we all have our moments.

A "Skinny Bitch" is a woman who cares about what she's putting into her body. She cares about the small print. She's eager to re-channel our collective global frustrations to take a stand for what she believes in—even if her friends think she's nuts.

What will you do when you find out what's in your meat? Run to the golden arches and grab a cheeseburger or start working alternatives into your diet? What about when you find out your food travels an average of fifteen hundred miles to get to your plate? Will you start making more trips to your local farmers' market or continue supporting the system?

We all have a choice, ladies. But, Skinny Bitches don't just sit there and shrug. They make shit happen. They ask questions and they get answers.

Like everyone else, we splurge on a dessert occasionally that's got a few ingredients we're not proud of. We grab fast food here and there. We even screw up and buy produce that's not organic. But it doesn't matter. We're human. What matters is what we do with most of our days. We have a voice and we use it. The question is: What will you do?

Are you a Skinny Bitch?

....

THE SKINNY: PROCESSED FOODS

....

The 11 **Worst** Food Additives on the Market

....

Your local grocery store might as well be a land mine. The smiling checkout associates and god-awful elevator music are just disguises for the shopping cart of disease-causing crap you're pushing along like Suzie Freakin' Homemaker.

Remove the rose-colored glasses, honey. There is a reason the product labels on the back of the box look like an illiterate game of Scrabble. Food manufacturers are filling commercial foods with dangerous preservatives, sprays, and harmful chemicals to increase their shelf life, enhance the taste and texture, and make them look pretty. These very ingredients have been found to cause nervous system damage, immune system dysfunction, life-threatening disease, and a handful of other serious health conditions.[50]

Start reading your labels and familiarize yourself with what not to buy. Here is the *Skinny Bitch* Cheat Sheet of the 11 Worst Food Additives on the market.

ARTIFICIAL COLORS (RED, BLUE, GREEN, YELLOW, FD&C COLORS)

Most of the cheap, low-grade products in the grocery store contain artificial colors simply for visual appeal. Though it sounds harmless, artificial colors are made from petroleum, coal tars, acetone, or cochineal bugs. Yes, bugs. Some colorings are acquired by boiling dried insects in water to extract carminic acid.[51] Research has shown food coloring to cause hyperactivity and behavioral issues (ADHD, ODD and OCD), adrenal gland, brain and kidney tumors, cancer, asthma and severe allergies.[52] Some countries have been smart enough to ban them but not our friends at FDA! Ingredients to look for: Blue 1, Blue 2, Red 3 (erythrosine), Green 3, Yellow 5 (tartrazine) and Yellow 6.

ARTIFICIAL SWEETENERS

Commonly found in chewing gums, diet soda, and sugar-free foods, artificial sweeteners claim to reduce the number of calories, but they're taking your health hostage in the meantime. They disguise themselves under such aliases as Acesulfame-K, saccharin, Equal, Splenda, NutraSweet, Sweet'N Low, sucralose, sorbitol, and aspartame. Aspartame—a common artificial sweetener that is still on my shit list—is one of the most controversial ingredients on grocery shelves. By 1998, eighty percent of complaints brought to the FDA about food additives were focused on aspartame products. Its running list of negative side effects makes pill popping look saintly: blurred vision, memory loss, anxiety attacks, seizures, migraines, dizziness, depression, vomiting, nausea, abdominal pain and cramps, and various forms of cancer.[53] There are even aspartame victim support groups. Sucralose, another modified sugar mentioned above, is 600 times as sweet as sugar. Not a difficult one to figure out.

BENZOATE PRESERVATIVES: BHA (BUTYLATED HYDROXYANISOLE) AND BHT (BUTYLATED HYDROXYTOLUENE)

BHA and BHT are oxidants, lovely preservatives that food companies use to preserve fats and prevent foods from going rancid. Hello, cancer! They also have been known to affect estrogen levels, while causing asthma, rhinitis, dermatitis, tumors, and urticaria.[54] BHT has been banned in England but, again, the U.S. says it's a-okay.[55]

BROMINATED VEGETABLE OIL (BVO)

A chemical that enhances flavor in citrus-based fruit drinks and soft drinks, BVO increases triglycerides and cholesterol and can cause serious damage to the liver, testicles, thyroid, heart, and kidneys. No refills, please.[56]

POTASSIUM BROMATE

Bromate has been banned throughout most of the world, and California requires a cancer warning on the label if this additive is an ingredient. But the FDA hasn't illegalized it.[57] They just encourage bakers not to use it. Smart move, geniuses. That's going to stop them. While we're at it, let's encourage them not to put gasoline in our muffins, either.

Often found in white flour, breads, and rolls, potassium bromate can cause nervous system damage, kidney disorders, and gastrointestinal problems.[58]

PROPYLENE GLYCOL

The FDA claims propylene glycol is "generally safe" except when used in foods. Maybe that's because it's also a mineral oil found in automatic brake fluid, hydraulic fluid, and antifreeze.[59] But that's just a lucky guess. Propylene glycol is used to thicken dairy products and factory foods like soda pop and salad dressing.[60] Your safest bet is to keep it out of your pantry.

PROPYL GALLATE

Often used in conjunction with BHA and BHT to keep fats and oils from going rotten, this synthetic preservative has prompted warnings of adverse side effects such as allergic reactions that constrict breathing.[61] Recall that you need to breathe to stay alive. It's used in everything from mayonnaise and soup to vitamins.

SODIUM NITRATE AND SODIUM NITRITE

Nitrates and nitrites produce cancer-causing agents in the stomach and can cause death but have not been banned by the FDA because they prevent botulism.[62] Big red flag. Commonly used to prevent bacteria growth in meats and preserve its color and flavor. Yet another reason to cut meat out of your diet.

MONOSODIUM GLUTAMATE (MSG)

A flavor enhancer most often found in packaged foods, MSG might as well be radioactive. It can cause headaches, chest pain, high blood pressure, nausea, and nervous system and reproductive disorders.[63] According to author and neurosurgeon Dr. Russell Blaylock, there is a link between sudden cardiac arrest (aka death) and excitotoxic damage evoked by MSG and artificial sweeteners.[64] Food manufacturers have even found ways to downplay it in infant formulas and over-the-counter medications by labeling it under common nicknames such as hydrolyzed protein, autolyzed yeast, free glutamate, and yeast extract. Some companies are kind enough to warn expectant mothers, lactating mothers, infants, and children to stay clear. How nice of them, right?[65]

OLESTRA

Olestra is a synthetic fat that prevents your digestive system from absorbing fat. It also *prevents* the healthy absorption of fat-soluble vitamins A, D, E, and K, which reduce the risk of cancer and heart disease and play a role in vision health. Olestra also leads to severe diarrhea or "anal leakage," abdominal cramps, flatulence, and gas.[66]

HIGH-FRUCTOSE CORN SYRUP (HFCS)

High-fructose corn syrup is on my shit list. Sure, it maintains sweetness, but it also increases your risk for Type-2 diabetes, coronary heart disease, cancer, and stroke. Your liver doesn't like it, either. Surprise, surprise![67]

I know this is a lot to digest (pun intended), but changes don't happen overnight. The first step is to pick specific ingredients that are the most important for you to cut down on, and work toward healthier options. You will find plenty of recipes to help you choose the right path in this cookbook.

THE SKINNY: SUGARS

Sweet-Tooth Approved Sugar Alternatives

In America, we're all on a sugar high. But no matter how many candy bars we snub and Pop Tarts we pity, it's the most unusual of suspects that inject our veins with liquid crack. From white breads and rice to microwavable meals and even spaghetti sauce, these processed foods are draining our immune systems, raising our insulin levels, making us fat, and pumping us with diseases.

And you thought you were on a diet? How sweet.

The truth is, even when we're consciously limiting our sugar intake, the average American consumes about two to three pounds of sugar a week. Over the last two decades, food manufacturers have increased sugar consumption in the U.S. from twenty-six to one hundred-thirty-five pounds per person.[68] Bummed? Yeah, so was I. Nobody can deny that we need sugar to boost our energy levels and fuel our bodies. But not the kind we're eating. The sweeteners that are sneaking into our diets—high-fructose corn syrup and refined sugar—cause our blood sugar to dramatically spike and dip. You think that's what your body needs to survive? Think again.

Nobody in his or her right mind expects you to kiss sugar goodbye. It tastes good. It makes you happy. It keeps you from locking yourself in your bedroom and watching Barbra Streisand classics during that wonderful time of the month. I get it. You just need to know where it's coming from—whether it's nature or the assembly line.

The key is to become buddy-buddy with healthier sugars if you need a fix. There are a handful on the market—yes, even at your friendly local grocer—that feed your body the essential minerals it needs to run efficiently, rather than treat it like a chew toy. The raw, unprocessed sugars are the ones that are better for your health, and even better to your taste buds. Use these natural sugars as replacements in recipes and home-cooked meals, where you control what the hell you're putting into your body.

Five Healthier Sweeteners

EVAPORATED CANE SUGAR

This is the closest sweetener to commercial refined white sugar, but it doesn't undergo the same degree of processing. As a result, it retains more of the nutrients found in sugar cane due to the retention of molasses.[69] The crystals are a bit larger, but they can be used the same way as white sugar in everything from baked goods to iced tea. Gaining in popularity, evaporated cane sugar is available at health food stores and has taken over most major grocery retailers.

STEVIA

Of all the natural sweeteners, this one's the most likely to sit tableside at your favorite restaurants with the likes of Equal, Sweet'N Low, and Splenda. The healthy restaurants, that is. Extracted from a plant found in China and South America, Stevia is 100 percent natural, and boasts no glycemic index so it won't mess with your blood-sugar levels. Plus, it has zero calories. Now I have your attention. As far as health benefits, Stevia helps regulate your digestive tract, and acts as an anti-inflammatory and anti-fungal. Keep in mind: It is three hundred times sweeter than refined sugar so you only need a pinch to get the job done.

AGAVE NECTAR

Sounds familiar, right? That's likely because the very plant agave nectar comes from is the same succulent plant used to make tequila in Mexico. (This is either a pleasant surprise, or it makes you think of those wretched nights when you worshipped the porcelain god.) Organic raw and unprocessed agave nectar is very similar to honey with a good dose of vitamins and minerals. But the most important thing to consider is agave nectar has a low glycemic index. This means it absorbs slowly into the bloodstream, rather than flooding it, so it doesn't send your blood-sugar levels into adrenaline shock. You don't want that. Nobody wants that.

BITCHWORTHY: Agave nectar and Stevia are safe for diabetics due to a low glycemic index.

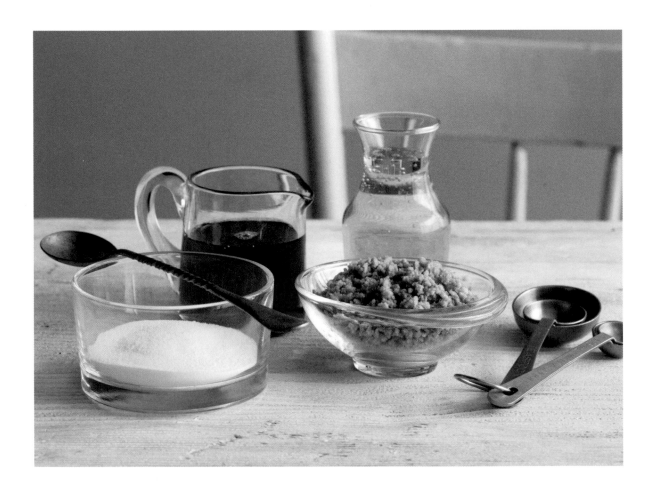

SUCANAT

Often used as a substitute for brown sugar, Sucanat is an organic, unrefined cane sugar. Though noticeably milder than other natural sugars, Sucanat does retain some molasses, thus giving it a very distinctive flavor. Like evaporated cane juice, it is minimally processed so it retains some vitamins and minerals. Think of it as an all-purpose sweetener for cooking, baking, and beverages.

MAPLE SYRUP

Yes, it's the stuff you used to drizzle all over your pancakes, and it's still got cool factor. Sweeter than sugar and with fewer calories, maple syrup is simply the sap from maple trees. It lends to a healthier heart and immune system, and boosts male reproductive glands. (That's what I'm talking about.) Surprisingly, maple syrup is also packed with manganese and zinc, and has twice as much calcium as milk.[70] Damn! When buying at the store, make sure to look for pure organic maple syrup and avoid maple syrup "flavors," which are overused in commercial pancake syrups and don't bring you the same health benefits or quality. Grade A versions are light, medium, and dark amber; the lighter the color the more subtle the flavor. Grade A maple syrup is best to enjoy straight-up when serving, while Grade B versions carry the most prominent taste and are best for cooking.

All of these natural sweetener alternatives can be found at specialty health food stores and some major grocery retailers. Call your local grocer to inquire.

THE SKINNY: MEAT

Awesome Meat and Protein Substitutes

Carnivores just love to take pity on vegans. They assume that because we don't chow down on meat or dairy, we are missing out on life. But we do just fine. Actually, we do more than fine. We are freakin' dandy. Though it comes as a raging surprise to some, we do the same things meat-eaters do. We love a hot shower. We watch funny movies and laugh. And sometimes, we even forget to return our library books. Crazy, huh?

The truth of the matter is vegans really don't miss out on anything, and you don't have to, either. If you're ready to take a meatless diet for a test drive or even just start cooking up a few meat-free meals each week, there are plenty of substitutes that taste and feel like the real deal—but are a better deal in the end. Below, I've rounded up some of the most common substitutes, their health benefits, and the best way to serve them up. Now, if only I could figure out how to return those damn library books on time.

Filling "Meat" Substitutes

TEMPEH

A primary ingredient in the Indonesian diet for more than two thousand years, tempeh has a tender, chewy, and nutty texture, yet a delicious mild flavor. Made from fermented soybeans and pressed into a solid cake, tempeh is an ideal alternative for those who have trouble digesting plant-based or high-protein foods like beans, legumes, or soy. (The fermentation process greatly reduces oligosaccharides, the very thing that makes beans hard to digest for some people.) Plus, tempeh contains an enzyme that breaks down phytates (see page 41), thus increasing the absorption of such kick-ass minerals as zinc (immunity builder), iron, and calcium. One serving of tempeh contains more fiber than most get in one day! Bring it on.[71]

Best Results: Season or marinate for 30 minutes prior to cooking to enhance the flavor. Tempeh is a pro at absorbing the flavor of the foods or spices it simmers with. I recommend stir-frying, grilling, sautéing, or adding to soups, stews, or chilis as a substitute for meat.

SEITAN

If your burger or Sloppy Joe cravings are too strong to resist, look no further. Seitan has the same chewy, meaty, and dense texture of meat when cooked. It is, however, missing things that meat is full of—saturated fat and bad cholesterol. Yuck. On the nutritional side, seitan, aka the "wheat meat," tips the scale. In both quality and quantity, it has a similar amount of protein as beef, and boasts twice as much protein as tofu and 40 percent more than what you would get from two medium eggs. To put it simply, seitan is the cat's pajamas.[72]

Best Results: Truth be told, raw seitan can be bland. Just a little seasoning or marinade gives it the flavor punch it needs to make your taste buds go buck wild. Seitan is superb when cooked in red wine or vegetable stock, makes for a succulent bourguignon, grounds like chopped meat, and pan-fries or breads like cutlets. Just switch it out for ground beef next time you feel like making lasagna, Sloppy Joe, or some roll-up tacos and you'll have something to write home to Mom about.

QUICK TIP: Unseasoned seitan is low in one essential amino acid, lycine. No problemo. Just sauté or cook it in a broth seasoned with soy sauce or combine with lysine-rich foods like beans.

TOFU

A popular option among both vegetarians and vegans, tofu has reached grocery stores across mass America as one of the most accessible meat alternatives. You can get it in a silken or firm (solid) form, but no matter how you dice it, tofu has a much spongier consistency than meat. I heart tofu because it's packed with such vitamins as iron, calcium, and omega-3 fatty acids, but it trumps meat with zero cholesterol or saturated fat.

Best Results: Tofu's versatility is great for all kinds of dishes, from sweet to savory. Silken tofu is best used as an ingredient in dressings, sauces, and dairy-free desserts like ice cream or cheesecake. But firm tofu fills in the blanks as a fun substitute in stir-fried, grilled, scrambled, smoked, or barbecued dishes. Similar to other meat alternatives, it also soaks up the flavor of cooking or marinating liquids and seasonings.

BITCHWORTHY: Whenever possible, buy organic tofu. It greatly cuts down your exposure to harmful chemicals and genetic modification (GM).[73]

BEANS

You never thought of beans as an alternative to meat, right? Boy, did they have you fooled. One of the easiest foods to fit into a plant-based diet, beans are a fine source of protein, minerals, and vitamins. The anthocyanins in beans also act as a powerful antioxidant that help to ward off damage from free radicals.

Best Results: Pinto beans, black beans, chickpeas, and black-eyed peas are the easiest to digest. Simmer beans with a bay leaf or cumin to reduce gas. Nobody wants a stinky ass at dinner.

LEGUMES

Another simple alternative to getting your daily dose of protein, legumes are a class of veggies ranging from peas to peanuts to lentils. They are the most versatile and nutritious in the produce aisle, with "good" fats, antioxidants, and soluble and insoluble fiber. For those watching their weight, legumes are also low in fat and free of cholesterol. Kiss those pounds goodbye.

Best Results: Most supermarkets stock a wide variety of both dried and canned legumes. They are a perfect addition to stews, soups, casseroles, salads, or on their own as a side dish.

With the rise of vegetarians and vegans, most major grocery retailers are carrying soy- or vegetable-based proteins and meat alternatives now. You will find the best selection of product lines and brands at specialty health food stores. Use some of the recipes in this book to do a taste test and decide which proteins you and your family go gaga over. If you're not a veggie already, remember to work meat alternatives into your diet slowly and don't overdo it. Especially if you have a thing for soy. It's crawling with health benefits, but too much of something is never good.

THE SKINNY: SOY

The Balancing Act of Soy

Soy has such a mixed rap. With the rise of the plant-based diet, activists across the country have been quick to take a side, either bashing it or putting it on a pedestal. Where's a bitch to find the truth among all the hype?

The simple truth is that, when eaten in moderation, soy is a great alternative for those who are lactose-intolerant or skipping dairy for their own cause. Just ask the millions of people who love it right up.

Benefits of Soy

Low in fat and cholesterol and high in protein and fiber, soy is believed by many to be linked to the prevention of cancer. In 1999, the FDA authorized companies to label foods containing soy protein for their ability to reduce the risk of coronary heart disease, the number one cause of death in the U.S.[74]

THE SKINNY: DAIRY MILK

Yummy Dairy-Free Milk Substitutes

Milk doesn't do every body good. For the more than thirty million Americans who are lactose-intolerant, it's like a big glass of toxic. Not even David Beckham's rock-hard abs and five o'clock shadow could get us to nod our heads at those Got Milk? campaigns. But they sure make us smile.

Lactose intolerance is no funny business. It is the body's inability to digest a sugar called lactos

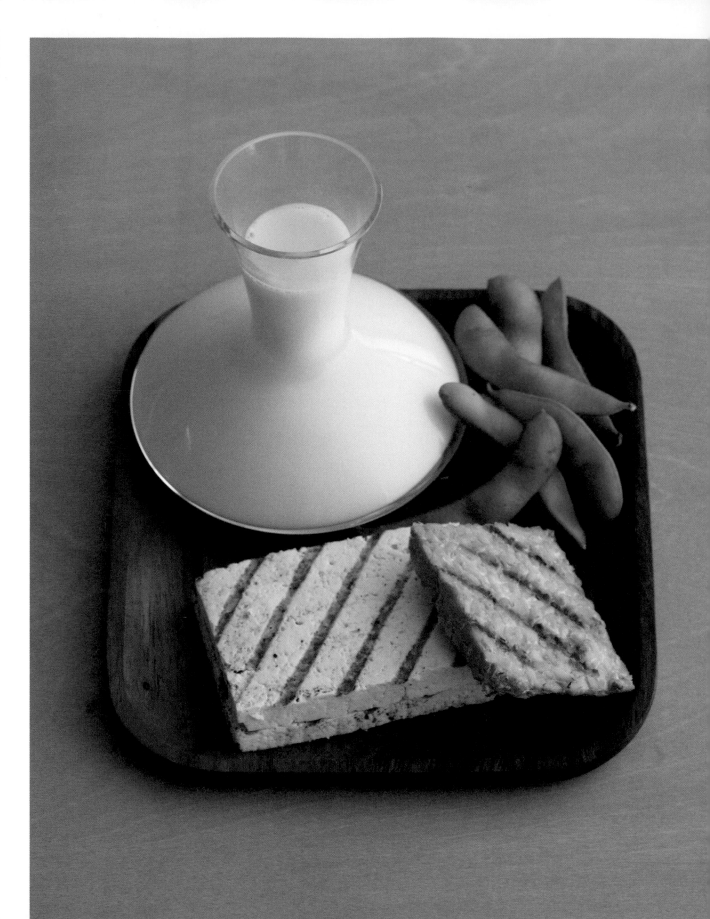

that is found in milk and other dairy products. Why do some people's bodies drink it right up and others reject it? The problem is due to a deficiency of lactase, the enzyme responsible for breaking down lactose into simple sugars to be absorbed into the bloodstream. An intolerance results in all sorts of nasty gastrointestinal problems when milk or milk products are ingested.[78]

Of course, an intolerance to cow's milk doesn't only apply to those with a lactose allergy. Some people just have an intolerance to dairy because of what it stands for—the mistreatment and slaughter of animals.

But just because you don't "got milk," doesn't mean you can't enjoy the same things dairy drinkers do. There are a handful of options below that still deliver your body wonderful nutrients, with no cholesterol or casein, and very little fat. Drink up.

SOY MILK

A great substitute for milk in cereals, oatmeal, and tea, soy milk is the most common dairy substitute available. A sign of the times, you can even buy it at major grocery retailers.

Tipping Points:

- Cholesterol-free with less saturated fat
- Higher dosage of iron and vitamins A and D than dairy milk
- Great source of potassium, riboflavin, zinc, vitamin B12, fiber, essential amino acids, and isoflavones
- Does not contain casein
- Loaded with bio-active components, which are thought to maintain healthy bones, relieve menopausal symptoms and hot flashes, and prevent prostate, breast, and colorectal cancers[79]

Bitchworthy Brand: Silk soy milk comes in vanilla and chocolate flavors.

www.silksoymilk.com

ALMOND MILK

....

Made from ground almonds, almond milk has a sweet, nutty taste and creamy consistency that is perfect for smoothies, beverages, and desserts. I prefer the unsweetened version, which tastes the closest to cow's milk, for savory dishes and baking.

Tipping Points:

- Cholesterol-, lactose- and casein-free with less saturated fat than cow's milk
- High in antioxidants and vitamin D, which aid in the absorption of calcium and help to build strong bones[80]
- Studies have shown that the balance of protein, "good" fats, and fiber found in almonds helps you lose weight

Bitchworthy Brand: Almond Breeze is light on calories and comes in original, lactose-free, and unsweetened. www.bluediamond.com

BITCHIONARY: CASEIN

A PROTEIN FOUND IN COW'S MILK AND USED INDEPENDENTLY IN MANY FOODS AS A BINDING AGENT. IN THE CHINA STUDY, T. COLIN CAMPBELL FOUND THAT THE PROTEIN—FOUND IN 87 PERCENT OF COW'S MILK—PROMOTED CANCER IN ALL STAGES OF DEVELOPMENT.[81]

RICE MILK

....

Another popular dairy substitute, rice milk is derived from brown rice. Generally sweet and fairly watery, rice milk has an almost translucent quality.

Tipping Points:

- Boasts very little fat
- Often fortified to be a good source of calcium
- Great source of carbohydrates but isn't rich in nutrients except when it's fortified

Bitchworthy Brand: Rice Dream Organic is fortified in calcium, and vitamins A and D. www.tastethedream.com

HEMP MILK

....

Calm down, pothead. Fairly new to the U.S., hemp milk is made from the seeds of the hemp plant, but it doesn't contain THC (the psychoactive element of marijuana). It is creamier than soy or almond milk and tends to be a bit thicker. The nutty flavor makes this substitute another good candidate for baking, smoothies, and desserts.

Tipping Points:

- Contains no soy, gluten, sugar, or cholesterol
- Concentrated in vitamins A, B12, D, and E; magnesium; iron; zinc; beta-carotene; phosphorus; riboflavin; and the omegas
- Studies have shown that hemp milk helps strengthen your immune system and heart, increase your mental capacity, and make for clearer skin, hair, and nails.
- May be more digestible than soy protein because it contains no oligosaccharides[82]

Bitchworthy Brand: Living Harvest Hempmilk is a great source of the omegas with less sugar. All five varieties are non-GMO and dairy-and soy-free. www.livingharvest.com

HUNGRY FOR CALCIUM?

SOME STUDIES HAVE SHOWN THAT WE ABSORB 75 PERCENT MORE CALCIUM FROM SOY MILK THAN DAIRY MILK [83]

THE SKINNY: CHEESE

New and Improved Vegan Cheese Alternatives

Becoming a vegan was an easy choice for me. But like most people who make the leap from vegetarian to vegan, giving up cheese was about as easy as helping a kid with his algebra homework (x + y = what?!). There is just something about the way cheese melts in your mouth that always makes it the last to bite the dust.

Here's the deal: Cheese was in every recipe I loved, every meal on the restaurant menu, and every drawer I opened in the fridge. *Would I like some cheese with my wine?* You bet your ass I would.

When I gave it up, I had a temporary meltdown, searching the Internet for addiction centers that catered to dairy abuse. (P.S. There are none to my knowledge.) Still, before I volunteered for an intervention, I made the decision to try to embrace my new lifestyle choice and find a way to still get my cheese fix. With the cow as my witness.

Then I discovered vegan cheese. And I cried. Not a good cry. It tasted like dirty feet. So, I continued the search with a relentless will to hang in there until I found what I was looking for. Eventually, I found what I was looking for. Boy, did I. In fact, I found three [Insert smile here].

Here they are, in no particular order, the three cheese alternatives that saved me from a life of Cheddar-free remorse. Amen.

DAIYA CHEESE

A welcomed addition to the vegan cheese market, Daiya is a plant-based, soy-free cheese that could hardly be considered an "alternative." It comes in block or shredded cheddar and Italian blends that melt like chocolate in 110-degree heat. Besides being loaded with vitamins B and B12, Daiya has gained the vegan blessing with no artificial ingredients, preservatives, or cholesterol. Did I mention it's low in fat? Say cheese, baby. Available at Whole Foods and natural health food stores.

www.daiyafoods.com

TEESE CHEESE

Someone pinch me. Teese is like a trip to the movie theater with the chips and cheese sauce, but oh so much better. Low-fat and made from non-GMO soybeans with no cholesterol, Teese comes in mozzarella and cheddar blocks, and cheddar and nacho cheese sauces. For those with allergies, Teese is made in an allergy-free facility with no egg, dairy, peanut, tree nut, or sesame. Available in restaurants nationwide and some natural health food stores.

www.teesecheese.com

SHEESE CHEESE

Ooh la la, the choices! The brainchild of three cute studs from Scotland, Sheese Cheese is soy-based and gluten-free. It comes in nine flavors of block cheese and five flavors of cream cheese called Creamy Sheese. Aside from the basics, they also offer blue cheese and Gouda. Genius!

Visit www.buteisland.com or purchase online at www.veganstore.com.

PART THREE

A PARTY IN YOUR KITCHEN

Your kitchen has been bad. *Very bad.* In fact, it's time you showed it just how bad it's been. Toss your hair into that cute little bun, push pause on your silly TV programs, get in the kitchen, and . . . *Cook.* You heard me. Get cooking. Use and abuse your stove. Flirt with your oven. Get frisky with your pantry. Quit playing hard to get.

Your kitchen should entertain you. If it does nothing to reel you in, do something about it. Let loose a little bit and cooking can actually be rewarding.

Cooking gives you an opportunity to challenge yourself, unwind from work, strengthen friendships, spark some romance, get laid, and get creative. The beauty of cooking is that you can create whatever the hell you want. There are no annoying referees blowing whistles telling you the oven was not done pre-heating. It's just you and the kitchen. What you do with it is entirely up to you.

Now, let's get this party started. Shall we? If only I remembered where I put my disco ball. . . .

WHERE'S THE PARTY AT, BITCHES?

Your kitchen is your playground. You're not five anymore. You can't climb the jungle gyms, rock on the squeaky pony, or slide down the shiny pole.

Okay, maybe the pole. Just make sure the kids aren't watching.

Hopefully you love spending as much time in the kitchen as I do. In that case, these tips may just give you new reason. Who knows? Hobbies turn into professions all the time. But if you're one of those that have tried to rent out your kitchen on Craigslist, then you need some help. Maybe more than I can offer. But I'm willing to give it a shot.

In this section, you will find a handful of ideas and tips that have helped my friends, family, and *Skinny Bitch* fans discover new ways to have fun in the kitchen. May they bring you some enjoyment, too.

GIVE YOUR KITCHEN SOME LIFE

A blender is not a decoration. It is an appliance, Einstein. If you are going to spend some time in your kitchen, then start making it a place you *want* to be. Breathe some life into it. Make sure there is good feng shui (See "Feng Shui" on page 110). Create an environment that is you. Don't be shy.

Small kitchens shouldn't hold you back either. I suffer from small kitchen*itis,* but I refuse to see it as an obstacle. I customized some cute curtains, found wall space to showcase my son's finger paintings, and covered my refrigerator with wedding invitations, baby photos, magnets from our travels, and a Polaroid of me when I shaved my head. (Yes, I was once a crazy bitch.) It may look disheveled, but it's mine.

CREATING A KITCHEN THAT IS *YOU*

If you lack a creative bone in your body, but want to get your kitchen cooking-worthy, here are some tips from my good friend and celebrity "green" interior designer Sarah Rosenhaus. Here's her philosophy: It's the little details in a room that help to create an ambiance that make us want to spend all of our time there.

"Every object you bring into your kitchen should make you feel good and inspire you to spend time cooking, socializing, or enjoying a meal by yourself," she says. "Beautiful things are nice, but it is important to create the energy in a space that draws you."

THE SKINNY: ORGANIZED BITCH
STACK PLATES AND BOWLS IN AN ORDERLY FASHION, AND KEEP GLASSES LINED UP NEATLY BY SIZE SO THAT EVERYTHING NOT ONLY LOOKS SEXY BUT IS ALSO A CINCH TO GET TO. DIGGING AROUND FOR WHAT YOU NEED ADDS STRESS TO YOUR KITCHEN TIME.

Play That Funky Music

I love nothing better than winding down in the kitchen with my favorite album. Music is perfect for creating different moods. Some days I just want to bake a pot pie and hum out to Sade. Other days, I feel like putting on my stonewashed jeans and making a mess with the Red Hot Chili Peppers screaming at the top of their lungs. I guess it just depends on

SHOW OFF YOUR FRUIT AND VEGGIES: Healthy bitches stock up on fruits and veggies. Rather than hide them, get a fun bowl to display on your kitchen counter or table that is piled high with your colorful produce. The beauty and accessibility of it will inspire you to munch on a healthy snack throughout the day.

APPEAL TO YOUR SENSES: One to two candles add instant ambiance to a kitchen. Choose a few lightly scented clean-burning soy candles that you can switch out depending on your mood. They also work wonders in covering up that unpleasant smell like something may have just died in your garbage disposal.

DIM THE LIGHTS: Bad fluorescent lighting is not going to entice you to cook. Consider hiring an electrician to install a dimmer switch on the existing light switch in your kitchen. This way, you can dim the lights to your liking and light a candle for a more romantic, sensual cooking experience. Dimming the light bulbs only costs about $100, and it's energy efficient.

START A FUN DINNERWARE COLLECTION: One of the best ways to encourage yourself to cook is to invest in dinnerware that makes you want to serve food on it. Have a blast collecting a mismatched array of quirky eclectic pieces that tell a story about where you've been and what you like(d). Or find different varieties of flatware that follow the same color scheme but wake up your kitchen with different textures, styles, and sizes.

Are you aching for some stylish, green touches in your kitchen? Let Sarah work her magic. Visit her website at www.sarahrosenhaus.com.

whether I have alone time, or if my son is hanging from my leg screaming that he just farted. [Sigh]

If cooking tends to be a winding down experience for you, as well, pour a glass of red wine or hot tea to add to the experience. Just keep in mind that if you're an easily distracted person and following a recipe, tunes can throw you off. Make sure you are paying attention to each step of the recipe or your lasagna may look like a cracked-out pizza.

MAKE PLAYLISTS: Let the cuisine take control by creating different playlists. Apple iTunes allows you to type in keywords to search for different genres (www.itunes.com). Pandora is a free music site that lets you type in what genre of music you are looking for, and then creates a continuous, alternating playlist of artists and songs that match your keyword (www.pandora.com).

MAKE IT A HOBBY

Cooking can be a little like doing it missionary style. In order to keep the passion alive and exciting, you have to change it up every once in a while. Swing from the chandelier! Experiment with new recipes and styles of cuisine. Cook with others who not only share your love for food, but your level of skill, too. Maybe your best friend has trouble boiling water while your fiancé is a personal chef to the stars. Find your happy medium.

COOKING CLUBS

If you are a self-confessed foodie, meeting people who share your interests is not difficult. There are foodies all over the country, in every city and every neighborhood, who are looking to find someone of their caliber. Ask around your networks, call the nearest cooking school or peruse online community forums. Another option is to start your own. Surf the Internet, online community forums, and Craigslist for tips on starting your own cooking club or joining one.

COOKING CLASSES

Whether you're learning the basics of Cooking 101 or you're a seasoned sous chef, there is a cooking class for every level. For those who have varying work schedules or travel frequently, classes can range from one-night to six-week courses. Many cooking schools offer private classes for one-on-one instruction or you can hire an instructor for a private party. (Perfect for bachelorettes and birthday parties!) If you have a friend who loves to dabble in the kitchen, gift certificates for a cooking class are the perfect gift. It is thoughtful, fairly inexpensive, and original.

THE ART OF SEDUCTION

If you think your relationship needs a little help behind closed doors, say no more. Relationships take work, sex kitten. Watching football with him on Sunday afternoons as a flirting method will *not* do the trick. Honey, the only thing on his mind is holding the quarterback for two more downs and what color the cheerleader's panties are. He doesn't even know you are home.

So, instead of catering to his chauvinistic needs, cater to your mutual needs. Give the kitchen a chance. Food is just oozing with sex. The hot flame on the stove, the big wooden spoons and the flour in your hair all remind him of just how messy things can get.

COOK TOGETHER: Cooking a romantic dinner for him is always a nice gesture. But you don't want nice. You want to get laid. Not tomorrow. Not over the weekend. *Tonight.* Spice things up. Plan ahead of time and tell him to block off a night for the two of you to cook one of his favorite recipes. Light some lavender candles in the kitchen, crack open a bottle of red wine, and work some aphrodisiacs into your main dish (see page 100, "The Love Chef"). This is probably not an ideal night for lentils or beans.

THE ALLURE OF THE APRON: Do not doubt the sexual prowess of the apron. Or more appropriately, do not doubt *your* sexual prowess in an apron. Consider surprising him in the kitchen one night. Slip into your apron, to reveal that you are wearing nothing underneath while still leaving a little to the imagination. Just remember, there is a fine line between a temptress and a hooker. Do not get them confused.

DINNER PARTIES

Take a look at your bank statements. If it looks more like a city guide for the hottest restaurants in town than your checking account, it's a good sign you are dining out too much. Settle down, hipster. If parties, dinners, and cocktail soirees are more your style, throw your own! This may sound like a lot of time and money, but it doesn't have to be.

Hosting a Dinner Party that Doesn't Break the Bank

TAPAS-STYLE DINNER: Rather than spending your monthly salary on a five-course dinner for ten guests, stick to the basics. Choose five to six hors d'oeuvres or appetizers and host a tapas dinner. I like to ask each of my friends to send me the recipe for their favorite tapas dish, and we all cook it together. You can still have the typical sit-down dinner setting, just inform guests prior to the invitation that it will be small plates.

AFTER-DINNER PARTY: Break the mold and host the most untraditional of dinner parties. Sweet tooth required. Invite guests over for a late-night tasting of your favorite healthy desserts. Show off your baking skills with a wide arrangement of confections that appeal to all invitees, and pair each with a beverage that complements the savory flavors. Set the arrival time for 9 p.m. and make it clear that you will not be serving dinner. You do not need your guests raiding the refrigerator for snacks.

MODERN-DAY POTLUCK: Instead of a hodgepodge of random dishes, a New-Age potluck is a sit-down dinner party focused on a single-style cuisine. This is not a cheesy awards banquet—no buffet tables allowed. First off, choose a cuisine style. Send each guest a recipe for a course that falls under the desired cuisine (scanned versions via e-mail are quick and eco-friendly), and tell them how many people to prepare for.

I hope your friends are not shy. Each guest will be asked to prepare the finishing touches and serve their dish to the table when it's their turn in the lineup. While they are at it, ask them to give a speech about the first time you both met, how pretty you looked, and why they love you so much. Hey, it's your party!

Eco Party Planning Tips

When planning a dinner party or small cocktail affair, keep in mind that you are a green-bitch-in-training. Anna Getty, a top-notch green living lifestyle educator and best-selling author of *Anna*

Getty's Easy Green Organic, offers up a few tips on throwing an eco-chic home affair. Give that green thumb a manicure. It's your party and the planet is invited.

BRING IN DECORATIONS FROM THE OUTDOORS. Decorate the table with branches, stones, and field flowers. Afterwards throw them into your composter or your yard for mulch.

GIFT POTTED HERBS. Give parting gifts that grow, like potted herbs (they can double as table decor at the party), packets of vegetables, or flower seeds.

THINK SEASONAL WITH THE MENU. When deciding on the menu, think local, seasonal, and organic. Skip the ingredients with large carbon footprints. That means no dishes with strawberries or asparagus in December. Head to your farmers' market instead of the supermarket. Connect with the growers of your food.

MAKE IT A FAMILY AFFAIR

Your kids are on the couch watching cartoons. Your other half is camping out in front of the computer screen. The dog is snoring in the corner. And, there you are, in the kitchen cooking a healthy three-course meal for the family to enjoy. Now, aren't you just a spitting image of Mrs. Cleaver? I'll bet you have a white picket fence and monogrammed bathroom towels, too.

Wake up, woman. This is a new millennium. Why are you waiting on your family hand-and-foot, like the goddamn Brady Bunch? Who do they think you are—their *bitch? Please.*

Get the whole gang involved! Cooking with your family is a great way to hear about everyone's day, encourage healthy interaction, coordinate schedules and plans, and most of all, laugh. With how busy our lives have gotten, this is sometimes the only time that all family members are gathered in one place. Research has shown that families who engage in shared activities like, say, cooking, have been shown to be less likely to have conflict five years down the road. That's a good enough reason for me.

Getting the Kids Involved

I could talk for days about why cooking is so beneficial for kids. But I'll spare you. In a nutshell, they are more likely to eat what they cook, it boosts their self-esteem, teaches them to work as a team, and stimulates their imagination and creativity. The best part is they don't even know they are learning life skills that are important to their health and future. Child obesity is not something we should be proud of.

The earlier you bring your children into the kitchen with you, the more it will feel like home to them. The last two months of my pregnancy, I was cooking up a storm for my husband and me, while Jack kicked in my stomach. Deep inside, I knew that I was doing something right. In his first few months out of the womb, I placed him in the Baby-Björn so he faced the kitchen while I washed lettuce for a salad. At the mere ages of one and two, my little sous chef was licking the chocolate frosting off of the electric beaters, and pouring the ingredients in a big wooden bowl for Sunday morning pancakes. Now my big boy has his own herb garden in our backyard. Jack digs through the soil, plants and replants seeds, waters them daily to watch them grow into edible vegetables, and picks them at dinnertime when they are ripe and ready.

He also has one of the most amazing palates a young man can have—courtesy of his father, a former French chef, and his mother, a neurotic, cooking-obsessed freak of nature. Because of his young "training," he doesn't like the traditional junk foods most kids enjoy. He is more refined than that.

When bringing your little tykes into the kitchen, keep tasks simple and time-consuming. And, of course, *safe*. Handing your two-year-old son a butcher knife and asking him to finely dice garlic will probably raise a red flag for Child Protective Services. Kids love washing vegetables, rolling out dough, or anything having to do with cakes, cookies, or decorating. Mixing and stirring, while tedious, is another popular task that still makes children feel a part of the cooking experience.

Crafty Activities for Kids in the Kitchen

DECORATE THE TABLE. The table is the focal point of meals. Assign nights when kids are responsible for making the centerpiece, name placeholders, or decorating the napkins. Have them set the table and choose the dinner topic. That's if you're willing to risk a half-hour discussion about Barbie's daily escapades in her Corvette. Man, that bitch has everything.

GIVE THEM THE REINS. Allow them to choose the menu one night a week. Do not kid yourself into assuming your little angels will choose healthy meals. Without fail, they will ask for cheeseburgers. To avoid temper tantrums, give them a handful of fun, healthy choices, and let them pick one meal. This will give you the chance to teach your children about the food groups and a well-balanced regimen.

PLAY WITH YOUR FOOD. Kids love eye candy. Offer them dipping sauces and attention grabbing shapes. Rather than cook conventional toast, give them cookie cutters to make their own star-shaped toast. You can also get creative with pasta noodles, which come in dozens of shapes and sizes.

You can have a field day with ideas, just remember to create a happy-go-lucky environment for children, and they will see food for what it is—fun.

BITCHIFYING YOUR PANTRY

There is nothing worse than getting halfway through a recipe—oven preheated and vegetables chopped on the cutting board—and realize you are missing an ingredient. There is no time to make a run to the store. (You're low on gas, too.) And your neighbors are out of town doing whatever people with stocked pantries do on the weekend. Jerks. All that work and all that planning for a romantic dinner-for-two, and you screwed it all up because you forgot you used the last of the soy cheese to sneak your dog his flea medication yesterday.

Time to get organized, bitch.

Cooking should be rewarding. Not a pain in the ass. In order to have some fun in the kitchen, you must know what you have at your disposal, and what you need at your disposal. This isn't always easy to figure out. So, I've prepared a Pantry Guide that outlines the standard foods in a *Skinny Bitch* kitchen and a grocery wish list.

THE EIGHT PANTRY STAPLES: WHAT TO BUY, WHAT TO AVOID, AND WHAT MAKES ME SWOON

Here are a few common kitchen must-haves (alongside their notorious alter-egos) to start you off on the right path. I make sure I have these guys stocked at all times, hell or high water, since they are versatile and most commonly used in the kitchen. (For sugar, meat, milk, and cheese alternatives, see pages 35-43.)

Breads

What to Buy: Whole grain bread

White bread may feel nice and fluffy, but it undergoes a bleaching process to ensure a longer shelf life in the grocery store. Bleaching strips bread of its essentials nutrients, leaving only fattening starches, refined sugars, and proteins with no helpful benefits.[84] Whole-grain bread endures minimal processing and maintains all of its healthy vitamins and minerals. It is much higher in fiber, vitamins B6 and E, magnesium, zinc, folic acid, and chromium. You can thank fiber for good digestive health, a healthy body weight, and lowering your risk of heart disease.[85]

Flour

What to Buy: Unbleached flour (organic)

Chemicals like potassium bromate and benzoyl peroxide are used to chemically whiten flours.[86] Unbleached "all-purpose," whole-wheat, and buckwheat (gluten-free) flours are all good choices and really depend on preference and food allergies.

Organic is always a good option since they are milled from crops grown without synthetic fertilizers and chemicals. I swear by King Arthur's unbleached all-purpose flour, while their 100-percent organic whole-wheat flour is the top seller. www.kingarthurflour.com

Butter

What to Buy: Earth Balance

If I could have Earth Balance's babies, I would. (Yes, I know butter can't procreate.) The buttery all-natural spread contains zero trans fats and is full of omega-3 fatty acids. Earth Balance has also been shown to increase HDL ("good") cholesterol while lowering LDL ("bad") cholesterol. www.earthbalancenatural.com

Eggs

What to Buy: Ener-G Egg Replacer

A must-have for the vegan baker, Ener-G is an egg replacer that is a piece of cake to use in recipes. The eggless product caters to all types of allergies, with no gluten, wheat, casein, dairy, egg, yeast, soy, nut, and rice. I owe my signature cookie recipes to this stuff. www.ener-g.com

Mayonnaise

What to Buy: Vegenaise by Follow Your Heart

An eggless mayonnaise substitute for vegans, Vegenaise has a diverse product line that is delicious and all-natural. The reduced-fat version, made with flaxseed and olive oil, has half the fat of regular mayonnaise and zero cholesterol. They also offer an organic option. www.followyourheart.com/vegenaise

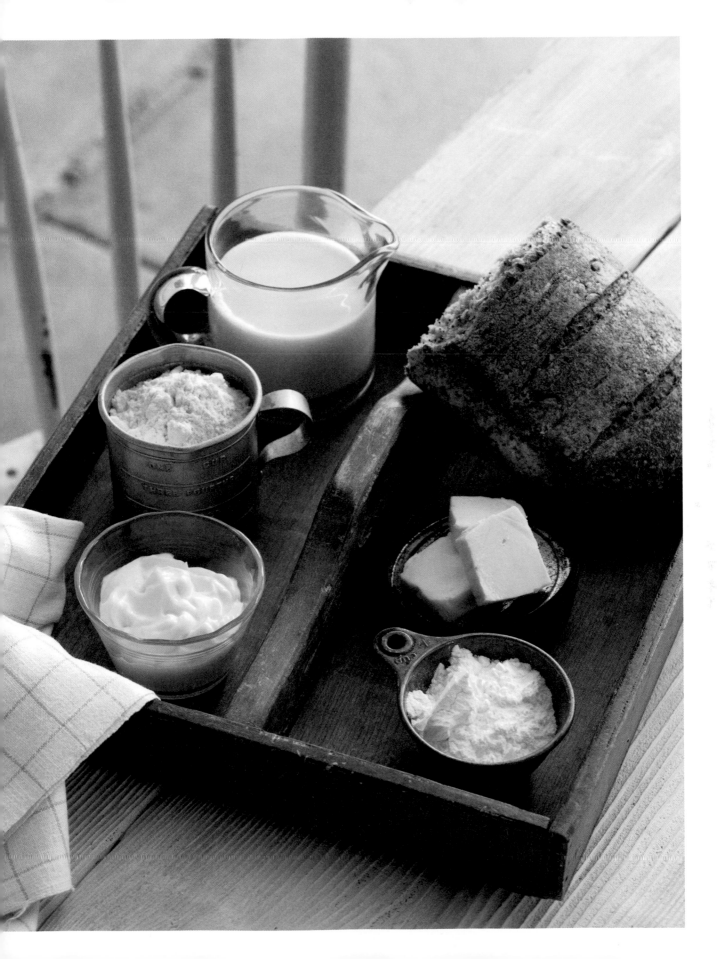

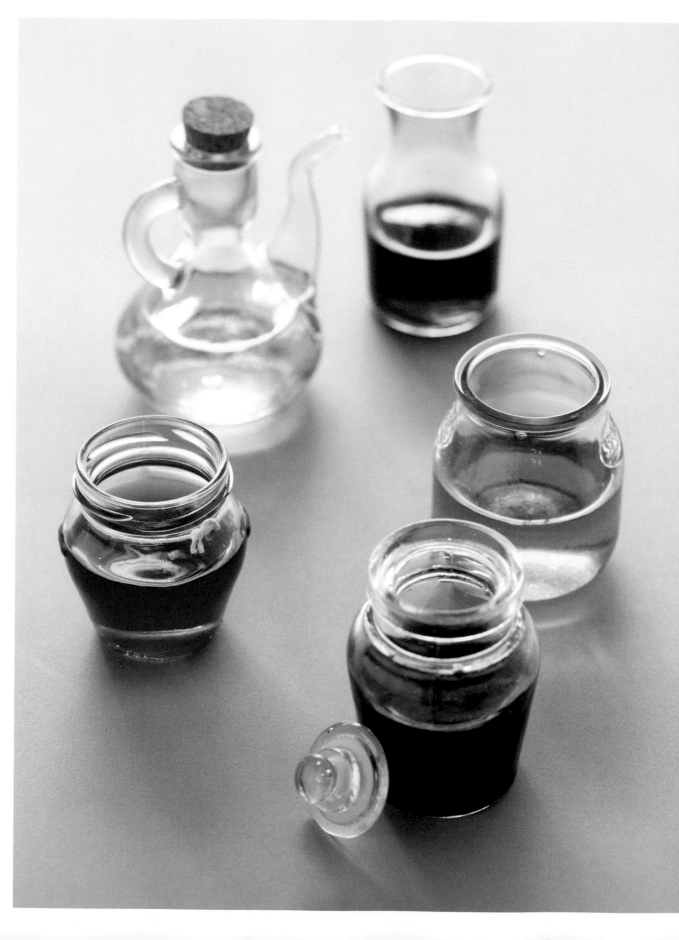

Oils

What to Buy: Grapeseed oil, extra-virgin olive oil, sesame oil, safflower oil, walnut oil, canola oil.

Cooking oils are essential to baking, salad dressings, marinades, and deep-frying. I use grapeseed oil for most of my cooking, because it has a high flash point, and has a light, neutral taste. But I do flirt with other oils too—they all have their own unique taste, and lend varying flavors to a recipe. You'll use all of the above-listed oil in this cookbook. Canola oil is one of the most popular cooking oils in the kitchen. It has a very mild, almost bland taste, which makes it a great all-purpose oil because it produces no interfering flavors. Safflower and sunflower oils can also withstand high heat and carries a very mild, nearly neutral flavor. Olive and sesame oils are good alternatives for cooking and stir-fry dishes.

BITCHWORTHY: WHEN CHOOSING A CANOLA OIL, ALWAYS GO ORGANIC. NON-ORGANIC CANOLA OIL CAN BE GENETICALLY MODIFIED (GM).[87]

There are some oils that are best used on foods already cooked, such as walnut, flaxseed, and hempseed oils. They are best on salads, pasta, grilled veggies, and in dressings and smoothies. For optimal flavor and quality, buy expeller and cold-pressed organic serving oils.

Vinegars

What to Buy: Apple cider vinegar, rice vinegar, balsamic vinegar, white-wine vinegar, white vinegar

They all get the *Skinny Bitch* stamp of approval. Apple cider vinegar and rice vinegar are both high in minerals and amino acids. Balsamic vinegar has a more pungent flavor and helps to prevent fatigue and anemia. White-wine vinegar can serve as a salt replacement and is ideal in sauces, marinades, and salads. Lastly, distilled white vinegar freshens wilted vegetables (and can clean your floors!).

Pasta

What to Buy: Whole grain pasta

Unlike white pasta, whole grain pasta still retains all the disease-fighting nutrients like folate, vitamin E, magnesium, potassium, selenium, and a whole army of other healthy powerhouses. It also contains more fiber and can contribute to weight loss. I am a fan of Eden Organic whole grain pastas (www.edenfoods.com) and I love, love, love Pappardelles. The online resource is great for amazing and unique varietals of pasta. I discovered them at a farmers' market in Florida, a few years ago and it changed my life. I order my favorites—lemon basil, lime cilantro, even dark chocolate—on a regular basis to give family meals an edge.

www.pappardellesonline.com

TIPS ON STORING OILS

OILS ARE VERY FICKLE. IF YOU DON'T GIVE THEM THE PROPER ATTENTION OR CARE, WELL, THEY'LL TURN THEIR BACK ON YOU. PISSED-OFF OILS ARE NOT FUN ENEMIES. FOR BEST RESULTS, STORE IN AIRTIGHT CONTAINERS IN A DARK, DRY AREA AWAY FROM LIGHT AND HEAT. IF YOU USE THE OILS ONLY OCCASIONALLY OR LIVE IN WARMER CLIMATES (HELLO, ARIZONA!), STORE IN THE REFRIGERATOR (NUT OILS TURN RANCID QUICKLY, SO ALWAYS STORE IN THE REFRIGERATOR.) YOU MAY NOTICE SOME OILS BECOME CLOUDY WHEN REFRIGERATED, BUT THEY WILL RETURN TO NORMAL ONCE AT ROOM TEMPERATURE AGAIN. LASTLY, LIKE YOU AND ME, OILS AGE, SO USE WITHIN A YEAR OF OPENING OR SUCK IT UP AND BUY A NEW BOTTLE .

THE SKINNY BITCH SHOPPING LIST

Ladies, what's the number-one rule in healthy shopping? That's right! Always go to the store with a grocery list. If you head down the aisles empty-handed, you are ten times more likely to purchase processed foods with hidden additives. Women with goals are hot. Make like Santa and compile that list, and then check it twice. Consider these pantry staples, and use this grocery list to guide you toward more healthful choices. Any questions? *Skinny Bitches*, dismissed.

Baking Goods

- Unbleached all-purpose flour
- Unbleached whole wheat flour
- Whole wheat pastry flour
- Spelt flour
- Baking powder
- Baking soda
- Cornstarch or arrowroot
- Evaporated cane sugar
- Agave nectar
- Maple syrup
- Molasses
- Brown sugar
- Non-hydrogenated vegetable shortening
- Wheat germ
- Nutritional yeast
- Dark cocoa powder
- Chocolate chips
- Vanilla extract
- Almond extract
- Panko breadcrumbs
- Oats

Condiments

- Ketchup (organic)
- Dijon mustard
- Earth Balance butter
- Vegan mayo
- Miso paste
- Tahini
- Organic peanut butter
- Almond butter (organic)
- Worcestershire sauce

Canned Goods

- Coconut milk
- Beans
- Chickpeas
- Black beans
- Kidney beans
- Pinto beans
- Black-eyed peas
- Adzuki beans

Oils and Vinegars

- Olive oil
- Grapeseed oil
- Canola oil
- Toasted sesame oil
- Safflower oil
- Walnut oil
- Apple cider vinegar
- Balsamic vinegar
- Rice vinegar
- White wine vinegar
- Distilled white vinegar

Nuts/Seeds

- Walnuts
- Almonds
- Sesame seeds
- Sunflower seeds
- Flaxseeds
- Pumpkin seeds

Pasta

- Whole grain pasta
- Brown rice pasta
- Soba pasta
- Spelt pasta
- Corn pasta
- Quinoa pasta
- Artichoke pasta
- Spinach pasta

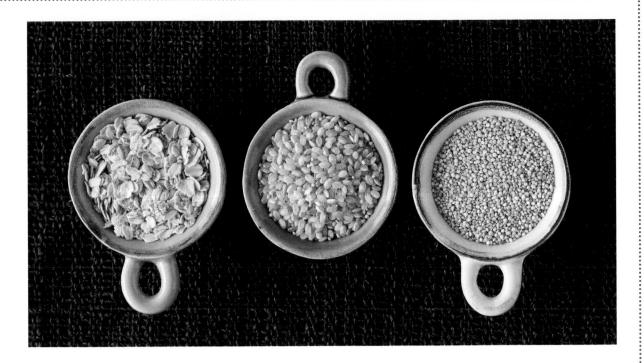

Grains

Quinoa
Lentils
Split peas
Couscous
Basmati rice
Brown rice
Wild rice
Jasmine rice
Barley
Millet

Refrigerator Arsenal

Almond milk
Rice milk
Soy milk
Hemp milk
Tempeh
Seitan
Tofu
Ener-G Foods egg replacer
Vegan cheese
Soy/coconut milk yogurt
Salsa
Hummus
Bean dip
Edamame
Applesauce (organic)

Dry Goods

Rice cakes
Whole grain crackers
Tortilla chips
Whole grain tortillas
Trail mix
Whole grain bagels
Tea
Green tea
Chamomile tea
White tea
Mint tea

THE SKINNY: WHOLE-GRAIN TORTILLAS

I HAVE AN ENTIRE DRAWER DEDICATED TO TORTILLAS IN MY REFRIGERATOR. IF THAT DRAWER IS HOME TO LESS THAN THREE BAGS, I DECLARE A STATE OF EMERGENCY. WE USE THEM FOR EVERYTHING IN THE BARNOUIN HOUSEHOLD: BURRITOS, ENCHILADAS, TACOS, QUESADILLAS, YOU NAME IT. AFTER I PUT JACK TO BED, I LIKE TO WARM THEM UP AND SPREAD SOME EARTH BALANCE, A SPRINKLE OF CINNAMON, AND EVAPORATED CANE SUGAR ON TOP. IT'S MY SPECIAL MOMMY TREAT.

NATURE'S SEASONINGS: HERBS AND SPICES

A Party in Your Mouth

Herbs and spices once served a very different role in my life. One that wasn't quite so honorable. One that was of pure decoration.

In my waitressing days, my herbs and spices vocabulary was limited to salt, pepper, and garlic powder. Oh, and parsley. Though I didn't know you could actually eat it. Nobody taught me the basics. My biggest concerns involved making sure salads arrived before entrees, and that the head bartender kept his distance from the underage hostess. As you can see, sweetheart, I had bigger fish to fry.

Those days are long behind me. Thanks to popular influences like the Food Network, a deep, understated love for cookbooks, a desire to explore my bare kitchen, and falling in love with a French chef, I'm a whole new woman. Through trials and tribulations, I have gained an utmost respect for herbs and spices to add a sublime dose of flavor, as well as essential vitamins and nutrients to a dish, without the added calories, sugar, and fat.

For the droves of moms and career-driven women out there, herbs and spices are your best friend. They will help you create a great-tasting, healthy meal with little preparation required . . . in no thyme. (Wink, wink)

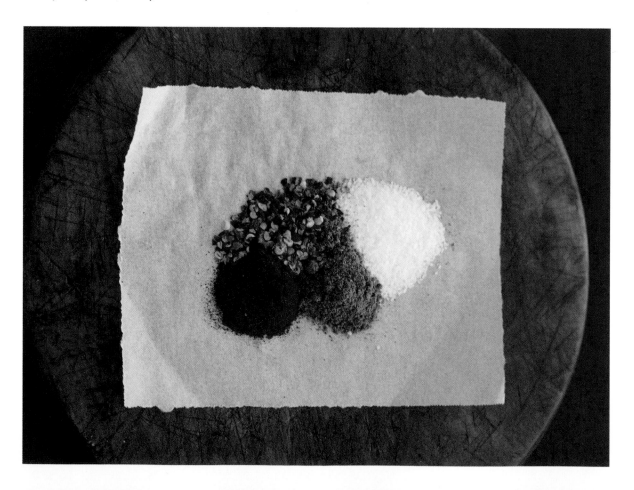

GET SPICY

Not all herbs and spices are created equal. While some are ground up into a powder, others are worked into the dish like they were just plucked from the plant. With that said, each one comes with a different set of rules.

Follow these simple guidelines to ensure you get the most from your seasoning of choice:

STORAGE: To help preserve the flavor of herbs and spices, store in a cool, dry place away from sunlight. Do not store them above the stove or dishwasher, where they may come in contact with increased levels of moisture and heat.

MOISTURE AND HEAT: Avoid adding spices and herbs directly from the jar into a steaming pot, pan, or skillet. Moisture and heat will take away from the flavor, and can cause the remaining product to cake. Measure into a spoon or a cup away from heat before adding to your recipe to retain optimal flavor and consistency.

GROUND SPICES: These guys, such as cayenne pepper and saffron, release their flavor quickly so they are best used in quick-fix recipes. If they cook along with the food for a while, they have a bad habit of turning bitter.

SEEDS: Toast seeds— sesame, cumin, and peppercorns—in the oven or on the stove, prior to serving. This enhances their natural aroma and flavor. When toasting on the stove, stir occasionally.

DRIED HERBS: There's a little trick to getting the most bang from your dried herbs: Brush the leaves with your fingers to release volatile oils and increase the flavor. Try it! Dried whole spices and herbs, such as bay leaves and whole allspice, release flavor more slowly than ground or crumbled. So, they are best used in dishes that require longer durations to simmer like soups and stews.

FRESH HERBS: The more delicate herbs, such as basil, chives, parsley and cilantro, should be added toward the end of the cooking cycle to preserve their fresh flavor. For best results, sprinkle a dash of seasoning a minute or two before the dish is ready, or when the food is served. When substituting fresh herbs in a recipe, use three times as much as you would a dried herb. They shrink when cooked.

LESS DELICATE HERBS: I make it sound like herbs have feelings, but hopefully, you get my drift. Add less delicate herbs, such as oregano, rosemary, tarragon, and thyme, during the final twenty minutes of preparation.

THE SKINNY: HOW TO WASH FRESH HERBS

WASH HERBS WHEN YOU ARE READY TO USE THEM. JUST RINSE A SMALL HANDFUL UNDER COOL, RUNNING WATER. SHAKE OFF MOISTURE OR DRY IN A SALAD SPINNER. PAT DRY WITH CLEAN PAPER TOWELS. IF WASHING A LARGE AMOUNT AT ONCE, PLACE IN A CLEAN SINK OR BOWL FILLED WITH COLD WATER AND SWISH AROUND LIKE A HULA HOOP. LATHER, RINSE, AND REPEAT IN ANOTHER BOWL OF CLEAN WATER.

The Herb + Spices Chart O' Fun

There are hundreds of delicious herbs and spices out there, but I've decided to narrow it down for you. The ones listed below not only add natural flavor, they also deliver a dose of heart protecting, cancer-preventing, bacteria-fending healthy benefits. This nifty chart outlines which herbs and spices work best with what dishes. Copy and display on your fridge as a cooking tool.

	BEST PAIRINGS	BEST RESULTS
Basil	The ultimate pairing for Italian dishes, basil adds a special touch to tomatoes, onions, garlic, and olives. It is an ideal seasoning for pasta sauce, fresh pesto, salads, gazpacho, eggplant, and zucchini.	Fresh basil. You won't obtain full flavor from dried basil. If you're in a pinch and only have dried basil, use one-third the amount of fresh.
Bay Leaves	Enhance the flavor of beans and soups with one or two whole dried leaves; a superb pairing for spaghetti sauce, casseroles, and stews.	Crinkle the leaves just before using to release the potent flavor. Replenish this herb often, as old, dried leaves tend to lose their flavor with age. Add to water while cooking vegetables or pasta.
Cinnamon	An excellent baking tool, cinnamon spruces up apple and pumpkin pies, and is a delicious topping for oatmeal, hot cocoa, pancakes, or applesauce. Cinnamon also adds a nice touch to chili and pasta sauce.	It is one of the few spices that deliver the best results with the "cheapest stuff."
Cumin	The second bestselling spice in the world, cumin is the essential ingredient in curries. A good companion to asparagus, grains, chili, salsa, peas, potatoes, and spinach; adds some kick to lentils or fries nicely with onions.	Buy whole cumin seeds instead of ground powder since the latter tends to lose its flavor sooner. Toast the whole seed in a skillet to enhance the flavor.
Garlic	Garlic goes well with everything (some even use it in ice cream). The best pairings are pasta, tomato-based dishes, roasted vegetables, potatoes, dips, sauces, and breads.	For maximum flavor and health benefits, use fresh garlic, crushed or chopped.
Turmeric	A strong spice that evolves in flavor as it cooks, turmeric is best with soups, stews, rice, and curry dishes; also good with lentils, cauliflower, potatoes, green beans, and onions.	Widely used in cooking as a dried, powder form, but some prefer the fresh turmeric root. A little goes a long way so use sparingly.
Rosemary	A common ingredient in marinades, oils, vinegars, stews, and soups, rosemary also complements mushrooms, squash, eggplant, lasagna, tomatoes, roasted potatoes, breads, and fruits.	Use your fingers or a knife to break up or chop the dried leaves before adding to a recipe.
Paprika	Tasty with potatoes, pasta sauce, stews, soups, and chili.	Stir into a tablespoon of oil before adding to a recipe. Paprika releases its color and flavor when heated.
Ginger	An Asian favorite, ginger is used in baking sweets, ice creams, stir-fries, sauces, and curries; it's also a great complement to garlic.	Opt for fresh ginger over dry ginger powder. Most recipes call for grating or mincing into a fine consistency.

Oregano	Greek oregano is traditionally used in Italian and Mediterranean dishes, including pasta, peppers, tomato sauces, and pizza. Mexican oregano is a fine touch in chili. Add to a container of olive oil to jump-start its flavor.	While fresh oregano has a distinct, complex flavor, it's among only a handful that work best dried.
Nutmeg	A sweet pairing with cinnamon and ginger, nutmeg is a flavor savor for muffins, pies, soups, spinach, squashes, broccoli, lentils, onions, and eggplant; adds zing to mashed potatoes and sweet potatoes.	Best when freshly grated. **NOTE:** Not recommended for expectant or nursing mothers.
Sage	Sprinkle in olive oil with some fresh, ground pepper, use as a dip for breads, and add to salads and dressings. Also good with onions, cabbage, corn, eggplant, squash, stuffings, and tomatoes.	Fresh, raw sage is said to be higher in nutrients and exudes a bolder flavor. Still, both dried and fresh have their place in the kitchen. When using fresh, whole leaves, use sparingly. **NOTE:** Experts say sage should not be taken during pregnancy.
Peppermint	This holiday favorite works well in teas, tabouli, tomato-based or gazpacho soups, desserts, salads, or puréed with yogurt and fruit.	Whenever possible, choose fresh mint over the dried form. Fresh mint is superior in flavor.
Thyme	Crush into soups, sauces, stocks, marinades, pasta, bean dishes, summer squash, casseroles, mushrooms, potatoes, tomatoes, and carrots.	Choose fresh, raw thyme over the dried form since it's a cut above in flavor and preserves the vital nutrients. Buy organically to ensure it hasn't been irradiated.
Parsley	The world's most popular herb, parsley is most commonly paired with pasta dishes, soups, salads, tomato and pesto sauces, tabouli, potato salad, and vegetable sauté dishes.	Choose fresh parsley over the dried form for a superior flavor. There are two types, curly and Italian flat leaf. Italian flat leaf is more fragrant and less bitter than curly. Buy organically to ensure it hasn't been irradiated.
Cilantro (Coriander)	A fine ingredient for Mexican, Asian, and Caribbean dishes, including rice, pasta, vegetables, salsa, taco fillings, guacamole, black beans and corn salad, and lentils.	Best when purchased fresh. When possible, buy whole coriander seeds instead of ground powder since the latter loses its flavor quickly. Coriander seeds can be easily ground with a mortar and pestle.
Dill	Pairs well with Russian, German, and Greek dishes; adds a sweet flavor to such vegetables as beets, carrots, cucumbers, green beans, tomatoes, and potatoes.	Like most, use fresh dillweed over the dried form for best results.
Tarragon	Delicious in traditional French cuisine, tarragon boosts salad dressings and such earthy foods as green beans, fava beans, artichokes, asparagus, tomatoes, peas, and carrots.	When dried, the oils dissipate. Fresh tarragon has a more intense flavor and should be used sparingly.
Saffron	The priciest spice in the world, saffron is an exotic pairing for such tangy fruits as cranberries and grapefruit and such vegetables as mushrooms and peas.	Purchase saffron threads for best results. The powdered spice loses its flavor quickly. Threads also stay fresh longer.
Black Pepper	The world's most popular spice, pepper seems to complement every recipe under the sun.	Available in whole, crushed, or ground powder form. To ensure best flavor, purchase whole peppercorns and grind them in a mill just before adding to a dish. Fresh ground pepper has a more lively flavor.

Disease-Fighting Fats and Where to Get Them

Ever since the day you first tried on that bikini in the department store, you were convinced that *fat was the enemy*. Evil. Relentless. Nobody really had to persuade you. The visual of your body in that size 6 bikini, under those über-flattering fluorescent bulbs in a three-way mirror did the trick. Granted, the bubbly sales associate that continued to bring you variations of polka dots and zebra prints didn't soften the blow either. Bitter? No, never.

The problem here is we were lied to. If that sounds harsh, then call it an "accidental omission." Whatever helps you sleep at night.

Not all fats are bad for you. In fact, as you are hopefully well aware of at this stage in your life, some fats are [deep breath] *good* for you! Gasp. Eek.

There are a whole range of healthy fats that are actually essential to good health. While your body is superb at making its own fat and storing it in your tummy, thighs, and buttocks, there are a slew of "good" fatty acids that your body cannot produce. These building blocks of fat are essential to your overall health and have been proven to fight such diseases as diabetes, depression, dementia, cancer, joint and muscle pain, and heart disease.

These "good guys" in the fat family—monounsaturated and polyunsaturated fats—come in many forms. Monounsaturated shows off her good genes in olive oil—one of nature's richest sources of monounsaturated fat—canola oil, nuts, peanut oil, and avocados. Polyunsaturated gets its time to shine through its two main types of fats, omega-3 and omega-6 fatty acids. Walnuts, walnut oil, flaxseed, and flaxseed oil are good sources of omega-3s. Omega-6s flourish in corn, sunflower, safflower oil, and soybean oil. Together, a healthy diet of both can help you live a long and healthy life. Here are some of the disease-fighting benefits "good" fats carry:

CONTROL BLOOD SUGAR: Research shows that monounsaturated fats help safeguard you against Type-2 diabetes, by controlling blood sugar and levels of triglycerides (the fat your body stores).

REDUCE RISK OF BREAST CANCER: These healthy fats may also reduce the activity of a gene that triggers an aggressive form of breast cancer, and moreover, increases the effectiveness of transluzumab (Herceptin)—a drug used to treat breast cancer patients.

BEAT DEPRESSION: Individuals with higher levels of omega-3s are generally happier, and are less likely to experience mild depression.

FEED THE BRAIN: Docosahexaenoic acid (DHA), a major component of omega-3 fatty acids, helps build and repair brain cells to improve memory. Experts have also found that an omega-3 deficiency can lead to other cognitive problems, including Attention Deficit Hyperactivity Disorder (ADHD).

FIGHT INFLAMMATION: Though inflammation serves an essential purpose in treating infection and injury, it is the culprit behind a handful of other life-threatening problems, including increased risk of heart disease, asthma, diabetes, rheumatoid arthritis, thyroid disease, and inflammatory bowel disease. Omega-3s act as nature's own anti-inflammatories, helping to control and limit the destruction it can cause.[88]

All this research tells us something. Getting well acquainted with our "good" fats and omega-3s could ensure us a longer, happier, healthier life. But, for us non-fish eaters, this means tapping into the healing powers of healthy nuts and oils. Watch the benefits crack open.

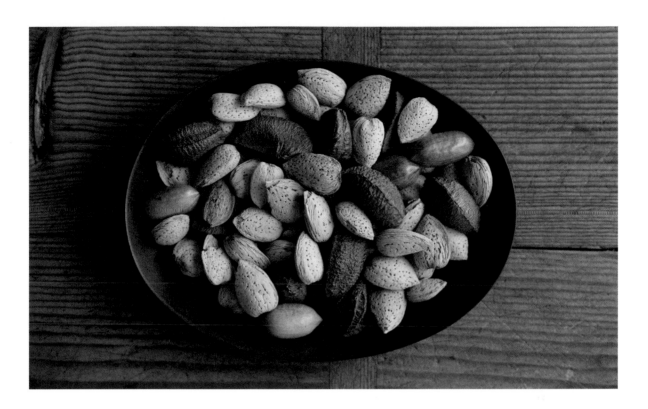

THE SKINNY: NUTS & SEEDS

....

Nuts and Seeds That Act as Natural Disease Fighters

Girl, start poppin' those kernels in your mouth like you're storing for the winter. Despite freak-outs that nuts pack extra calories and fats that make us prime candidates for Weight Watchers, the opposite is actually true. Research, like the Physicians' Follow-Up Study, has found that the unsaturated fats in these babies are actually body fat inhibitors and may help aid in weight loss. Because they take the place of more traditional protein sources, nuts and seeds actually reduce saturated fat and calories in the body for a well-balanced overall diet.

Aside from being a leading source of omega-3's, nuts bathe in protein, fiber, antioxidants, and phytonutrients. Prominent studies, including the Nurses' Healthy Study, the Iowa Women's Health Study, and the Adventist Study, have actually linked eating nuts to a 30- to 50-percent lower risk of heart disease and heart attack. Why? Experts suggest that arginine, an amino acid responsible for protecting the inner lining of arterial walls, might just be the hero in this story.[89]

Nuts and seeds are the ultimate simple, healthy snack for the girl on-the-go who wants to avoid fast food like an ex-boyfriend. Opt for unsalted and raw, and just store them in mini Tupperware containers or paper bags for a quick pick-me-up during the workday. You can also toss them in cereals, yogurts, smoothies, stir-fries, and salads for an extra boost of health benefits.

To gain the health benefits offered from our hard-shelled friends, you actually don't have to go overboard either. A one ounce serving (or five ounces per week) does the trick.

To Soak or Not To Soak? The Lowdown on Soaking Nuts and Seeds

It may sound nuts, but soaking nuts and seeds can enhance the nutrients and minerals you absorb from these little guys. Raw nuts and seeds contain enzyme inhibitors, which protect the food until its nutrient content is where it should be for adequate growth. Once proper conditions are met—sun, rain, wind—nature takes its course, allowing for the inhibitors and toxins to be naturally removed. Make sense? When you soak nuts and seeds, you take on the role of Mother Nature.

Follow this set of simple rules to get 'em wet:

STEP ONE: Look for raw, organic nuts and seeds, and fill a glass or stainless-steel bowl with clean, fresh water. Skip the plastics since they have been known to contain BPAs (Bisphenol-A), an icky chemical used in plastics. Rinse the seeds before you get rolling.

STEP TWO: Soak. Rinse. Repeat. Place the nuts and seeds in the bowl and cover with a paper towel or washcloth. How long you soak depends on the nut and seed (see below).

Drain and rinse two or three times, making sure you rinse until the water drains clear.

EXTRA CREDIT If you want to get fancy, you can rinse them with grapeseed oil or organic apple cider vinegar to be free and clear of bacteria. Don't worry, the nuts or seeds won't absorb the oil or vinegar.

The Benefits of Soaking

- Stimulates the process of germination, thereby increasing the vitamin B, C and carotenes (pre-vitamin A) content

- Counteracts phytic acid, a substance that can inhibit some absorption of calcium, magnesium, iron, copper, and zinc

- Breaks down gluten for smoother digestion

- Increases the amount of vitamins your body can absorb [90]

While you should generally dunk at room temperature, soaking durations will depend on the nut. For the most part, the more dense the nut, the longer the underwater time.

Nut/Seed	Soaking Time (hrs)
Almonds	8 to 12
Cashews	2 to 2½
Sesame seeds	8
Sunflower seeds	2
Walnuts	4
All other nuts	6 to 24

KITCHENWARE BASICS THAT ROCK MY WORLD

Even someone who lives on Top Ramen can appreciate the value of a can opener, veggie peeler, rubber spatula, and kitchen knife.

But rather than bore you with the most basic of utensils, I want to fill you in on a few of the cooking tools that are the bread to my Earth Balance. For those on a tight budget, you don't have to run to the cookware section and pull a supermarket sweep. In fact, one of the most exciting elements of cooking is giving yourself something to look forward to. Just gradually add items to your stockpile.

Pots and Pans

Though many of these are standards in kitchens across America, a few exude very special qualities. Some are planet-conscious and others promote healthier cooking. So, move over chemical-laden nonstick cookware. Mama's got some new pots and pans, and she's not afraid to use them.

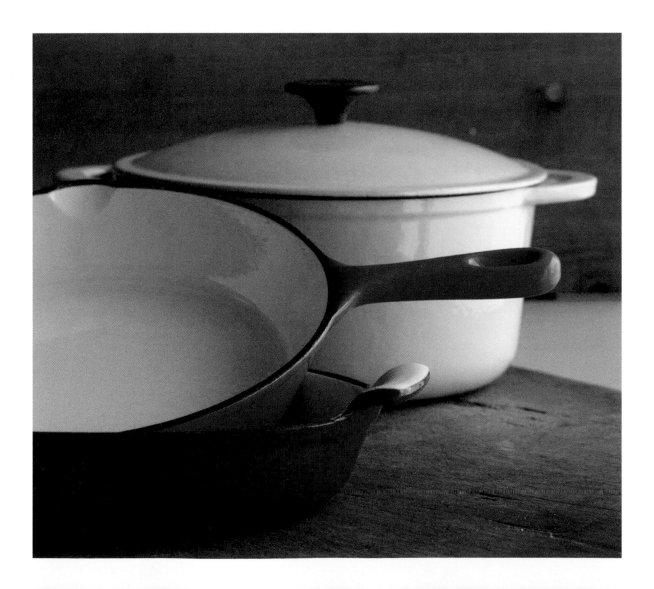

HOW TO SEASON A NEW PAN

PREHEAT OVEN TO 350°F. WASH THE PAN WELL WITH WARM WATER AND MILD DISHWASHING SOAP. DRY COMPLETELY WITH A TOWEL. SPREAD ABOUT ONE TABLESPOON OF A NEUTRAL OIL (GRAPESEED OIL WORKS WONDERS) IN THE PAN USING A KITCHEN BRUSH OR PAPER TOWEL. WARM THE PAN GENTLY OVER LOW HEAT ON THE STOVETOP. ONCE THE SURFACE IS COMPLETELY COVERED WITH NO EXCESS OIL, PUT THE PAN IN THE OVEN FOR APPROXIMATELY ONE HOUR. AFTER ONE HOUR, TURN OFF THE OVEN AND LEAVE THE PAN INSIDE UNTIL COOL.

CAST-IRON COOKWARE

This is a staple in any cook's kitchen—and for good reason. Cast iron promotes even heat distribution, and seeps off small amounts of iron into your food to ensure you are getting an appropriate amount in your diet. The real benefit is that cast iron pans last f-o-r-e-v-e-r. They can handle a beating or two, and are passed from generation to generation without ever losing their touch. As a new owner, make sure you season prior to using for the first time. Or purchase pre-seasoned from Lodge Cookware Company, www.lodgemfg.com.

ENAMELED CAST IRON

Enameled cast iron is a prettier alternative to bare cast iron. Its enamel glaze prevents rusting, so it doesn't have to be seasoned, and it is much easier to clean. The downside? You may have to shell out a few extra bucks. But the good things in life are far from free. While enameled cast iron cannot withstand the searing heats bare cast iron can, it absorbs heat and distributes it evenly. It's also energy-efficient, safe to use in the oven, and won't absorb the odors and flavors of food to pass on to your next meal.

Some of my favorite brands are:

GREEN COOKING POTS: The innovation of twin sisters and longtime healthy cooks, Mica and Café McMullen, Green Cooking Pots offer some color therapy while contributing to the betterment of our earth, all at once. The eco-friendly cookware come in bright, vibrant colors, and have the ability to add life to any meal. All pots are chemical-free and void of any toxic materials. Not only a healthier way to cook but a perfect opportunity to support cool female entrepreneurs.

www.greencookingpots.com

LE CREUSET: A standard in professional kitchens and restaurants around the world, industry giant Le Creuset carries everything from enameled cast iron and frying pans to textiles and kitchen accessories. Another great option for those who appreciate bright accents for cooking.

www.lecreuset.co.uk.

COPPER POTS

Perfect for quick warm-ups or foods that cook quickly like beans, lentils, soups, and sauces. They distribute heat evenly and are typically lined with tin or stainless steel so the copper doesn't find its way into the food. You will have to give copper pots a bit more TLC as the exterior really wears its age and use, but it's a great, safe choice in cookware. *Note:* Copper pots can contain nickel. If you have a nickel allergy, check with a retail associate or the company you're purchasing from to make sure you're in the clear.

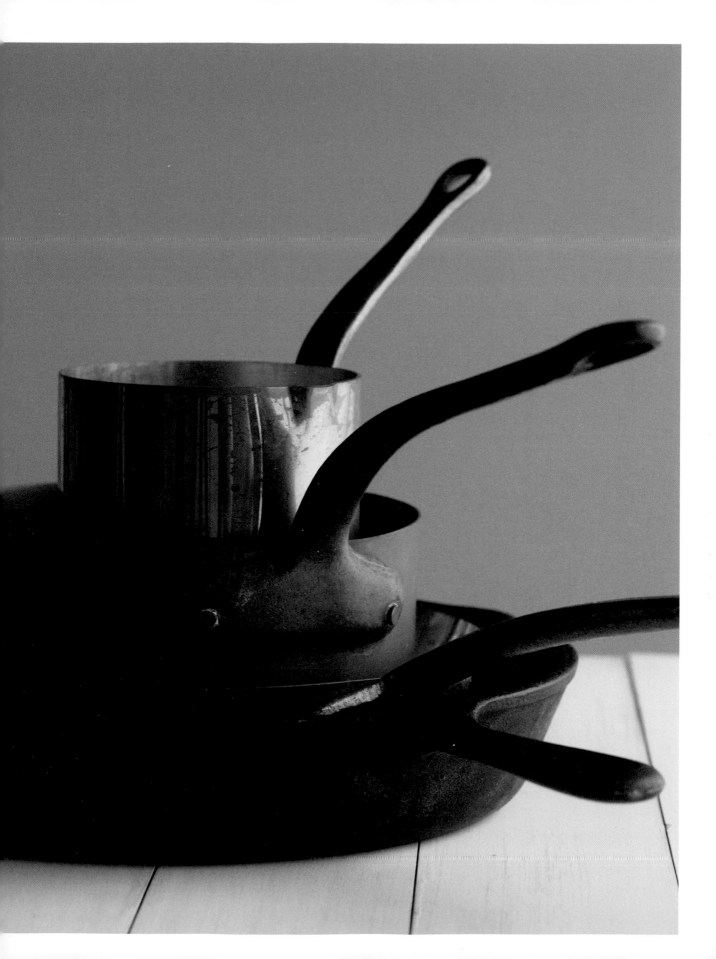

360 COOKWARE

I use this energy-efficient cookware line more than my blow-dryer. 360 Cookware uses vapor technology to heat food at lower temperatures without any excess water or added fats. Using food's natural moisture, it cooks evenly from all sides while preserving the flavor, texture, and healthy vitamins and nutrients. Because it cooks food so quickly, it continues to save my ass in a pinch.

QUICK TIP: IF YOU NEED TO WHIP UP SOMETHING QUICKLY, 360 COOKWARE IS A GODSEND. FOR AN EASY SIDE DISH, I HEAT UP TWO TABLESPOONS OF OLIVE OIL, TWO TABLESPOONS OF WHITE WINE, A TEASPOON OF EARTH BALANCE AND A PINCH OF SALT AND PEPPER. THROW IN SOME VEGGIES LIKE BROCCOLI OR CAULIFLOWER, COVER AND SIMMER FOR A FEW MINUTES. VOILÀ! YOU GOT YOURSELF A NUTRITIOUS DISH.

STAINLESS STEEL

Available at most grocery stores and cooking retailers, stainless steel pots and pans are durable, easy to clean, resistant to stains, chips and rust, and they don't affect the flavor of foods.

Cutting Boards

These aren't just any cutting boards. These are tree-huggin' cutting boards made for healthy living. Cut the shit and start cutting on something that doesn't wear down Mother Earth.

TERRA VERDE BAMBOO CUTTING BOARDS

This sexy, two-toned bamboo cutting board is chemical- and dye-free. The makers hand-select the bamboo to ensure they are not using varieties that are food sources nor habitats for the Giant Panda.

www.amazon.com

BITCHWORTHY: BAMBOO IS 16 PERCENT HARDER THAN MAPLE. THE STRONGER, DURABLE SURFACE EQUALS FEWER KNICKS, WHICH CAN HARBOR NASTY BACTERIA. BAMBOO'S NATURAL DENSITY IS ALSO WATERPROOF TO SCARE AWAY GERMS AND BACTERIA.

BLACK EPICUREAN CUTTING SURFACES

Made from an earth-friendly natural wood fiber laminate, Epicurean cutting boards are maintenance-free and heat resistant up to 350°F. Basic and nice on the wallet, they are a good choice for the beginner chef.

www.surlatable.com

PRESERVE PAPERSTONE RECYCLED PAPER CUTTING BOARD

Scraps put to good use. Designed with a petroleum-free coating and 100-percent post-consumer recycled paper, this board is a conversation starter. It's tough against use, dishwasher safe, non-porous, and affordable. Time to start planning your next dinner party.

www.bedbathandbeyond.com

THE SKINNY: CLEANING A CUTTING BOARD
YOU WEREN'T GOING TO LET IT SIT THERE ON THE COUNTER, COLLECTING DUST, FOOD BUILD-UP AND STAINS, WERE YOU? IF YOU WANT TO GET A LIFETIME OF USE OUT OF YOUR BEAUTIFUL BOARDS, WASH WITH CARE. DETERGENTS AND DISHWASHERS CAN BE ROUGH ON THESE GUYS AFTER CONTINUOUS WASHES. ALWAYS SCRUB WITH HOT WATER AND MILD SOAP, AND DRY WITH A CLEAN TOWEL. TO GO THE EXTRA MILE, CREATE YOUR OWN ANTIBACTERIAL SPRAY:

DO-IT-YOURSELF ANTIBACTERIAL SPRAY

1: GRAB A SPRAY BOTTLE OR SPRITZER

2: POUR IN TEN DROPS OF PURE LAVENDER ESSENTIAL OIL

3: ADD ONE CUP OF WATER

4: SHAKE WELL

5: SPRAY ON CUTTING BOARD AND DO NOT WASH OFF

Beyond the Essentials

Once you start getting the hang of things in the kitchen, cooking can get addictive. You spend your free time looking for new recipes and walking through the aisles of Sur La Table aimlessly. Before you know it, you're pulling all-nighters to make pistachio cookies for your husband's office. Um, hello? There are 750 employees, babe. And that's just the sales department.

Put your energy elsewhere. As you start to become a more refined cook or one who wants to leave most of the work to a machine, there are some nifty gadgets on the market for your ever-growing collection of cooking tools. Keep in mind that a handful of these are more high-tech tools, so it is reflected in the price.

You didn't need to pay the rent this month anyways, did you?

FOOD PROCESSOR

My food processor is my kitchen staple and my sanity. I am not sure I would have made it through the early stages of motherhood without it. Aside from being a dream for pureeing baby food, I quickly discovered its versatility and use it to chop veggies, nuts, and breadcrumbs; shred cheese blocks; and whip up homemade salad dressings, dips, and pesto. Now, years later, the thing is still in mint condition and has helped me find so many ways to get creative with food. Cuisinart, KitchenAid and Hamilton Beach are all popular and reliable brands for durable, long-lasting food processors. If you have limited space in your kitchen and want to limit the number of appliances, Cuisinart offers a duet blender and food processor that is perfect for preparing hors d'oeuvres or baby food with seven speeds.

MANDOLINE

A simple tool that simplifies your life, a mandoline is a hand-operated slicing machine for cutting veggies. It does its best work cutting juliennes, but with firmer veggies and fruits, it makes slices, and waffle and crinkle cuts. Dummy-proof, this utensil doesn't require much of a manual. Kyocera makes a lightweight mandoline with a hand guard that cuts in half the time while protecting your fingers from unnecessary roughness.

STANDING MIXER

This bad boy is more of a luxury than a standard, but it's a lifesaver for frequent cookers or those who love to make pastries and bread. (It makes the fluffiest frosting!) All you have to do is dump the ingredients in the bowl, adding more as you deem necessary, and it does all the work for you. You can focus on other parts of the recipe or paint your nails while you make a batch of cookies. Cuisinart, KitchenAid and Hamilton Beach are again the most dependable brands for standing mixers industry wide.

ZESTER

This compact tool allows you to remove the peel of citrus fruits to extract the zest for cooking, baking, and mixology. Zesters are most often used to remove the citrusy flavor from lemons, limes, and oranges, but many chefs are catching on to multi-purpose zesters-slash-graters to cut down their number of kitchen utensils. They can also be used to finely grate cheese, ginger, garlic, or chocolate. Microplane makes top-of-the-line yet affordable graters/zesters that get the job done.

BREAD MACHINE

This may sound a little granola for you hip cooks, but since we're learning how to be eco-friendly in this cookbook, let's chat about bread. When you make your own bread, you're in charge of what goes into it. You can choose to buy local, sustainable, and organic ingredients, and bake with the healthiest flours. Plus, you're reducing transportation costs and limiting materials required for store packaging. It's a win-win.

There are so many varieties of bread you can make with this little number. Zojirushi, Breadman, Cuisinart and Oster all make bread makers with different cycles for baking varying styles of bread—whole grain, sourdough, pizza, shaped loaves—and they are very easy to use. The trade-off is they take up a lot of room but can be stored in a pantry or supply closet when not in use.

FLOUR SIFTER

A sifter helps get the lumps and clumps out of flour, confectioners' sugar, baking soda, baking powder, and cocoa that may not otherwise break down with basic stirring. It works like a gem for recipes that call for a more even distribution in the mixture. They are typically made of stainless steel and come in several varieties like trigger action handle, small crank style, battery operated and the good ole' fashion mesh strainer. All varieties are fairly cheap. Some cooks swear by it while others don't think it's necessary. Personally, I love the softer, lighter, and fluffier texture it gives flour. Feel free to be your own judge.

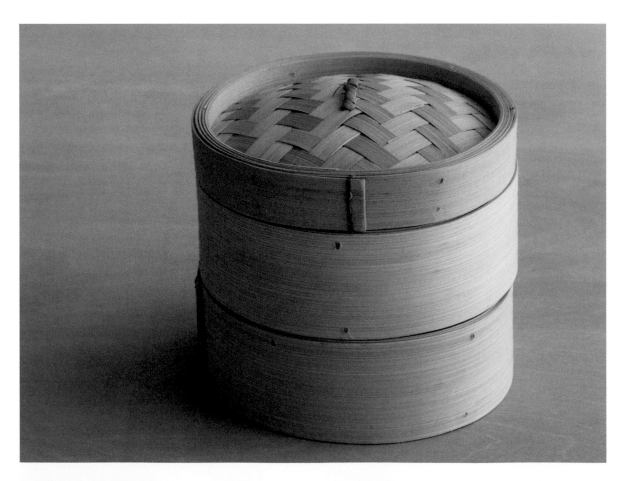

GLASS PIE PLATE

If you enjoy baking pies, this is a great investment. Because of its transparency, you can see the pie's progress as it bakes, and it doesn't absorb odors, flavors, or stains. It is also safe for the oven, microwave, freezer, or dishwasher. Pyrex is the most trusted name in glass cookware, but you can find these babies at grocery stores and any cooking retailer. I have the most kick-ass recipe for apple pie later in this cookbook (courtesy of my mother) so consider this purchase sooner than later.

QUICK TIP: WHEN USING A GLASS PIE PLATE, ADJUST THE OVEN TEMPERATURE TWENTY-FIVE DEGREES LOWER THAN WHAT THE RECIPE CALLS FOR. THIS WAY IT WON'T OVERCOOK THE BOTTOM OF THE PIE WHILE THE TOP BROWNS.

VEGETABLE STEAMER

A food steamer is a great addition to a healthy, low-calorie diet. Because it uses steam rather than boiling water to cook vegetables and fruits, it preserves the vitamins and minerals, and reduces fat intake. Steamers also don't hotbox the kitchen like an oven and require less energy to operate. They usually come as a steamer pot, bamboo steamer, three-tiered plug-in food steamer, stainless-steel insert that fits into a saucepan, or a small steamer with feet. The cook has many options here.

VITA-MIX

This incredible kitchen appliance turns whole foods into juice, cooks up soup from scratch, grinds grain, whips up peanut butter and can even make homemade ice cream! It is another one that is rather pricey, but the lovers of this wonder appliance have found countless ways (more than fifty) to use and abuse it. I don't actually own one yet, but have been advertising it at the top of my cooking wish list on the fridge for ages. Any day now, hubby....

Great Websites for Sustainable Cooking

Below are a few of my favorite home and living websites for finding the best sustainable, green brands for your cooking pleasure. As you'll see, it's not so tough being green.

BAMBU HOME: An online retailer that thinks outside-the-box with contemporary, colorful solutions for your kitchen and home. All materials used are derived from renewable resources, and packaging is made from 100-percent post-consumer recycled fibers. One percent of net sales are contributed to the preservation and restoration of the environment. Just what I like—a company with a conscience.
www.bambuhome.com

MODERN ECO HOMES: With beautiful goods for your kitchen and home, Modern Eco Homes acts as a green concierge service to help you locate products that meet your everyday needs. Their blog will keep you up-to-date with reviews on the newest and coolest products and services.
www.modernecohomes.com

ECO KITCHEN: This eco Internet store believes in practical, superior kitchens that are still energy efficient. You'll find thousands of products to choose from that don't sacrifice quality for the environment.
www.ecokitchen.com

PRISTINE PLANET: More of a one-stop shop for all your green needs, Pristine Planet goes beyond the kitchen basics with a superstore of meat alternatives, oils, sauces, spices, and snacks.
www.pristineplanet.com

PART FOUR

THE RECIPES

Nutritional Information Key:

Srv	▶	Serving Size
Cal	▶	Calories
Fat	▶	Fat
Sat Fat	▶	Saturated Fat
Col	▶	Cholesterol
Carb	▶	Carbohydrates
Fib	▶	Fiber
Pro	▶	Protein

BREAKFAST

Fresh Corn-off-the-Cob and Pepper Frittata

Shuck the corn off the cob for a healthy omelet that surprisingly tastes just like a traditional egg-based frittata. This is a fun breakfast for a Saturday morning when you have some extra time to play in the kitchen. Once you get it down pat, change up the recipe and toss in a piecrust for a tasty quiche.

MAKES 6 SERVINGS

1 tablespoon grapeseed oil
1 cup (160 g) diced onion
1 red pepper, diced
2 ears corn, kernels removed
1 (14-ounce/400 g) package extra-firm tofu, drained
½ teaspoon baking powder
⅓ cup (90 g) nutritional yeast
1 tablespoon soy sauce
2 tablespoons red wine vinegar
Salt and pepper, to taste

Preheat the oven to 350° F (180° C).

Heat the oil in a medium skillet on medium-high heat. Add the onion and sauté until translucent, about 3 minutes. Add the red pepper and corn kernels and sauté an additional 5 minutes. Set aside.

In a food processor or blender, add the tofu, baking powder, nutritional yeast, soy sauce, vinegar, and salt and pepper, to taste. Blend until the mixture is smooth and no tofu chunks are visible. Be sure to scrape the edges of the bowl a few times to incorporate all of the ingredients.

In a large bowl, combine the tofu mixture with the vegetables until well incorporated. Transfer to a 9-inch (23 x 3.5-cm) round pie pan and press evenly into the pan. Bake, uncovered, 50 to 60 minutes, or until the top is golden brown.

Srv: 1 Slice (171 g) | Cal: 150 | Fat: 6 g | Sat Fat: 1 g | Col: 0 mg | Carb: 15 g | Fib: 4 g | Pro: 11 g

BITCHWORTHY: Once you get the hang of this recipe, you can switch out corn and peppers with a handful of other veggies and spices. Try a few variations: sweet tomatoes, vegan mozzarella, and basil; baby spinach, mushroom, onion, vegan cheddar, and thyme; and asparagus and tarragon.

Orange Scones

I must admit this recipe is one of my greatest achievements in this book. Growing up, my mom and I used to have tea parties and she always made the best scones. But once I went vegan, I was broken-hearted that I would never taste them again. But, I spoke too soon. Here they are—light and flavorful with the perfect texture—and I am not scared to look my mother in the eye and say they are just as good as hers.

MAKES 8 SCONES

2 cups (255 g) unbleached all-purpose flour

½ cup (100 g) evaporated cane sugar, plus
    1 tablespoon

1 tablespoon baking powder

½ teaspoon baking soda

1 teaspoon salt

½ teaspoon ground nutmeg

½ cup (120 ml) orange juice, plus 1 tablespoon

1 teaspoon orange extract

1 tablespoon orange zest, grated

½ cup (115 g) Earth Balance, at room temperature

Preheat the oven to 350° F (180° C).

In a large bowl, mix together the flour, ½ cup (100 g) of the sugar, the baking powder, baking soda, salt, and nutmeg. In a separate bowl, whisk together ½ cup (120 ml) of the orange juice, the orange extract, and orange zest. Add to the flour mixture and mix until well combined. Add the Earth Balance and mix well.

Lightly flour a flat surface and knead the dough for about a minute. Form the dough into a ball and then shape into a small pizza crust shape, lightly flattening down the dough into the desired thickness. (I like mine about 1-inch/2.5 cm thick.) Cut the dough with a large knife into four wedges, just like you would a pizza. Place each pie wedge onto a baking sheet. Using a pastry brush or your fingers, cover the dough with the remaining 1 tablespoon of orange juice. Sprinkle with the remaining 1 tablespoon of sugar. Bake 15 minutes. Remove from the oven and place on a wire rack to cool. Serve with your favorite jam.

Srv: 1 Scone | Cal: 260 | Fat: 11 g | Sat Fat: 3 g | Col: 0 mg |
Carb: 36 g | Fib: 1 g | Pro: 3 g

> **BITCHWORTHY:** ADD ½ CUP (120 G) CRANBERRIES FOR SOME ADDED FLAVOR AND COLOR.

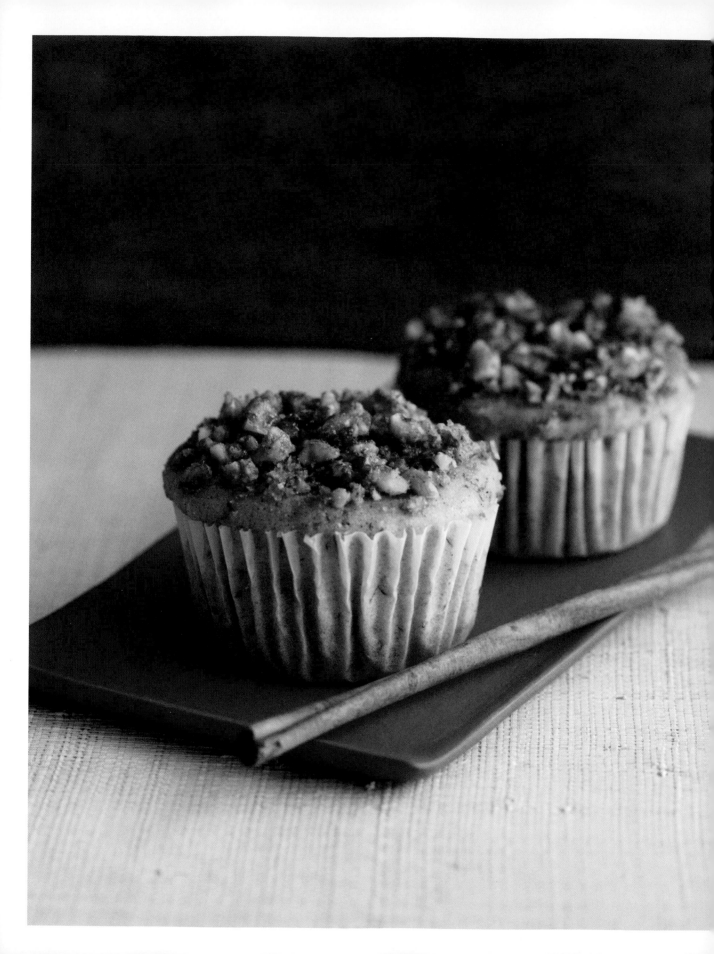

Banana and Cinnamon Muffins

I love the efficiency of muffins as a nutritional, grab-and-go breakfast. They are fitting for almost any occasion, and practical for passing around the office or a last-minute bake sale at school. Bananas are a dynamite ingredient since they are a morning superfood that helps to stimulate the brain for optimal learning and memory. The crunchy topping on the muffins is just my special touch. You're welcome.

MAKES 12 MUFFINS

1½ cups (360 ml) almond milk

2 teaspoons apple cider vinegar

2⅔ cups (335 g) unbleached all-purpose flour

1½ teaspoons baking powder

½ teaspoon baking soda

¾ teaspoon salt

2½ teaspoons ground cinnamon, divided

⅓ cup (80 g) Earth Balance, at room temperature

¾ cup (150 g) evaporated cane sugar

¼ cup (60 ml) vanilla soy yogurt

1 teaspoon pure vanilla extract

2 large bananas, mashed

⅓ cup (35 g) chopped walnuts

¼ cup (50 g) firmly packed brown sugar

Preheat the oven 325° F (165° C).

In a small bowl, mix the milk and vinegar and let sit until curdled. In a large bowl, mix together the flour, baking powder, baking soda, salt, and 2 teaspoons of the cinnamon.

In a separate large bowl, beat the Earth Balance and sugar with an electric mixer until fluffy, 1 to 2 minutes. Add the yogurt, milk mixture, and vanilla. Beat until mixed well. Pour the wet mixture into the flour mixture and stir with a wooden spoon until just incorporated. Stir in the bananas.

In a small bowl, add the walnuts, brown sugar, and the remaining ½ teaspoon of cinnamon. Set aside. Spoon the batter into paper muffin liners in a muffin pan until they are about two-thirds full.

Bake 10 minutes. Remove from the oven and add the walnut mixture to each muffin. Return to the oven and bake 10 to 15 minutes, or until a toothpick inserted in the center comes out clean. Place on a wire rack to cool.

Srv: 1 Muffin | Cal: 300 | Fat: 14 g | Sat Fat: 5 g | Col: 0 mg | Carb: 40 g | Fib: 2 g | Pro: 4 g

> **THE SKINNY: BANANAS, THE ANTI-WRINKLE FRUIT**
>
> BANANAS ARE THE FOUNTAIN OF YOUTH. MASH UP ONE RIPE BANANA AND APPLY TO YOUR FACE. LEAVE ON FOR TWENTY MINUTES TO FIGHT WRINKLES. REPEAT SEVERAL TIMES A WEEK.

Breakfast Bake

This recipe is nostalgic of something my dad used to make on Sunday mornings when I was young, except for one teensy difference. My dad wouldn't be caught dead eating tempeh. And something tells me he wouldn't even know what to do with rosemary and thyme. Your loss, pops. My version of the Breakfast Bake is a hearty, comfort breakfast that's easy to prepare and reminds me of my carefree days living at home with the folks.

MAKES 6 SERVINGS

2 tablespoons grapeseed oil

½ onion, minced

2 garlic cloves, minced

2 medium russet potatoes, peeled and diced into small cubes

12 ounces (340 g) soy sausage or tempeh, chopped

½ cup (35 g) chopped mushrooms

½ teaspoon dried thyme

1 sprig of rosemary, chopped

½ teaspoon salt

⅛ teaspoon pepper

½ cup (60 g) shredded vegan Cheddar

Preheat the oven to 400° F (200° C).

Heat the oil in a large sauté pan. Add the onion and cook over medium-high heat until soft, about 3 minutes. Add the garlic and cook about 1 minute. Add the potatoes, soy sausage or tempeh, and the mushrooms. Sauté 5 minutes. Add the thyme, rosemary, salt, and pepper. Sauté for 2 minutes.

Pour the mixture into a 13 x 9-inch (33 x 23 cm) baking dish. Bake 30 minutes, or until the potatoes are soft. During the last few minutes of baking, sprinkle the vegan cheese over the potato mixture and bake until the cheese melts.

Srv: 166 g | Cal: 270 | Fat: 14 g | Sat Fat: 1.5 g | Col: 0 mg | Carb: 21 g | Fib: 4 g | Pro: 15 g

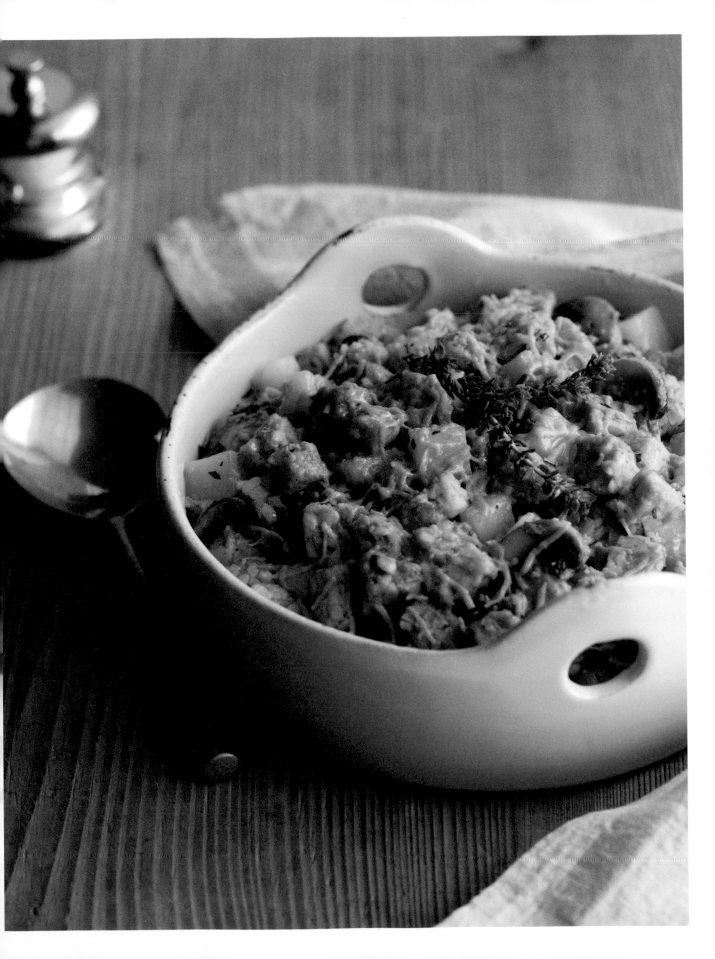

Dill and Chive Biscuits

There's nothing like the smell of biscuits in the morning. I remember my mom with her box of Bisquick, whipping up a batch for our Saturday breakfast. These dill and chive biscuits are a terrific variation on that classic, and can even be a great side for dinner.

MAKES 8 BISCUITS

2 cups (255 g) unbleached all-purpose flour

1 tablespoon baking powder

1 teaspoon evaporated cane sugar

1 teaspoon salt

½ teaspoon dry mustard

8 tablespoons (115 g) Earth Balance, sliced and cold

¾ cup (180 ml) almond milk

2 tablespoons chopped fresh chives

1 tablespoon chopped fresh dill

Preheat the oven to 400° F (200° C).

In a large bowl, mix together the flour, baking powder, sugar, salt, and mustard. Add the Earth Balance and mix with a pastry cutter (or a fork). The batter will look crumbly. Pour in the milk, chives, and dill. Stir until just combined. Lightly flour a flat surface and knead the dough with your hands. Reflour the surface, if necessary, so the dough doesn't stick. Be careful not to over mix. Lightly flatten the dough with your hands so it forms a circle about ½-inch (12 mm) or 1-inch (2.5 cm) thick. Use a round cookie cutter or a round drinking glass turned upside down to cut out the dough.

Place the dough on a baking sheet. You will need to remold the dough pieces back into another shape to cut the rest of it. Bake 10 to 15 minutes.

Srv: 1 Biscuit | Cal: 230 | Fat: 12 g | Sat Fat: 4.5 g | Col: 0 mg | Carb: 26 g | Fib: 1 g | Pro: 3 g

> **BITCHWORTHY:** WHEN YOU ARE BAKING, COLD INGREDIENTS WILL AFFECT THE OVERALL TEMPERATURE, LEAVING PARTS OF THE BATTER TO BAKE FASTER THAN OTHERS. SO SET OUT THE REFRIGERATED ITEMS AHEAD OF TIME AND ALLOW THEM TO REACH ROOM TEMPERATURE BEFORE YOU BEGIN TO BAKE. WORKS LIKE A CHARM.

Maple and Apple Cinnamon Pancakes

I make these a few times a week with my son sitting on the counter stirring the batter in a bowl between his legs. Together, we make the most heavenly and fluffy batch that you would never imagine they are dairy-free. The maple and apple topping is the perfect touch to jazz up regular pancakes for a family brunch or morning tea with girlfriends.

MAKES 8 PANCAKES

1 cup (130 g) unbleached all-purpose flour
3 tablespoons evaporated cane sugar
2 teaspoons baking powder
½ teaspoon baking soda
¼ teaspoon salt
1¼ teaspoons ground cinnamon, divided
1 cup (240 ml) almond milk
1 teaspoon vanilla extract
2 tablespoons canola oil
3 tablespoons Earth Balance, divided
2 Granny Smith apples, peeled and thinly sliced
⅓ cup (75 ml) pure maple syrup
¼ teaspoon ground nutmeg

In a medium bowl, stir together the flour, sugar, baking powder, baking soda, salt, and ¼ teaspoon of the cinnamon. In a separate bowl, whisk together the milk, vanilla extract, and oil. Combine the milk mixture and the flour mixture, and whisk until smooth. If the batter is too thick, add more of the milk, 1 tablespoon at a time. Heat 1 tablespoon of the Earth Balance in a large skillet or griddle over medium heat. Pour about ¼ cup (60 ml) of the batter into the hot pan and cook until the batter starts to bubble. Flip with a spatula and cook until the other side is golden brown.

In a medium sauté pan, melt the remaining Earth Balance. Add the apples and sauté about 2 minutes. Add the maple syrup, the remaining cinnamon, and the nutmeg. Stir and cook 2 minutes. Place the maple apples on top of the pancakes.

Srv: 1 Pancake | Cal: 110 g | Fat: 4 g | Sat Fat: 0 g | Col: 0 mg | Carb: 17 g | Fib: 1 g | Pro: 2 g

Maple-Apple Topping: Srv: 54 g | Cal: 60 | Fat: 1.5 g | Sat Fat: 0 g | Col: 0 mg | Carb: 12 g | Fib: 1 g | Pro: 0 g

Brain Boosters

Everyone seems to have an excuse for missing breakfast. I can't, I'll be late for work. I'm not hungry. That damn Lucky Charms leprechaun still haunts my dreams at night. Yada, yada, yada.

Grow the hell up. Studies have found that breakfast is needed more for the brain than the stomach. The decision to eat a meal before kicking off your day has a radical impact on your mood, memory, concentration, and learning capabilities. This is even more important for children. Kids who eat breakfast have proven to score higher on standardized tests, exude better behavior and focus in the classroom.[91] Give it up for the most important meal of the day.

BREAKFAST IMPROVES YOUR MEMORY: Food supplies your body with a steady supply of glucose. When you neglect to feed your body, it has to dig into its energy and protein sources to get it. This is a much slower process than converting food directly into fuel, and results in your brain working about as well as a car running on fumes. Fill 'er up! Remember the last meal you had prior to breakfast was dinner. It's been a whopping eight to twelve hours, genius.

BREAKFAST IMPROVES YOUR CONCENTRATION: Having food in your system in the morning affects your level of alertness and ability to focus on one thing. You also think faster on your feet to process and solve problems.

BREAKFAST PUTS YOU IN A BETTER MOOD: Your body needs a sufficient amount of vitamin B, such as niacin, riboflavin, thiamin, and folic acid to maintain serotonin levels. Serotonin is what makes you all happy and bushy-tailed. If you are hungry and crabby, you're more likely to head for the vending machine at lunch. Dumb move, grouchy ass.[92]

BREAKFAST IMPROVES YOUR VERBAL COMMUNICATION: Getting stuck on the first sentence in a client presentation isn't going to earn you a promotion. Research shows that eating breakfast can have an effect on your semantics.

Skinny Bitch 101: Breakfast Superfoods for the Brain

Do some foods make you smarter than others? Answer: Yes. Though any breakfast is better than skipping a morning meal, some foods contribute more to brain health than others. Think *healthy,* bitches.

A well-balanced breakfast of protein, complex carbs, and fiber-dense nutrients takes longer to digest, stabilizes energy, improves coordination, and enhances memory for increased learning.[93] These food groups also satisfy your hunger so you stay fuller longer. Get your fiber fix from whole grains, vegetables, and fruits. Foods high in protein include oatmeal, oats, fortified cereal with soymilk, soy yogurt, nuts, and other whole grains.

What to Avoid: Keep away from sugary cereals, donuts, syrups, white breads, and pastries at all costs. They make you feel hungry again quicker and put your brain and body to sleep. Naptime is for babies.

What to Eat:

WHOLE GRAINS: Breads (non-white) and fortified cereal provide the body with folate, which delivers oxygen-rich blood to the brain, along with such key nutrients as vitamin B6 and thiamine. Whole-grain foods help to sustain energy levels, stabilize blood sugar levels, and enhance memory and focus.

BERRIES: The ellagic acid in such berries as strawberries, blueberries and blackberries protects and encourages communication between brain cells and improves cognitive skills and memory.

BANANAS: Juiced with such nutrients as vitamin B6, potassium, and folic acid, bananas increase serotonin levels and mood. Scarf one in the car on the drive to work, or give to the kids to eat on the school bus. Bananas are also delish in smoothies, cereals, and soy yogurts.

WALNUTS, ALMONDS AND PECANS: A handful of nuts can power your brain like a Nascar vehicle. Pecans have a healthy serving of *choline*, which improves memory and brain development. Almonds kick up your memory drive, while the omega-3 and omega-6 fatty acids in walnuts work to equalize the brain's serotonin levels so you don't crash by lunch. Add to cereals, smoothies, and oatmeal.

AVOCADOS: Rich in monounsaturated fats, avocados help to maintain focus and concentration while assisting in healthy blood flow. Add a side of avocado to an omelet using Ener-G Egg Replacer or other vegan substitute.

GREEN TEA: Skip the morning latte and opt for a mug of green tea while you curl your hair. Concentrated in catechins and polyphenols, green tea helps the brain to relax and energize dopamine levels. It also helps with maintaining concentration and increasing memory capability.[94]

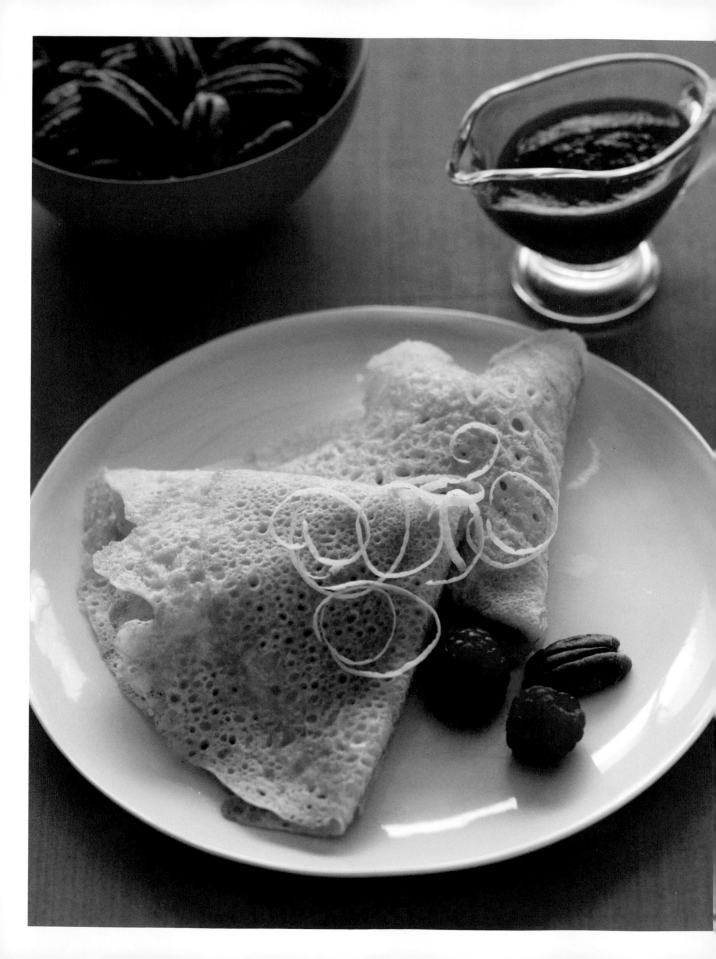

Crêpes with Raspberry Sauce

Crêpes aren't the easiest recipe to pull off in a vegan kitchen, but when you do, boy is it worth it. Thin and lighter than pancakes, they make me feel like I am getting away with a savory dessert at eight o'clock in the morning. Shhh . . . if you don't tell, I won't.

MAKES 6 SERVINGS

1 cup (130 g) unbleached all-purpose flour

½ teaspoon baking powder

½ teaspoon baking soda

3 tablespoons evaporated cane sugar,
  plus ½ cup (100 g)

¼ teaspoon salt

1 cup (240 ml) almond milk

1 teaspoon vanilla extract

1 cup (125 g) fresh or frozen raspberries

¼ cup (60 ml) water

2 tablespoons Earth Balance

In a medium bowl, combine the flour, baking powder, baking soda, 3 tablespoons of the sugar, and the salt. Whisk in the milk and the vanilla extract until smooth.

In a blender or food processor, add the raspberries, the remaining ½ cup (100 g) of the sugar, and the water and blend until puréed, for the sauce. Set aside.

Heat the Earth Balance in a skillet over medium heat. Pour about ¼ cup (60 ml) of the batter mix into the skillet, swirling to coat the bottom of the skillet as evenly as possible with the batter. Cook until the edges are lightly browned and the crêpe is almost dry on the top. Loosen the edges with a thin spatula and flip the crêpe over with your fingers. Cook crêpe an additional 15 seconds. Transfer to a plate and continue cooking the remaining batter. Pour the raspberry sauce over the cooked crêpes. Serve hot.

1 Crepe | Srv: 69 g | Cal: 140 | Fat: 4.5 g | Sat Fat: 1.5 g | Col: 0 mg | Carb: 22 g | Fib: 1 g | Pro: 2 g

Raspberry Sauce | Srv: 36 g (about 3 tbsp) | Cal: 50 | Fat: 0 g | Sat Fat: 0 g | Col: 0 mg | Carb: 13 g | Fib: 0 g | Pro: 0 g

Tofu Mexicali Scramble

A staple for any vegan or anyone who wants to change up their morning routine, a tofu scramble is a fast and easy meal to whip up. This one in particular just comes alive with the use of exotic spices and cilantro. I have seen it convert tofu-haters into abusers, first-hand. Try it for yourself.

MAKES 4 SERVINGS

1 (14-ounce/400 g) package extra-firm tofu, drained

¼ cup (60 ml) salsa

2 tablespoons grapeseed oil

½ small onion, chopped

1 garlic clove, chopped

1 small red bell pepper, chopped

1 small green bell pepper, chopped

½ teaspoon salt

¼ teaspoon ground cumin

Pinch of chili powder

1 cup (240 g) canned refried beans

4 whole wheat tortillas

Freshly ground pepper, to taste

2 tablespoons chopped fresh cilantro

Preheat the oven to 200° F (95° C).

In a medium bowl, crumble the tofu and add the salsa. Set aside to marinate. In a large sauté pan, heat the oil over medium-high heat and then add the onion. Sauté until soft, about 4 minutes. Add the garlic and cook about 30 seconds. Add the bell peppers, salt, and cumin. Cook an additional 3 to 4 minutes. Add the tofu mixture and chili powder and cook 5 minutes.

In a small saucepan, heat the refried beans over medium heat until warm. Place the tortillas on a cookie sheet and bake until warm, about 4 minutes. Spread ¼ cup (60 g) of the refried beans on each tortilla and top with the tofu and vegetable mixture. Add the pepper and sprinkle with cilantro.

Srv: 251 g | Cal: 300 g | Fat: 12 g | Sat Fat: 1 g | Col: 0 mg | Carb: 33 g | Fib: 6 g | Pro: 15 g

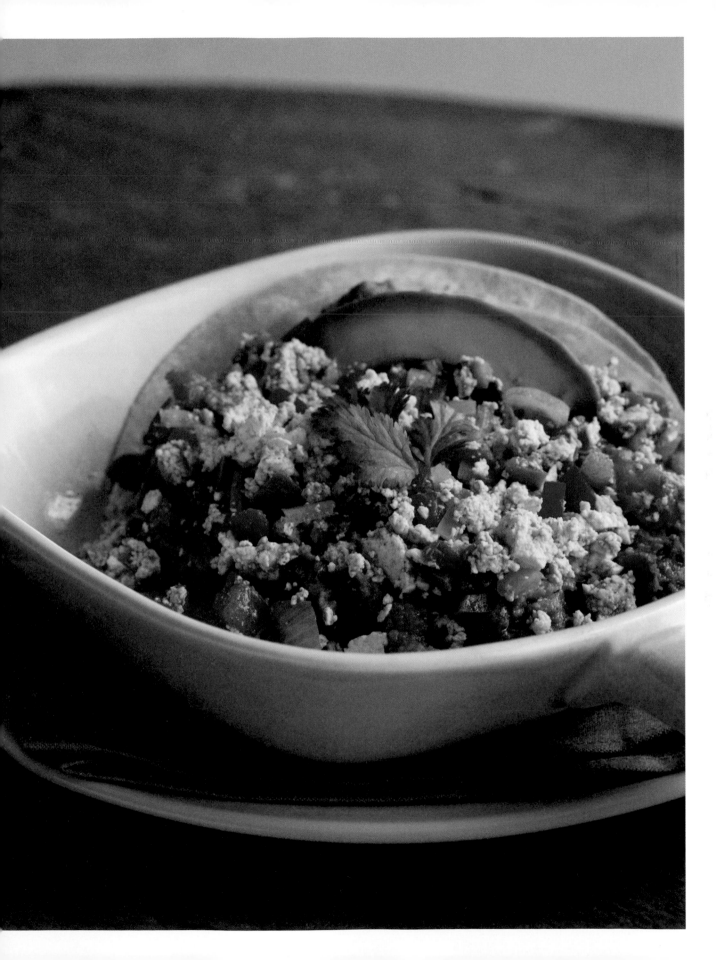

Coconut Banana French Toast

While it is true that pancakes stole my heart before I could walk, I have secretly been cheating with French toast. My guilty pleasure turned into a love affair when I became a waitress. Any waiter who's worked a weekend brunch shift knows it's a living hell. I'd rather give my cat a bath. But knowing the sous chef would make me a delicious batch of French toast post-shift was the only thing that got me through it. Thank heavens.

MAKES 6 SERVINGS

1 banana
½ cup (120 ml) light coconut milk
1 cup (240 ml) almond milk
2 tablespoons evaporated cane sugar
¼ teaspoon ground cinnamon
¼ teaspoon ground nutmeg
¼ teaspoon pure vanilla extract
6 slices whole grain bread
2 tablespoons Earth Balance

In a blender or food processor, add the banana, coconut milk, almond milk, sugar, cinnamon, nutmeg, and vanilla extract. Purée until the ingredients are mixed well and the mixture is smooth. Pour the batter into a shallow bowl and dip both sides of the bread into the batter.

Heat the Earth Balance in a skillet or griddle over medium heat. Place the slices of bread onto the skillet and cook in batches until lightly golden brown on both sides. Serve with maple syrup.

Srv: 1 Slice of French Toast | Cal: 100 | Fat: 1.5 g | Sat Fat: 0 g | Col: 0 mg | Carb: 17 g | Fib: 2 g | Pro: 4 g

Southwestern Griddle Cakes

I don't have a particular preference when it comes to sweet over savory. I love them both, often one right after the other. This recipe beautifully caters to both at the same time. An old-school name for pancakes, these griddle cakes get their savoriness from cornmeal, a slight heat from cayenne, and a touch of sweetness from sugar. Bring it on.

MAKES 8 GRIDDLE CAKES

1 cup (140 g) yellow cornmeal

½ cup (65 g) unbleached all-purpose flour

1 teaspoon baking soda

¼ cup (50 g) evaporated cane sugar

¼ teaspoon salt

1½ cups (360 ml) almond milk

¼ cup (55 g) silken tofu, drained

4 tablespoons (55 g) Earth Balance, at room temperature, divided

1 tablespoon pure maple syrup

Pinch of cayenne pepper

In a medium bowl, combine the cornmeal, flour, baking soda, sugar, and salt. In a blender or food processor, blend the milk, tofu, 2 tablespoons of the Earth Balance, the maple syrup, and cayenne pepper until creamy. Add to the flour mixture and stir until they are mixed well.

Heat the remaining Earth Balance in a skillet over medium heat. Pour about ¼ cup (60 ml) of the batter onto the skillet. When bubbles appear on the surface of the cakes, flip over and cook 1 to 2 minutes. Serve hot.

Srv: 1 Griddle Cake | Cal: 140 | Fat: 4 g | Sat Fat: 1 g | Col: 0 mg | Carb: 25 g | Fib: 1 g | Pro: 2 g

Pumpkin Pecan Banana Bread

This recipe is inspired by a pumpkin bread I used to buy every Sunday at the Lincoln Road Farmers' Market in South Beach. It was hands-down one of the best breads I have ever had. With that said, years ago my BFF Keesha snagged her dad's banana bread recipe for me—also out of this world. So I decided to combine the two and veganize it.

MAKES 10 SERVINGS

2 cups (255 g) unbleached all-purpose flour

¼ teaspoon baking powder

1 teaspoon baking soda

½ teaspoon cinnamon

1 teaspoon nutmeg

¼ teaspoon allspice

1 teaspoon salt

1½ cups (370 g) pumpkin purée

½ cup (120 ml) canola oil

½ cup (120 ml) almond milk

1 cup (200 g) evaporated cane sugar

½ cup (100 g) packed dark brown sugar

1 teaspoon vanilla extract

1 banana, mashed

⅔ cup (80 g) chopped pecans

Preheat the oven to 350° F (180° C). Lightly oil a large loaf pan and dust with flour.

In a large bowl, mix together the flour, baking powder, baking soda, cinnamon, nutmeg, allspice, and salt. In a separate large bowl, beat together the pumpkin purée, oil, and milk with an electric mixer until well combined. Add the sugars, vanilla extract, and banana, and beat until creamy. Stir in the pecans. Add the flour mixture to the pumpkin mixture and stir until all of the ingredients are well combined.

Pour the batter into the prepared pan and bake 1 hour. Remove from the oven and put on a wire rack to cool completely.

Srv: 1 Slice | Cal: 350 | Fat: 17 g | Sat Fat: 1.5 g | Col: 0 mg | Carb: 50 g | Fib: 3 g | Pro: 4 g

Skinny Bitch Recipe Winners

This part brings tears to my eyes. There's no better feeling than getting a recipe from a diehard *Skinny Bitch* fan. So, my girls and I at HealthyBitchDaily.com came up with an online recipe contest for the chance to be featured in this book. It gives me no better pleasure than to announce the reigning bitches, Sonja Pavlov and Carrie Dawley. Wear that crown well, ladies.

Apple-Cinnamon Granola

RECIPE WINNER: SONJA PAVLOV

A self-admitted gym rat, Sonja is up bright and early every morning in Los Angeles getting her ass in gear. When it came to a source of energy, she still hadn't found that quintessential healthy breakfast. Until now. Sonja is taking baby steps to living *la vida veggie*, but she knows the journey is well worth it.

MAKES 6 SERVINGS

1 cup (85 g) rolled oats

¼ cup (30 g) chopped almonds

½ cup (55 g) chopped pecans

3 tablespoons flaxseed

½ cup (50 g) unsweetened coconut

½ cup (45 g) dried apples, chopped

⅔ cup (165 ml) apple juice

⅓ cup (75 ml) unsweetened applesauce

½ cup (120 ml) brown rice syrup

1 tablespoon coconut oil

1 teaspoon ground cinnamon

1 teaspoon vanilla extract

Preheat the oven to 350°F (180° C).

In a large bowl, combine the oats, almonds, pecans, flaxseed, and coconut. Mix together and then spoon onto a cookie sheet. Bake 10 minutes. Remove from the heat and set aside to cool.

Decrease the oven temperature to 250°F (120° C). In a medium saucepan, combine the dried apples, apple juice, applesauce, brown rice syrup, cinnamon oil, and cinnamon. Bring to a light boil and simmer 15 minutes, or until the mixture starts to thicken. Remove from heat and stir in the vanilla.

In a large bowl, combine the oat mixture and the liquid mixture and stir until all of the ingredients are well coated. Transfer back to the cookie sheet and bake 40 minutes, or until lightly browned. Every 10 minutes, remove the cookie sheet from the oven and stir to make sure the mixture doesn't burn. When done, place on a wire rack to cool.

Srv: 130 g | Cal: 420 | Fat: 20 g | Sat Fat: 9 g | Col: 0 mg | Carb: 57 g | Fib: 10 g | Pro: 6 g

Blueberry Streusel Cake

RECIPE WINNER: CARRIE DAWLEY

Carrie comes to us from the heartland of Omaha, Nebraska, where she is using her newest *Skinny Bitch* purchase, *Bun in the Oven,* to coach her through her first pregnancy. A vegetarian for four years, Carrie recently stepped into vegan territory just in time to hear the big news. Congratulations on your new venture into motherhood, Carrie. There's no greater treasure in life.

MAKES 8 SERVINGS

2 cups (255 g) unbleached all-purpose flour, plus ¼ cup (30 g)

1 ½ teaspoons baking soda

½ teaspoon salt

2 teaspoons ground cinnamon, divided

¾ cup (150 g) evaporated cane sugar, plus ¼ cup (50 g)

⅓ cup (75 ml) canola oil

1 cup (240 ml) almond milk

1 tablespoon distilled white vinegar

½ teaspoon lemon extract

1 cup (150 g) fresh or frozen blueberries

2 tablespoons Earth Balance

Preheat the oven to 350° F (180° C).

In a medium bowl, mix together 2 cups (255 g) of the flour, the baking soda, the salt, 1 teaspoon of the cinnamon, and ¾ cup (150 g) of the sugar. Set aside.

In a large bowl, whisk together the oil, milk, vinegar, and lemon extract. Stir in the flour mixture until well combined. Add the blueberries and mix together. Pour the batter into an 8 x 8-inch (20 x 20 cm) baking dish.

In a separate small bowl, combine the remaining ¼ cup (30 g) of the flour, ¼ cup (50 g) of the sugar, 1 teaspoon of the cinnamon, and the Earth Balance (the mixture will be crumbly). Sprinkle the flour mixture over the batter in the pan. Bake 40 to 45 minutes. Remove from the oven and transfer to a wire rack to cool.

Srv: 1 Slice of Cake | Cal: 320 | Fat: 13 g | Sat Fat: 2 g | Col: 0 mg | Carb: 49 g | Fib: 2 g | Pro: 4 g

SOUPS

Sweet Pea Soup

This was my favorite soup when I was little. I made some slight additions to jazz up the flavor, like adding coconut milk, but it's still the same comforting classic. One of the best traits of pea soup is that it's just as good chilled.

MAKES 4 SERVINGS

½ cup (120 ml) almond milk

½ cup (120 ml) light coconut milk

1 pound (455 g) frozen sweet peas, thawed, rinsed, and drained

Salt and pepper, to taste

2 bunches fresh mint, stems removed

¼ cup (60 ml) olive oil

¼ cup (60 ml) soy yogurt, divided

In a small saucepan, bring the almond milk and coconut milk just barely to a boil. Remove from the heat immediately and set aside. Put the peas in a blender or food processor and add half of the milk mixture. Blend until smooth. Add the remaining milk mixture and blend until smooth. Return the mixture to the saucepan and simmer until hot. Season with salt and pepper to taste.

Combine the mint and oil in a blender or food processor and blend until smooth. Strain the mixture through a fine mesh strainer.

Divide the soup among four bowls. Place a small scoop of yogurt on each serving. Drizzle with the mint oil, for garnish.

Srv: 369 g | Cal: 300 | Fat: 15 g | Sat Fat: 1.5 g | Col: 0 mg | Carb: 30 g | Fib: 10 g | Pro: 10 g

Pasta, Navy Bean, and Spinach Soup

This comfort soup is like my partner in life, sticking by my side in sickness and in health. It's super-healthy and includes the entire range of food groups. Getting my son to eat pasta and beans has always been a huge ordeal, but this hearty soup is packed with so much flavor, it tricks him every time. Hey, a mom's gotta do what a mom's gotta do.

MAKES 6 SERVINGS

2 tablespoons grapeseed oil

1 small onion, chopped

2 garlic cloves, chopped

1 medium potato, peeled and cubed

2 medium tomatoes, seeded and chopped

2 cups (60 g) chopped fresh spinach

1 (15-ounce/430 g) can navy beans, drained and rinsed

1 (32-ounce/960 ml) carton vegetable broth

2 cups (480 ml) water

1 teaspoon salt

Sprig of fresh thyme or rosemary

1 cup (140 ml) cooked pasta, small shape

2 tablespoons chopped fresh basil

Pinch of freshly ground pepper

Heat the oil in a large saucepan over medium-high heat. Add the onion and sauté until translucent, for 3 to 4 minutes. Add the garlic and stir 30 seconds. Add the potato, tomatoes, and spinach, and sauté 2 minutes. Add the beans, broth, water, salt, and thyme or rosemary and stir to combine ingredients. Reduce the heat to medium and cook about 20 minutes, or until the potato is soft. Add the cooked pasta to the soup and cook 5 minutes. Garnish each serving with basil and freshly ground pepper.

Srv: 378 g | Cal: 240 | Fat: 6 g | Sat Fat: 0.5 g | Col: 0 mg | Carb: 40 g | Fib: 6 g | Pro: 10 g

THE SKINNY: SPINACH AND VITAMIN K
SPINACH CONTAINS PHYLLOQUINONE, A POPULAR FORM OF VITAMIN K, KNOWN TO HELP PRESERVE AND BUILD HEALTHIER BONES.[95] YOU CAN ALSO USE SPINACH IN LASAGNA TO REPLACE MEAT.

Thai Coconut Soup

Some soups taste just as good on a hot summer day as they do on a rainy afternoon. Thai Coconut Soup is one of those that swings both ways. It tastes unbelievably fresh, and opens up your sinuses thanks to the lemongrass, jalapeño pepper, and red pepper, which give it a spicy kick. It is one of my favorite soups because it's out of the norm, and full of vegetables for your daily dose of nutrients.

MAKES 4 SERVINGS

1 tablespoon grapeseed oil

2 garlic cloves, minced

2 tablespoons chopped fresh ginger

2 lemongrass stalks, lightly chopped

1 teaspoon chopped jalapeño pepper

1 (13.5-ounce/385 g) can light coconut milk

3 cups (720 ml) vegetable broth

1 tablespoon sugar

3 tablespoons chopped fresh cilantro

4 kaffir lime leaves

1 tablespoon white miso paste

1 tablespoon soy sauce

½ cup (35 g) sliced shiitake mushrooms

½ cup (30 g) peeled and sliced carrots

½ cup (45 g) small-cut broccoli florets

1 cup (225 g) firm tofu, drained and cubed

¼ cup (60 ml) lime juice

1 cup (100 g) bean sprouts

1 teaspoon pepper chili flakes

1 tablespoon chopped fresh basil

Salt and pepper, to taste

Heat the oil in a large pot over medium-high heat. Add the garlic, ginger, lemongrass, and jalapeño, and cook 1 minute. Add the coconut milk, broth, sugar, cilantro, kaffir lime leaves, and white miso and simmer 30 to 40 minutes. Place a strainer over a large bowl and pour in the soup; discard the strained ingredients and add the strained soup back to the pot. Cook again over medium heat and add the soy sauce, mushrooms, carrots, broccoli, and tofu. Simmer until the vegetables are soft, about 15 minutes. Add the lime juice, bean sprouts, red pepper flakes, and basil. Remove from heat. Add salt and pepper, to taste. Serve warm.

Srv: 434 g | Cal: 170 | Fat: 7 g | Sat Fat: 1 g | Col: 0 mg |
Carb: 18 g | Fib: 4 g | Pro: 10 g

> **BITCHWORTHY:** LEMONGRASS IS KNOWN FOR ITS CALMING EFFECTS IN RELIEVING INSOMNIA AND STRESS. IT'S ALSO A RECOGNIZED DETOXIFIER, HELPING TO CLEANSE THE LIVER, PANCREAS, KIDNEY, BLADDER, AND THE DIGESTIVE TRACT.[96]

Black Bean and Tomato Soup

A low-fat and hearty option, Black Bean and Tomato Soup is filling for lunch and ideal for dinner with a side salad. While it pairs well with any dish, it complements a grilled (vegan) cheese sandwich or veggie burger like nothing else.

MAKES 6 SERVINGS

2 tablespoons grapeseed oil

1 small onion, chopped

2 garlic cloves, chopped

1 large red bell pepper, chopped

1 teaspoon chili powder

1 teaspoon cumin

2 (15-ounce/430 g) cans black beans, drained and rinsed

1 (28-ounce/800 g) can stewed tomatoes

½ cup (70 g) corn, fresh or frozen

3 cups (720 ml) vegetable broth

1 cup (240 ml) water

1 teaspoon dried oregano

¼ teaspoon red pepper flakes

2 teaspoons Worcestershire sauce

Juice of half a lime

½ teaspoon salt

1 tablespoon chopped green onions

1 tablespoon chopped fresh cilantro

Heat the oil in a large pot over medium heat. Add the onion and sauté 3 to 4 minutes. Add the garlic and red bell pepper, and sauté about 30 seconds. Add the chili powder and cumin, and stir until well combined. Add the black beans, tomatoes, corn, water, oregano, red pepper flakes, and Worcestershire sauce. Stir and simmer about 15 minutes. Transfer half of the soup to a blender or a food processor. Let sit about 10 minutes to cool, and then blend until creamy before returning to the pan. Add the lime juice and salt. Stir and simmer 5 minutes. Garnish with the green onions and cilantro.

Srv: 372 g | Cal: 180 | Fat: 5 g | Sat Fat: 0 g | Col: 0 mg | Carb: 31 g | Fib: 9 g | Pro: 7 g

The Love Chef

Getting in the mood for foreplay can be tough sometimes. After a long day at the office and sitting in rush-hour traffic, all you want to do is put on your Granny panties and apply your green mud mask. I'll bet you just scream *sex*.

But a little one-on-one lovin' is just what the chef ordered. According to experts, some foods have a direct impact on your sex life, affecting your hormones, brain chemistry, and energy and stress levels. While some have psychoactive properties, others can even increase blood flow to the land down under.

Start cooking up some of these delicious ingredients and prepare to get busy, sister. *Bow-Chicka-Bow-Wow.*

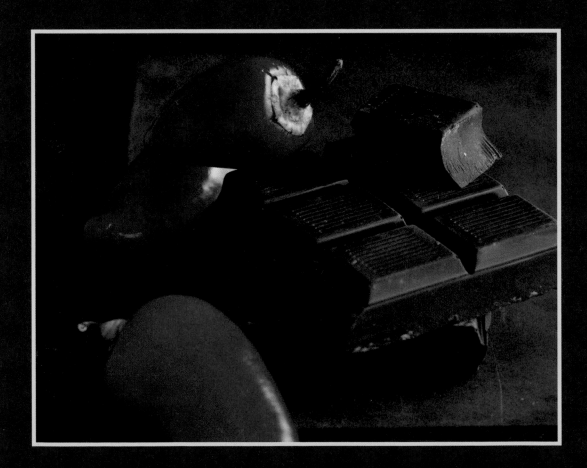

ASPARAGUS: Dating back to the seventeenth century, scholars have believed that asparagus "stirs up lust in a man and a woman." The Vegetarian Society suggests eating asparagus for three days for the most powerful effect. It is also a great source of folate, which boosts histamine production essential to pleasure for both sexes. Just expect smelly pee.

CARROTS: Carrots have been believed to be a stimulant dating back to ancient times, when early Middle Eastern royalty used them as a male aid in the seduction process. Think of it as an ancient Viagra.

SWEET BASIL: This member of the mint family has an alluring aroma, and a warming effect on the body, which promotes circulation and stimulates sexual drive.

ALMONDS: The nut has been symbolic of fertility throughout the ages, and the aroma is believed to arouse passion in females.[97]

CHILE PEPPERS: Chile peppers contain capsaicin, which stimulates our nerve endings and evokes physiological responses in our bodies that are reminiscent of sex. Spicy foods are also believed by some to trigger the release of endorphins, body chemicals that give us a natural high.[98]

GARLIC: Yes, your breath alone could be a bit of a buzzkill on a first date, but garlic contains allicin, an ingredient that increases blood flow.

BANANAS: Its shape alone could lead to some heavy petting. Bananas are rich in potassium and vitamin B, both necessities for hormone production. Bananas also contain bromelian enzyme, said to enhance male libido.

DARK CHOCOLATE: The king of aphrodisiacs, pure chocolate exudes phenylethylamine (PEA), which releases dopamine in the pleasure centers of the brain and helps induce feelings of excitement. Another major ingredient, *anandamide*, is said to be the psychoactive " feel-good" chemical.[99]

FIGS: The Greeks held them sacred as symbols of love and fertility, and rumors suggest they gained aphrodisiac status because of their close resemblance to the female sexual organs. They are packed with amino acids that improve sexual stamina, and their heady sweetness and creamy consistency are said to induce *amore*.

VANILLA: The tantalizing scent of vanilla is said to increase lust and cure male impotency. The aroma of vanilla also triggers the release of serotonin, a " feel-good" neurotransmitter.[100]

ARUGULA, AVOCADO, PINE NUTS, GINGER, AND CARDAMOM are a few other natural stimulants that are believed to entice some heat between the sheets. Is it getting hot in here, or is it just me?

Butternut Squash Soup with Poppy Seeds

Sometimes you want soup. Sometimes you want a filling meal. With the Butternut Squash Soup, you get both. My dear friend Julie May made more then a few dozen tweaks to this recipe before she finally nailed it. From the sweet apple and cinnamon to the hot spice of the ginger, the ingredients blend together like they were meant to be. I prefer this soup with a thicker consistency, but if you want to thin it out, just add an extra cup of vegetable stock.

MAKES 6 SERVINGS

1 large butternut squash

2 tablespoons olive oil

2 garlic cloves

1 teaspoon salt

½ teaspoon pepper

2 tablespoons grapeseed oil

1 large yellow onion, chopped

1 quart (960 ml) vegetable stock

½ cup (120 ml) water

1 large red apple, chopped

1 teaspoon ground ginger

1 teaspoon agave nectar

1 teaspoon cinnamon

½ teaspoon ground nutmeg

½ teaspoon dried sage

¼ cup (35 g) poppy seeds, for garnish

Preheat the oven to 375° F (190° C).

Cut the butternut squash in half lengthwise, creating two equal halves. Scoop the seeds, and place squash, cut-side up, on the baking sheet. Drizzle each squash half with 1 tablespoon of the olive oil to create a small pool of oil in the cavity. Put 1 garlic clove in each cavity. Sprinkle with salt and pepper. Put the squash in the oven and bake 45 minutes, or until squash is tender when pierced with a fork. Remove from the oven and let cool. When cooled, peel off the squash skin and cut the squash into large chunks. Reserve the garlic cloves.

In a large pot, heat the grapeseed oil on medium heat. Add the onion, stirring until softened, about 5 minutes. Pour in the vegetable stock and the water. Add in the butternut squash, apple, and the two baked garlic cloves. Cover and simmer 20 minutes, or until the apple is very tender. The squash should already be tender. Remove from the heat and pour half of the soup into a food processor or blender. Let cool for 10 minutes. Leave the remaining soup in the pan to cool. Purée the soup until smooth. Add the remaining soup and blend together until creamy. Pour the soup back into the pot and add the ginger, agave nectar, cinnamon, nutmeg, and sage. Season with additional salt and pepper, if needed. Garnish with the poppy seeds.

Srv: 378 g | Cal: 190 | Fat: 10 g | Sat Fat: 1 g | Col: 0 mg | Carb: 27 g | Fib: 5 g | Pro: 3 g

Corn Chowder

Growing up in Rhode Island, I practically lived on New England clam chowder. This version loses the clams and brings in the corn, but it's no less creamy and filling. Every time I prepare this chowder, it just brings me back to childhood.

MAKES 8 SERVINGS

2 tablespoons grapeseed oil

1 small onion, chopped

½ cup (50 g) chopped celery

2 garlic cloves, chopped

6 small red potatoes, cut into medium-size chunks

2 cups (280 g) corn, fresh or frozen

4 cups (960 liters) vegetable broth

2 sprigs fresh thyme

2 cups (480 ml) almond milk

1 tablespoon unbleached all-purpose flour

3 tablespoons water

1 teaspoon salt

Freshly ground pepper, to taste

2 teaspoons chopped fresh dill, for garnish

In a large saucepan, heat the oil and sauté the onion and celery until soft, about 4 minutes. Add the garlic and sauté 30 seconds. Add the potatoes, corn, broth, thyme, and almond milk. Simmer 20 minutes, or until the potatoes are tender.

In a small bowl whisk together the flour and water until smooth. Add to the soup. Simmer 5 minutes. Add the salt and pepper. Garnish with the dill.

Srv: 343 g | Cal: 180 | Fat: 5 g | Sat Fat: 0.5 g | Col: 0 mg | Carb: 21 g | Fib: 4 g: Pro: 4 g

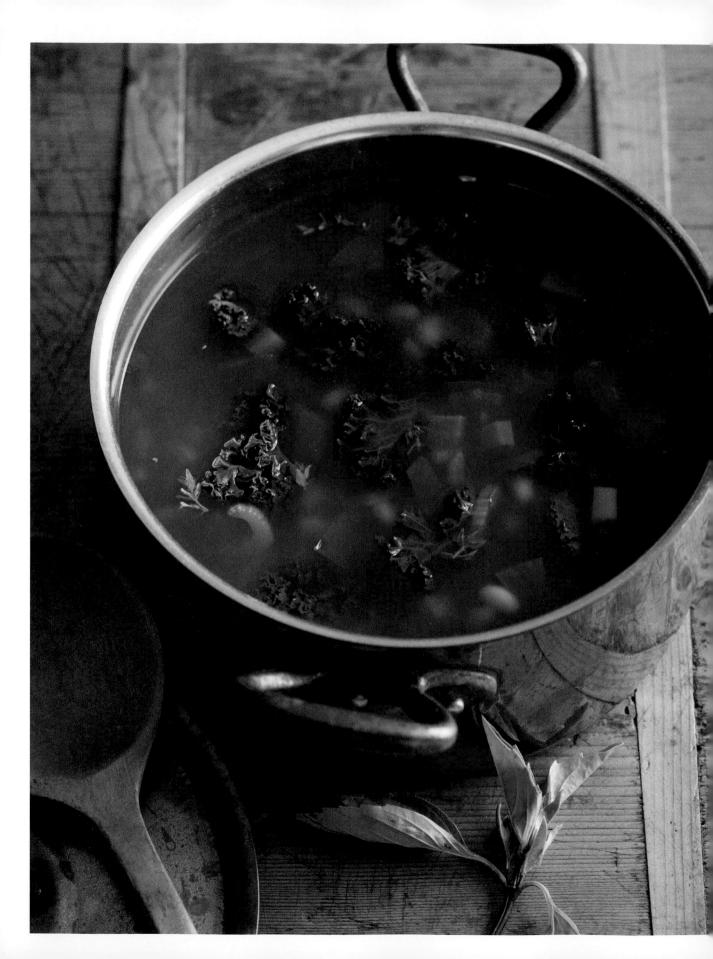

Kale and White Bean Soup

While this might be a nourishing winter soup, it makes me feel good any time of year. I am a big fan of kale because it is high in fiber, acts as a powerful detoxifier, and is packed with nutrients that may help fight cancer. For my Skinny Bitches, it also helps fight fat. Bingo!

MAKES 6 SERVINGS

2 tablespoons grapeseed oil

½ onion, finely chopped

1 garlic clove, chopped

1 cup (130 g) peeled and chopped carrots

1 celery stalk, chopped

½ cup (75 g) peeled and cubed potatoes

2 tablespoons tomato paste

6 cups (1.4 l) water

2 tablespoons white miso paste

1 teaspoon ground cumin

1 teaspoon ground coriander

¼ teaspoon salt

2 cups (135 g) chopped kale, with hard spine removed

1 (14-ounce/400 g) can white beans, drained and rinsed

¼ teaspoon dried thyme

1 tablespoon chopped fresh basil

Pinch of pepper

Heat the oil in a large saucepan over medium heat. Add the onion and sauté until golden brown, about 4 minutes. Add the garlic, carrots, celery, potatoes, and tomato paste, and sauté until the ingredients are well combined. Add the water, white miso, cumin, coriander, and salt and bring to a boil. Lower the heat and simmer 30 minutes. Add the kale, white beans, and thyme and simmer another half hour. Garnish with basil and pepper before serving.

Srv: 395 g | Cal: 150 | Fat: 5 g | Sat Fat: 0 g | Col: 0 mg | Carb: 21 g | Fib: 5 g | Pro: 5 g

> **BITCHWORTHY:** IF YOU HAVE LEFTOVER COOKED WHITE BEANS, SAVE THEM IN AN AIRTIGHT CONTAINER AND CARRY THEM OVER FOR THE WEEK'S LUNCHES. FROM A QUICK BEAN PASTA TO A BEAN AND SPINACH SALAD TO BEAN AND VEGAN CHEESE DIP, THE WHITE BEAN IS A VERSATILE LITTLE GUY.

Curried Sweet Potato and Parsnip Soup

This is the type of soup that has such an intense, rich flavor, it reminds you exactly why you never have to touch meat again. Good friend and chef Noriyuki Sugie created this delightful combo, which warms you up and wakes up the taste buds instantly. The curry spice accentuates the flavor of one of my favorite traditional vegetables, the parsnip.

MAKES 4 SERVINGS

2 tablespoons coconut oil

1 large sweet potato, peeled and cut into chucks

2 large parsnips, peeled and cut into chunks

Pinch of salt

1 tablespoon curry powder

6 cups (1.4 l) water

1 tablespoon sweet white miso paste

3 tablespoons hot water

Handful of chopped fresh parsley or cilantro,
   for garnish

> **BITCHWORTHY:** WHITE OR RED MISO PASTE IS AVAILABLE AT MOST WHOLE FOODS MARKETS OR SPECIALTY HEALTH FOOD STORES.

Heat the oil in large saucepan over medium heat. Add the sweet potato, parsnips, and a pinch of salt and sauté 3 minutes. Add the curry powder and sauté until well coated. Add the 6 cups (1.4 l) of water and bring to a boil. Cover and simmer 15 minutes, or until the vegetables are soft.

Transfer half of the soup to a food processor or blender and let it sit 10 minutes to cool. Keep the remaining soup in the pan and set aside to cool. Purée the soup until smooth, and then add the remaining soup and blend until creamy. Return the soup to the pan. In a small bowl, dissolve the miso paste in hot water and stir into the soup. Simmer 3 to 4 minutes. Garnish with parsley or cilantro. Serve hot.

Srv: 310 g | Cal: 100 | Fat: 5 g | Sat Fat: 4 g | Col: 0 mg | Carb: 13 g | Fib: 3 g | Pro: 1 g

> **THE SKINNY: SWEET POTATOES—AN AESTHETICIAN'S DREAM**
> SKINCARE SPECIALIST SARA ELIZABETH OF SARA ELIZABETH SKINCARE IN SAN DIEGO, CALIFORNIA, CITES SWEET POTATOES AS ONE OF HER FAVORITE VEGGIES FOR HEALTHY SKIN. ONE MEDIUM-SIZE POTATO CONTAINS 120 PERCENT OF THE DAILY VALUE OF VITAMIN A, A NUTRIENT THAT IS ESSENTIAL TO HEALING. VITAMIN A ALSO HELPS WITH ACNE, STRETCH MARKS, ECZEMA, AND MENSTRUATION CRAMPS. I THINK I MIGHT JUST KEEP ONE UNDER MY PILLOW FOR NOW ON.

Tony and Sage Robbins's Raw Green Soup

We dedicated *Skinny Bitch* to Tony Robbins and, personally, I just wouldn't feel right if this cookbook didn't boast one of his favorite recipes. Tony has been one of the most influential persons in my life for the past decade. He even cheered me on as I walked across hot coals during one of his seminars.

So, where does Tony get all of his energy? The ingredients to his success are below. Tony and his wonderful wife, Sage, have coined this recipe their secret weapon in awakening the giant within. Quick and easy, they prepare it with their Vitamix, which they schlep all around the world with them.

MAKES 4 SERVINGS

7 cups (210 g) organic baby spinach
2 carrots, peeled and cut in half
2 garlic cloves, roasted
3 tablespoons chopped onion
1 potato, steamed
1 red bell pepper, seeded and roughly chopped
3 chopped celery stalks
1 teaspoon "Better Than Bouillon" seasoning
1 teaspoon Italian seasoning
Salt and pepper, to taste
1 tablespoon pine nuts, for garnish

Add all of the ingredients to the Vitamix and turn on high. The centrifugal force of the machine heats the ingredients so you have a hot, healthy soup within five minutes. Top with pine nuts.

Srv: 205 g | Cal: 100 | Fat: 0 g | Sat Fat: 0 g | Col: 0 mg | Carb: 22 g | Fib: 5 g | Pro: 3 g

BITCHWORTHY: IN THE VITAMIX, "PULSE" ABOUT ½ CUP (118 ML) OF CORN OR STEAMED CAULIFLOWER TO ADD BODY TO THE SOUP. ONCE THE SOUP IS PIPING HOT, ADD YOUR CORN OR ANY STEAMED VEGGIES.

Curried Pumpkin Soup

This is the perfect fall soup. It reminds me of multicolored leaves, a slight chill forming in the air, and adorable trick-or-treaters. High in vitamin C, pumpkin is also a great immune system builder for flu season.

MAKES 6 SERVINGS

3 tablespoons Earth Balance

2 Granny Smith apples, peeled, cored, and roughly chopped

1 onion, roughly chopped

2 cups (500 g) pumpkin purée (not pie filling)

1 tablespoon curry powder

¼ cup (50 g) evaporated cane sugar

1 tablespoons dark brown sugar

3 cups (720 ml) vegetable stock

½ cup (120 ml) dry white wine

1½ cups (360 ml) almond milk

Salt and freshly ground pepper, to taste

2 tablespoons chopped toasted pumpkin seeds

In a large pot, add the Earth Balance and melt over medium heat. Add the apples and onion. Cook until the onion is soft, about 8 minutes. Add the pumpkin purée, curry, and both sugars, and cook 2 minutes. Add the stock and wine. Increase the heat to medium-high and bring to a boil. Then reduce the heat to low, partially cover, and cook about 20 minutes. Remove from heat and transfer half of the soup to a food processor or blender. Let it sit 10 minutes to cool. Keep the remaining soup in the pot and set aside to cool. Purée the soup in a blender or food processor until smooth. Pour into a large bowl. Transfer the remaining soup to the blender or food processor and purée until smooth. Return all the soup to the pan and cook gently over medium-low heat until heated through. Pour in the milk and stir until hot. Add the salt and pepper, to taste. Garnish with the pumpkin seeds.

Srv: 358 g | Cal: 190 | Fat: 7 g | Sat Fat: 2.5 g | Col: 0 mg | Carb: 28 g | Fib: 4 g | Pro: 2 g

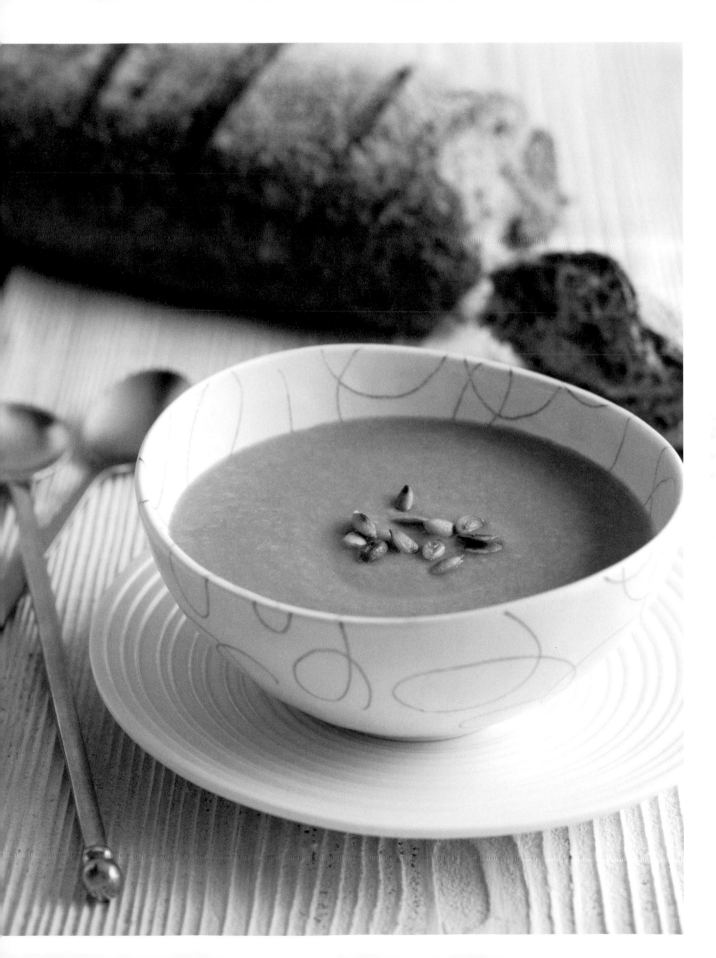

Practice Good Kitchen Etiquette: Feng Shui

Just like food gives you energy, feng shui is the idea that a given space gives a room its energy. The coolest part is that you are in control of this positive balance of *ch'i*, aka energy, to ensure nature can follow a proper ebb and flow. In feng shui terms, the kitchen is thought to be the most important area of your home. It is the part that nourishes and sustains life, and is a symbol of prosperity. The more you cook, the more opportunities you will have for wealth, good health, and romance.

While it may be new to us, feng shui is by no means a *new* design fad. It is an ancient system developed more than three thousand years ago by the Chinese. If you haven't noticed, the Chinese know what's up. They built the Great Wall, for heaven's sake.[101]

Feng Shui: The Color Diet

• White/Light Green/Orange/Yellow: These colors speed up metabolism and promote good digestion.[104]

• Red: A passionate color, red stimulates appetite.

• Blue: Blue helps keep your weight in check, helping to suppress your appetite. Use blue sparingly as a tablecloth, placemat or cloth napkins.[105]

KEEP YOUR KITCHEN CLUTTER-FREE

K.I.S.S. Keep it simple, stupid. Manage one junk drawer, keep it organized, and make sure it opens and closes easily. Too many gadgets or appliances manifests as excess weight. Ask yourself if you really need three types of blenders. Your home is *not* a Jamba Juice.

DON'T PLACE THE STOVE UNDER A WINDOW

A stove under a window allows the *ch'i* to escape and fly out the window, dragging with it your family's wealth and happiness. Wow. That's harsh. If you can't move the stove, just create a reflection around the window. A wind chime will work, too. Disaster averted.

DON'T POSITION STOVES AGAINST A WALL OR IN THE CORNER

Your stove should not be jammed up against the wall, nor should it be stuck in a corner. This restricts the free flow of positive *ch'i*. The cook should have full view of the doorway, and anyone entering the room to avoid surprise. If you face this problem, hang a mirror over the stove to get rid of blind spots.[102]

LIGHTEN UP

Well-lit and ventilated kitchen areas boost energy levels and provide important health benefits.[103]

THE SKINNY: KEEP BROOMS AND MOPS HIDDEN

EXPOSED BROOMS AND MOPS ARE THOUGHT TO SWEEP AWAY THE FAMILY'S LIVELIHOOD. POSITION BROOMS AND MOPS UPSIDE DOWN AGAINST THE WALL, FACING THE FRONT DOOR. THIS WARDS OFF INTRUDERS AND UNWANTED VISITORS. LIKE BILL COLLECTORS AND GIRL SCOUTS. THOSE DAMN THIN MINTS GET ME EVERY TIME.

Cream of Cauliflower Soup

I can't get enough of creamy soups, especially during the colder months. The smooth texture of this cauliflower soup drives my taste buds wild, but you may prefer to use larger pieces of cauliflower for a chunkier soup. Yummy.

MAKES 6 SERVINGS

3 cups (720 ml) water

4 cups (530 g) large-cut cauliflower pieces, with large stems removed

1 large potato, peeled and cut into medium-size chunks

1 tablespoon olive oil

2 tablespoons Earth Balance

1 onion, chopped

3 garlic cloves, finely chopped

1 quart (960 ml) vegetable broth

½ cup (120 ml) almond milk

Salt and white pepper, to taste

1 teaspoon celery salt

Preheat the oven to 450° F (230° C).

In a large saucepan, bring the water to a boil. Add half of the cauliflower and the potato. Reduce the heat and simmer 20 to 25 minutes, or until soft. Turn off the heat but keep the pan on the stovetop.

In a medium-size baking pan, add the remaining cauliflower, drizzle with olive oil, and add a pinch of salt. Bake 20 minutes, or until soft. In a separate sauté pan, add the Earth Balance and cook over medium-high heat until it melts. Add the onion and sauté 10 minutes, or until golden. Add the garlic and sauté 2 minutes. Remove the cauliflower from the oven. Transfer the onions and the roasted cauliflower into the saucepan with the boiled potatoes and cauliflower. Turn the heat back to medium-high and add the vegetable broth. Cook 10 minutes. Transfer half of the soup to a blender or food processor and let it sit 10 minutes to cool. Keep the remaining soup in the saucepan and set aside to cool. Purée until smooth. Transfer to a large bowl, and purée the remaining soup. Return all soup to the saucepan, stir in the almond milk, and cook on medium heat 5 minutes. Add the salt, white pepper, and celery salt. Serve hot.

Srv: 406 g | Cal: 100 | Fat: 4.5 g | Sat Fat: 1.5 g | Col: 0 mg | Carb: 13 g | Fib: 3 g | Pro: 3 g

THE SKINNY: WHITE PEPPER VS. BLACK PEPPER

I USE WHITE PEPPER BECAUSE IT HAS A MILDER FLAVOR, BUT IT'S ESPECIALLY IMPORTANT WHEN MAKING CAULIFLOWER SOUP. SINCE THE SOUP IS WHITE, YOU DON'T WANT TO RUIN THE PURITY OF THE COLOR OR PRESENTATION WITH BLACK FLECKS FLOATING AROUND IN THE SOUP.

SALADS

Watermelon and Heirloom Tomato Salad

Hands down, this is one of my favorite summer salads. It offers the best of both worlds—the sweet, refreshing flavor of a juicy watermelon and the taste of a succulent, ripe tomato pulled right from the soil. It's a fine example of why it is so important to buy organic and in season. You just don't get the same flavors otherwise. You can create a different variety of this salad by switching out red tomatoes with yellow tomatoes. The yellow tomatoes just sweeten the color scheme.

MAKES 4 SERVINGS

¾ cup (180 ml) balsamic vinegar

½ cup (100 g) evaporated cane sugar

2 tablespoons agave nectar

½ small seedless watermelon (about 3 to 4 pounds), cut into 1-inch (12 mm) cubes

2 large heirloom tomatoes, each cut into 8 wedges

2 tablespoons Champagne vinegar

½ cup (115 g) firm tofu, crumbled, for garnish

In a small saucepan, add the balsamic vinegar, evaporated cane sugar, and agave nectar for the dressing. Simmer until the liquid has reduced by half. Allow to cool completely before using. Place the watermelon and tomatoes in a large bowl and toss with Champagne vinegar. Drizzle with the dressing. Garnish with the tofu.

Srv: 465 g | Cal: 240 | Fat: 2 g | Sat Fat: 0 g | Col: 0 mg | Carb: 53 g | Fib: 2 g | Pro: 5 g

> ### THE SKINNY: FAMILY HEIRLOOM
> THE SEEDS OF HEIRLOOM TOMATOES HAVE BEEN PASSED DOWN FROM GENERATION TO GENERATION. THICK-SKINNED AND EXTREMELY FLAVORFUL, HEIRLOOM VARIETIES HAVE AN INHERENT RESISTANCE TO DISEASE. YOU CAN FIND THEM DURING SUMMER AND EARLY FALL, WHILE THEY GAIN A SWEETER FLAVOR IN HOT WEATHER. GREEN GRAPE, GREEN ZEBRA, AND STUPICE ARE MOST SAVVY TO FOGGY, COOLER CLIMATES, AND HAVE A THICKER SKIN. WATERMELONS DO THEIR BEST WORK IN SUMMER. MATCH MADE IN SOIL.

Edamame Salad

Why just stick with a bowl of edamame when you can dress it up as a salad with some bell peppers and sweet miso? Light and über fresh, this is a delicious snack that can be made up to four hours ahead of time. Just cover and chill.

MAKES 4 SERVINGS

3 cups (450 g) cooked and shelled edamame
1 cup (130 g) thinly sliced bamboo shoots
½ cup (70 g) diced water chestnuts
1 cup (150 g) diced red bell pepper
½ cup (120 ml) White Miso Dressing (see recipe on page 150)
1 tablespoon sliced green onions, for garnish

In a large bowl, combine the edamame, bamboo shoots, water chestnuts, bell pepper, and dressing. Toss thoroughly. Garnish with the green onions.

Srv: 205 g | Cal: 390 | Fat: 23 g | Sat Fat: 3 g | Col: 0 mg | Carb: 26 g | Fib: 4 g | Pro: 18 g

Beet & Cheese Napoleon Salad with Candied Pecans and Shallot-Balsamic Vinaigrette

The Beet & Cheese Napoleon Salad is ideal for a Sunday afternoon—when you have the time to prepare it and the appetite to enjoy it. Don't be intimidated by the length of the recipe. Unique, fun, and fancy, it may require a little more work than the average salad, but always proves worthy in the end. Invite girlfriends over and make it an afternoon to cook together and catch up for old times-sake.

MAKES 4 SERVINGS

3 medium-size beets, tails trimmed and tops removed

¼ cup (50 g) dark brown sugar

2 tablespoons water

¼ teaspoon salt, plus pinch, to taste

1 cup (115 g) chopped pecans

1 (8-ounce/225 g) container of vegan cream cheese, cold

½ teaspoon garlic powder

1 (10-ounce/280 g) bag of mixed baby greens

3 green onions, thinly sliced, with white and green parts

2 Persian cucumbers, thinly sliced

1 medium avocado, sliced

⅓ cup (75 ml) olive oil

2 tablespoons balsamic vinegar

2 medium shallots, finely minced

⅓ cup (65 g) evaporated cane sugar

2 tablespoons Dijon mustard

1 tablespoon Italian seasoning Mix

Salt and pepper, to taste

Preheat the oven to 375° F (190° C).

In a shallow baking pan, add the beets and enough water to fill the pan ¼ inch (6 mm). Cover tightly with aluminum foil and bake 45 to 55 minutes, or until soft. Remove from the oven and set aside to cool. Once cooled, use a paper towel to rub off the skins. Slice the beets into ¼-inch (6 mm) rounds. Reduce oven temperature to 350° F.

In a small bowl, mix together the brown sugar, water, ¼ teaspoon of the salt, and the pecans. Transfer the nuts in a single layer to a cookie sheet and bake 7 to 9 minutes, or until brown and crispy. Be careful not to burn them.

In a medium bowl, mix the cream cheese and garlic powder. Roll the cheese into 1-inch (2.5 cm) balls and place in a zip-top plastic bag. Lightly press to flatten out the cheese, to about ¼-inch (6 mm) thick. Remove from the bag and create a tower by starting with one beet round and then gently topping with a slice of the cheese round. Add another beet slice on top and continue alternating until you have three layers of the beets with two to three layers of the cheese. Wipe the knife in between each slice to minimize the bleeding from the beets onto the cheese.

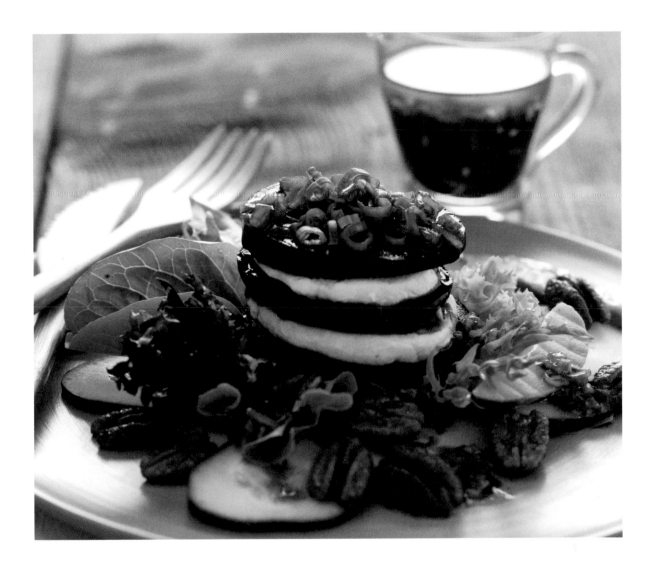

Put the baby greens on a large plate or platter and add the green onions, cucumbers, and avocado. In a medium bowl, prepare the dressing by whisking together the oil, balsamic vinegar, shallots, evaporated cane sugar, mustard, Italian seasoning Mix, and a pinch of salt and pepper. Gently place the beet cheese towers on the plate atop the greens. Drizzle with the dressing and top with the pecans.

Srv: 332 g | Cal: 470 | Fat: 34 g | Sat Fat: 3.5 g | Col: 0 mg | Carb: 38 g | Fib: 6 g | Pro: 10 g

THE SKINNY: THE NAPOLEON COMPLEX

WHAT THE HELL IS A NAPOLEON DOING IN YOUR SALAD? RELAX. A NAPOLEON IS SIMPLY SALAD INGREDIENTS SUCH AS VEGETABLES, CHEESE, AND GREENS STACKED IN A TOWER OR SKEWER-LIKE FASHION. IN THIS CASE, I'VE STACKED BEETS AND CHEESE, BUT YOU CAN PILE JUST ABOUT ANYTHING YOU FANCY.

Jicama, Papaya, and Grapefruit Salad

A juicy salad you can prepare in minutes. The crisp jicama paired with the butter-like consistency of papaya is an unbeatable combo that's ideal for a midday snack.

MAKES 4 SERVINGS

½ head jicama (about 4 ounces/115 g), peeled and julienned

1 papaya, peeled and julienned

2 grapefruits, peeled and sections removed

½ cup (120 ml) Citrus Mint Vinaigrette (see recipe page 151)

Coconut, shredded and toasted, for garnish

In a large bowl, add the jicama, papaya, and grapefruit. Gently toss to combine. Drizzle with the Citrus Mint Vinaigrette. Garnish with sprinkles of coconut.

Srv: 252 g | Cal: 230 | Fat: 11 g | Sat Fat: 1.5 g | Col: 0 mg | Carb: 31 g | Fib: 10 g | Pro: 3 g

---

THE SKINNY: HOW TO JULIENNE VEGETABLES

A JULIENNE CUT IS ESSENTIALLY A LONG, THIN STRIP THAT LOOKS ELEGANT IN SALADS AND OTHER DISHES. A MANDOLINE WILL DO THE JOB FOR YOU IN SECONDS, BUT IT ISN'T TOUGH TO DO ON YOUR OWN. TAKE A STAB AT IT.

1: CUT THE VEGETABLE IN HALF LENGTHWISE: CUT STRAIGHT DOWN THE CENTER OF THE VEGETABLE. THIS WILL LEAVE YOU WITH TWO PIECES ON THE CUTTING BOARD.

2: SLICE THE VEGETABLE: TAKE EACH SLICE, AND CUT INTO SLENDER STRIPS ABOUT ¼-INCH (6 MM) THICK. AT THIS POINT, THE PIECES SHOULD BE THIN LIKE MATCHSTICKS.

3: CUT THE PIECES IN HALF: GATHER ALL OF THE SLENDER STRIPS IN A BUNCH, AND CUT THEM IN HALF TO MAKE SHORTER STRIPS. FOR LONGER VEGGIES, SUCH AS ZUCCHINI OR CUCUMBERS, YOU MAY HAVE TO CUT INTO THIRDS. THE GOAL IS A GROUP OF STRIPS ABOUT ¼-INCH (6 MM) WIDE BY 1½-INCHES (4 CM) LONG.

Creamy Potato Salad

Someone grab my Daisy Dukes. I believe it's time for an outdoor barbecue! Sure, potato salad is good any time of the year, but it always reminds me of family reunions in the park with the whole gang. I decided to develop a homemade recipe as an alternative to the unhealthy tubs of potato salad in the store. You can easily build on this recipe by adding diced carrots, celery, or fennel.

MAKES 4 SERVINGS

1 pound (455 g) baby red potatoes
⅔ cup (165 ml) vegan mayonnaise
1½ tablespoons Dijon mustard
1½ tablespoons apple cider vinegar
Salt and pepper, to taste
¼ cup (15 g) thinly sliced green onions

Bring a large pot of water to a boil. Add the potatoes and return to a boil. Reduce the heat to medium and gently boil until soft, about 15 minutes.

In a large bowl, add the mayonnaise, mustard, and vinegar and whisk to combine. Season with salt and pepper to taste. Drain and rinse the potatoes and set aside to cool. Once cooled, cut the potatoes into quarters and add to the dressing, along with the green onions, gently tossing to coat. Cover and chill for at least an hour before serving. Serve cold.

Srv: 183 g | Cal: 360 | Fat: 24 g | Sat Fat: 2.5 g | Col: 0 mg | Carb: 28 g | Fib: 1 g | Pro: 3 g

Tangy Spinach and Strawberry Salad

There is so much deliciousness in this recipe, I don't know where to start. It was originally developed by food stylist and a fantastic friend of mine, Denise Vivaldo. But I stole it. Actually, I made her give it to me. When fresh strawberries and spinach are involved, a little threatening is necessary. Rest assured, you will soon understand why.

MAKES 2 SERVINGS

4 cups (120 g) baby spinach, loosely packed

1 cup (155 g) thinly sliced strawberries, stems removed

¼ cup (60 ml) Champagne Vinaigrette (see recipe on page 149)

⅓ cup (45 g) raw sunflower seeds

Pepper, to taste

In a large mixing bowl, combine the spinach and strawberries. Add the Champagne Vinaigrette and gently toss to combine. Add the sunflower seeds and sprinkle with the pepper.

Srv: 152 g | Cal: 290 | Fat: 22 g | Sat Fat: 3.5 g | Col: 0 mg | Carb: 21 g | Fib: 6 g | Pro: 6 g

Tabouli

My husband is from the south of France, where the cuisine has absorbed flavors and influences from Mediterranean countries like Italy, Spain, Turkey, and Lebanon. This light tabouli recipe is a dish born of this classic marriage of cultures. Typically, we make this for lunch, and end up snacking on the leftovers for another few days.

MAKES 4 SERVINGS

1¼ (300 ml) cups water

½ teaspoon salt, plus pinch, to taste

1 cup (175 g) uncooked whole wheat couscous (equals 3 cups cooked)

1 (15-ounce/430 g) can white beans, drained and rinsed

½ cup (40 g) shaved fennel, including some of the green part

½ cup (50 g) shaved radishes

½ cup (30 g) chopped Oven-Dried Tomatoes (see recipe on page 128)

2½ tablespoons finely chopped fresh parsley

2½ tablespoons finely chopped fresh basil

2½ tablespoons finely chopped fresh cilantro

¼ cup (20 g) finely chopped red cabbage, steamed

¼ cup (35 g) peeled and finely chopped carrot, steamed

2 tablespoons finely chopped red onion

¼ cup (60 ml) olive oil

¼ cup (60 ml) lemon juice

1 tablespoon lemon zest

½ teaspoon ground cumin

Pepper, to taste

In a medium saucepan bring the water and ½ teaspoon salt to a boil over high heat. Stir in the couscous, and turn off the heat. Cover immediately and move the saucepan to a cool burner. Let sit 5 minutes. Remove the cover and fluff with a fork. Set aside.

In a large mixing bowl, add the beans, fennel, radishes, tomatoes, parsley, basil, cilantro, cabbage, carrot, and onion. Stir until well combined. In a small bowl, whisk together the oil, lemon juice, lemon zest, cumin, pinch of salt, and pepper. Add the cooled couscous to the bowl of vegetables and stir together. Pour in the oil mixture and stir together. Chill and serve cold.

Srv: 216 g | Cal: 340 | Fat: 15 g | Sat Fat: 2 g | Col: 0 mg | Carb: 47 g | Fib: 11 g | Pro: 12 g

BITCHWORTHY: MEYER LEMONS

WITH THE TANG OF REGULAR LEMONS BUT NOT THE BITTER PUCKER, MEYER LEMONS ROCK MY FRUIT BOWL. THEY ARE GREAT IN SOUFFLÉS AND MAKE AN UNBELIEVABLE VINAIGRETTE DRESSING. FOR DESSERTS, THEIR PEEL IS SLIGHTLY SWEETER THAN OTHER LEMONS AND THE COLOR AND JUICE JUST POP. LOOK FOR THEM IN SEASON FROM NOVEMBER TO APRIL.

The Chronicles of the Common Flu

THE CAUSES OF AND CURES FOR A WEAK IMMUNE SYSTEM

Some hussy sneezes on you at the movie theater. Kleenex is on back order at your local grocer. Your friends are dropping like flies, their sick days slipping away faster than their youth. Then you start to feel it coming on. The body aches, itchy throat, splitting headache. *Damn it. I can't afford to get sick right now.*

You, my friend, actually play a bigger role than you think. Try to picture your immune system as an army—a big, bad, don't-take-shit-from-nobody army. That army's primary goal is to fight and destroy the scum that invades the body. When that army is sluggish, it leaves our bodies open to attack. Now, why in the world would the immune system go and do that? I thought you would never ask.

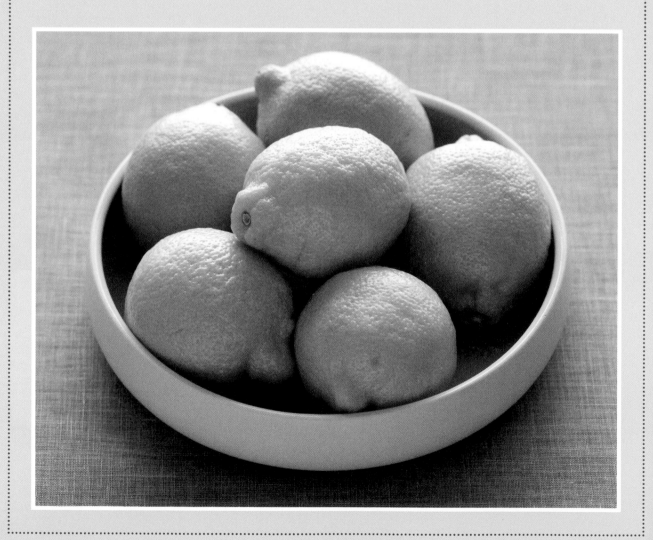

Exhibit A, please:

SUGAR HIGH: When you overdose on sugar, it reduces the ability of infection-fighting white blood cells to kill germs and invades the immune system. Even just two sodas a day can lower the power of your cold-busting immune system by 40 percent. Treat sugar like your ex-boyfriend. Tell yourself the relationship is over; dump it and move on.

OBESITY: Your pot belly and cankles can lead to a depressed immune system. This means your white blood cells are so busy throwing a pity party for one, they forgot to multiply and produce antibodies. Oh, spare me the melodrama!

DRINKING: Chugging one too many cocktails not only packs on more cushion for the pushin' but too much can also produce an overall nutritional deficiency.

STRESS: Chill out! Overwhelming evidence shows that stress negatively impacts your health. No shit.

POOR DIET: Your body needs a daily boost of antioxidants, vitamins, minerals, fiber, and enzymes to protect the immune system. What are you eating? [106]

Exhibit B:
Eat Your Way to Good Health

LEMONS: Lemons are the ideal food for restoring acid-alkali balance in the body. It helps maintain the body's natural pH levels, which support healthy bacteria instead of the viruses and harmful bacteria that thrive in acidic conditions. Yet another reason to drink water, too.

GREEN TEA AND WHITE TEA: Grab the scones and crumpets. Let's get this tea party started! Green tea stimulates the immune system to fight disease, while white tea can destroy the organisms that cause disease.

MUSHROOMS, BROCCOLI AND BLUE-BERRIES: Mushrooms, such as Reishi, Maitake, and Shiitake, and fruits and veggies, such as broccoli and blueberries, help de-stress the immune system so it doesn't have to work so hard.

KIDNEY BEANS, CHICKPEAS AND GARBANZO BEANS: You need about three to four ounces of protein twice a day to get the nutrients essential to a strong immune system. Toss them on salads, add them to pasta dishes, or enjoy them as their own side dish.

PUMPKIN SEEDS: Pumpkin seeds are high in zinc, the most critical nutrient to boost your immunity. Roast some seeds with a teaspoon of olive oil for a quick snack.

BRAZIL NUTS: Go nuts! Brazil nuts are the number one source for selenium, an antioxidant that the immune system loves to pieces. Selenium helps rejuvenate our bodies to kill off germs and protects cells from free radical damage.

GARLIC: You may have some stank-ass breath, but garlic, primarily when raw, seems to cure everything. It is an edible antibiotic that fights virus. Experts recommend chopping a clove and letting it sit for fifteen minutes to release the full health benefits. [107]

BITCHWORTHY: YOUR IMMUNE SYSTEM HAS AN APPETITE FOR INDIAN FOOD. COOK UP SOME MEALS HEAVY WITH LENTILS, DARK GREEN VEGGIES, AND CUMIN TO FEND OFF COLDS AND VIRUSES. [108]

Orange-Kissed Beet and Arugula Salad

This salad is pure eye candy. I make it primarily to impress houseguests or to show up other mothers at Mommy Playtime. The juxtaposition of beets paired with apples and a tangy orange vinaigrette make my eyes roll into the back of my head. Seconds, please.

MAKES 4 SERVINGS

4 beets, peeled, stems removed, and cut in half
Salt, to taste
1 bunch of arugula, washed and chopped
1 apple, cored and sliced
¼ cup (30 g) walnuts, toasted
1 orange, zested and juiced
1 tablespoon olive oil
1 tablespoon agave nectar
1 tablespoon sherry vinegar
Salt and pepper, to taste

Bring a large pot of water to boil over high heat. Add the beets and a pinch of salt, return to a boil. Reduce the heat to medium and gently boil until tender, 20 to 30 minutes. Drain and rinse with cold water. Cut the beets into large cubes and place in a medium-size bowl. Add the arugula, apple, and walnuts. Heat a small sauté pan over medium-high heat and toast the walnuts 3 to 5 minutes, stirring constantly. Remove from the heat and set aside. In a separate small bowl, mix and combine the orange juice and zest, oil, agave nectar, and vinegar for the salad dressing. Toss the dressing with the salad ingredients. Add salt and pepper, to taste. Serve immediately.

Srv: 204 g | Cal: 180 | Fat: 9 g | Sat Fat: 1 g | Col: 0 mg | Carb: 25 g | Fib: 5 g | Pro: 3 g

Curried Rice Salad

With some cultural Indian flair, this one's a clever entrée to bring along to a fun potluck. The perfumed aroma and nutty flavor of Basmati rice peps up any dinner and makes my house smell like a foreign marketplace.

MAKES 4 SERVINGS

1 cup (215 g) brown Basmati rice

1 cup (130 g) diced cucumber

1 carrot, julienned or grated

1 cup (135 g) frozen peas

8 basil leaves, minced

½ cup (120 ml) vegan mayonnaise

1 tablespoon soy sauce

1 tablespoon agave nectar

1 teaspoon rice vinegar

1 teaspoon curry powder

1 teaspoon sesame oil, toasted

½ cup (50 g) shredded unsweetened coconut

Salt and pepper, to taste

Fill a medium-size saucepan with water and bring to a boil. Stir in the rice. Return to a boil and reduce the heat to medium. Cover and simmer 25 to 35 minutes, or until done. Drain and return the rice to the saucepan. Cover and set aside. In a medium size bowl, combine the cucumber, carrot, peas, and basil.

In a separate bowl, whisk together the mayonnaise, soy sauce, agave nectar, vinegar, curry powder, and oil for the dressing. When done, combine the rice, dressing and vegetables, and toss the rice salad with a wooden spoon. Garnish with the coconut. Add salt and pepper, to taste.

Srv: 208 g | Cal: 490 | Fat: 28 g | Sat Fat: 10 g | Col: 0 mg | Carb: 53 g | Fib: 7 g | Pro: 7 g

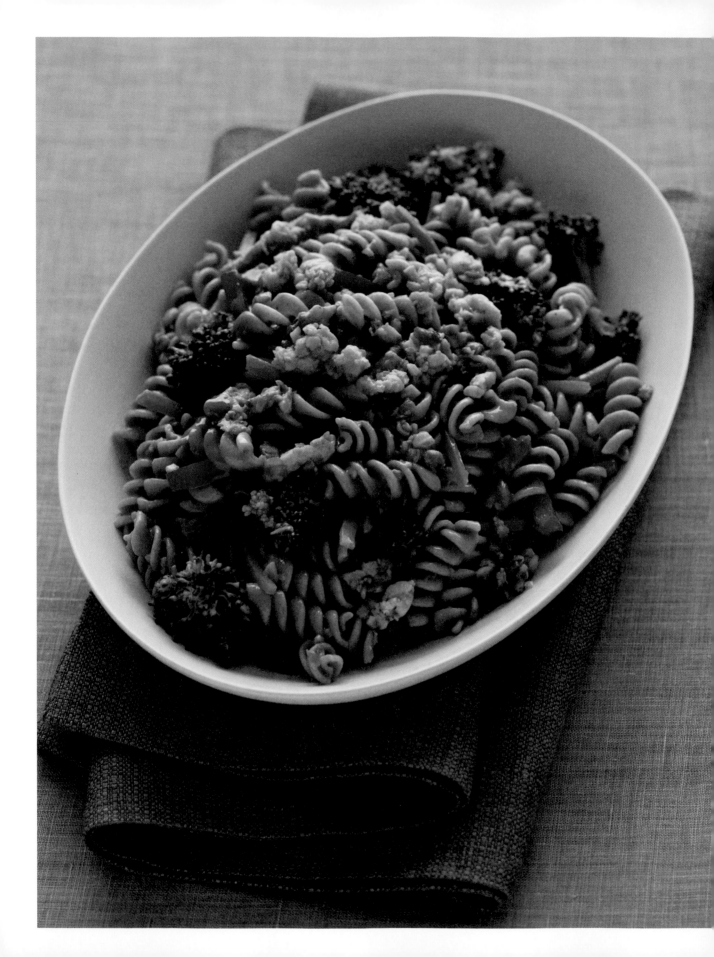

Peanut Pasta Salad with Fried Tempeh Bits

You put a peanut in anything and I'm sold. Especially a pasta salad topped with tempeh. The textures and different flavors competing in this salad are like a party in your mouth. The best part is the kids love it, too. It is a complete meal in itself with the recommended daily servings of whole grains, protein, and vegetables. Store any leftover pasta salad in a reusable container in the fridge to hit the spot for lunch the next day.

MAKES 4 SERVINGS

4 tablespoons (60 ml) sesame oil, divided

1 (8-ounce/225 g) block of tempeh, crumbled

1 large carrot, julienned

3 cups (275 g) broccoli florets, cut into bite-size pieces

1 red bell pepper, julienned

1 (8-ounce/225 g) package of brown rice pasta spirals (or any other pasta)

3 tablespoons organic peanut butter

¼ cup (60 ml) water

2 tablespoons soy sauce, to taste

1 tablespoon agave nectar

1 tablespoon apple cider vinegar

2 teaspoons minced fresh ginger

Sesame seeds, for garnish

Heat 3 tablespoons of the oil in a skillet over high heat. Fry the tempeh until slightly crispy, about 10 minutes, stirring occasionally. Bring a large pot of water to a boil. Blanch the carrots, broccoli, and red pepper separately until they turn bright in color, or about 30 seconds. Do not overcook. Drain, rinse under cold water, and set aside. Cook the pasta, according to the directions on the package. Drain and set aside. In a small bowl, whisk together the peanut butter, the remaining sesame oil, the water, soy sauce, agave nectar, vinegar, and ginger. Toss the vegetables, pasta, and sauce together. Garnish with the sesame seeds.

Srv: 346 g | Cal: 580 | Fat: 25 g | Sat Fat: 4 g | Col: 0 mg | Carb: 69 g | Fib: 7 g | Pro: 22 g

---

THE SKINNY: WHAT IS BLANCHING?

BLANCHING HELPS LOOSEN THE PEELS OR SHELLS OF VEGETABLES AND BEANS SO THEY CAN EASILY BE PEELED OFF. IT ALSO WORKS TO ENHANCE THE FLAVOR AND COLOR OF YOUR VEGGIES. IT'S SIMPLE: JUST GIVE THEM THE SHOCK TREATMENT. QUICKLY STEAM OR COOK THEM IN BOILING WATER, AND THEN PLUNGE THEM INTO A COLD BATH. REMEMBER WHEN YOU USED TO JUMP FROM THE HOT TUB INTO THE SWIMMING POOL IN THE MIDDLE OF WINTER? IT'S JUST LIKE THAT, YOU CRAZY BITCH.

Oven-Dried Tomatoes

This rustic mini-dish is great to toss into salads, dressings, pasta dishes, or grilled vegetables. In our household, we make a few pounds and store in the refrigerator for all types of meals. They are the tomatoes that keep on giving.

MAKES 4 CUPS (220 GRAMS)

2 pounds (910 g) Roma tomatoes, stems removed
⅓ cup (75 ml) olive oil
½ teaspoon dried thyme
Salt and pepper, to taste

Preheat the oven to 200° F (95° C).

Bring a large pot of water to a boil over high heat. Fill a large mixing bowl with very cold water, adding a few ice cubes. At the bottom of the tomatoes, slice an X-shape with a sharp knife, cutting about ¼ inch (6 mm) into the tomato. Drop the tomatoes in the boiling water about 30 seconds. Drain and then immediately drop into the bowl of ice water. Let the tomatoes cool down for a couple of minutes. Remove from bowl of water and peel off the skins. They should come off easily just using your fingers. Cut the peeled tomatoes into 4 wedges and remove the seeds.

Transfer the tomatoes to a large mixing bowl and coat with the oil, thyme, salt, and pepper. Place the tomatoes on a cookie sheet or large baking dish, being careful that they do not overlap. Bake the tomatoes on the top rack of the oven 45 minutes to 1 hour, checking frequently to ensure the tomatoes do not burn. When cooled, store in an airtight container in the refrigerator.

Srv: 60 g (1 tomato) | Cal: 40 | Fat: 3.5 g | Sat Fat: 0.5 g | Col: 0 mg | Carb: 2 g | Fib: 0 g | Pro: 1 g

Greek Salad with Tzatziki Sauce

In addition to all the other great things the Greeks have contributed to civilization, they also came up with Tzatziki Sauce! This tangy, light dressing goes well with just about everything—including, of course, a Greek Salad with pita bread. Opah! (That's like "Cheers!" in Greek.)

MAKES 8 SERVINGS

¼ cup (60 ml) olive oil

⅓ cup (75 ml) red wine vinegar

2 tablespoons Greek seasoning mix, divided

1 teaspoon oregano, preferably Greek

1 tablespoon, plus 1 teaspoon lemon juice

Pinch of salt, plus 1 teaspoon

½ cucumber, peeled, sliced thinly, and then cut into ¼-inch (6 mm) dice

1¼ cups (145 g) thinly sliced red onion, divided

⅔ cup (165 ml) coconut or soy plain yogurt

½ teaspoon white pepper

2 pounds (910 g) tomatoes, chopped into medium chunks

1 cup (150 g) sliced or chopped Greek olives

2 Persian cucumbers, cut into ½-inch (12 mm) chunks

4 whole pita breads whole, cut into triangle wedges, warmed

Preheat the oven to 350° F (175° C).

In a small bowl, prepare the dressing by whisking together the oil, vinegar, 1 tablespoon of the Greek seasoning mix, the oregano, 1 teaspoon of the lemon juice, and a pinch of salt.

In a separate bowl, prepare the Tzatziki Sauce by mixing the cucumber, ¼ cup (30 g) of the red onion, the coconut or soy yogurt, the remaining 1 teaspoon of salt, the remaining 1 tablespoon of lemon juice, the remaining 1 tablespoon Greek seasoning mix, and the white pepper.

In a separate medium-size bowl, combine the tomatoes, olives, Persian cucumbers, and remaining 1 cup (115 g) of red onion. Pour the dressing over the tomato salad and toss. Place the pita wedges on a cookie sheet and warm for 5 minutes, or until soft. Top each serving of the tomato salad with a large dollop of the Tzatziki Sauce. Serve with the warmed pita triangles.

Srv: 323 g | Cal: 280 | Fat: 16 g | Sat Fat: 2 g | Col: 0 mg | Carb: 31 g | Fib: 4 g | Pro: 6 g

THE SKINNY: MAKE YOUR OWN GREEK SEASONING MIX

THIS SEASONING IS AVAILABLE IN THE SPICE SECTION AT MOST MAJOR GROCERY RETAILERS. BUT, IF YOU HAVE NO LUCK, FOLLOW THIS QUICK RECIPE:

IN A SMALL BOWL, MIX ALL OF THE INGREDIENTS. VOILÀ! THE SEASONING WILL LAST FOR MONTHS AS LONG AS YOU STORE IN AN AIRTIGHT CONTAINER. REMEMBER TO STORE IN A DARK, DRY PLACE AT ROOM TEMPERATURE.

Makes 2½ Tablespoons

1½ teaspoon dried oregano

1 teaspoon dried mint

1 teaspoon paprika

1 teaspoon dried thyme

½ teaspoon dried basil

½ teaspoon dried marjoram

½ teaspoon garlic powder

½ teaspoon onion powder

½ teaspoon black pepper

½ teaspoon salt

Pomegranate and Brussels Sprout Salad

....

This salad has such a mild, unique flavor. The tart pomegranate bits add some unexpected zing to the clean taste of the shaved Brussels sprouts. It is very light on the belly and works wonders in cleansing your palate prior to dinner.

MAKES 4 SERVINGS

3 cups (725 ml) Brussels sprouts

1 cup (237 ml) thinly sliced radicchio

2 cups (500 ml) chopped romaine lettuce

¼ cup (59 ml) pomegranate seeds

½ cup (118 ml) mandarin oranges, or tangerine wedges

1 cup (225 g) firm tofu, drained and cubed

¼ cup (30 g) roasted hazelnuts

¼ cup (60 ml) balsamic vinegar

1 tablespoon soy sauce

2 teaspoons mirin

¼ cup (60 ml) olive oil

1 garlic clove, minced

½ teaspoon dried rosemary

Pepper, to taste

Steam the Brussels sprouts 3 to 5 minutes, or until soft. Place in a colander and rinse with cold water to stop the cooking. Cut them into quarters. In a large bowl, toss together the Brussels sprouts, radicchio, romaine, pomegranate seeds, oranges, tofu, and hazelnuts.

In a medium bowl, whisk together the balsamic vinegar, soy sauce, mirin, oil, garlic, and rosemary, for the dressing. Heat a small frying pan over medium heat and pour in the dressing, cooking until the mixture starts to bubble. Add to the salad and toss. Season with pepper, to taste.

....

Srv: 219 g | Cal: 160 | Fat: 7 g | Sat Fat: 1 g | Col: 0 mg | Carb: 16 g | Fib: 5 g | Pro: 9 g

---

THE SKINNY: DE-SEEDING A POMEGRANATE

CUTTING INTO A POMEGRANATE IS MESSY BUSINESS. THE FIRST TIME I TOOK A SHOT AT DE-SEEDING ONE, MY KITCHEN LOOKED LIKE A CRIME SCENE. FOLLOW THESE STEPS TO AVOID A COOKING MASSACRE.

1: CUT THE CROWN OFF THE POMEGRANATE.

2: SLICE THE RIND IN FOUR PLACES BUT AVOID CUTTING ALL THE WAY THROUGH.

3: SOAK THE POMEGRANATE IN COLD WATER UPSIDE-DOWN FOR APPROXIMATELY 7 MINUTES.

4: BREAK APART THE RIND OF THE POMEGRANATE AND REMOVE THE SEEDS FROM THE MEMBRANE. THE SEEDS SHOULD SINK TO THE BOTTOM OF THE BOWL.

5: USING A SIEVE, REMOVE THE RIND AND MEMBRANES FROM THE BOWL.

6: DRAIN THE SEEDS. PAT DRY WITH A PAPER TOWEL.

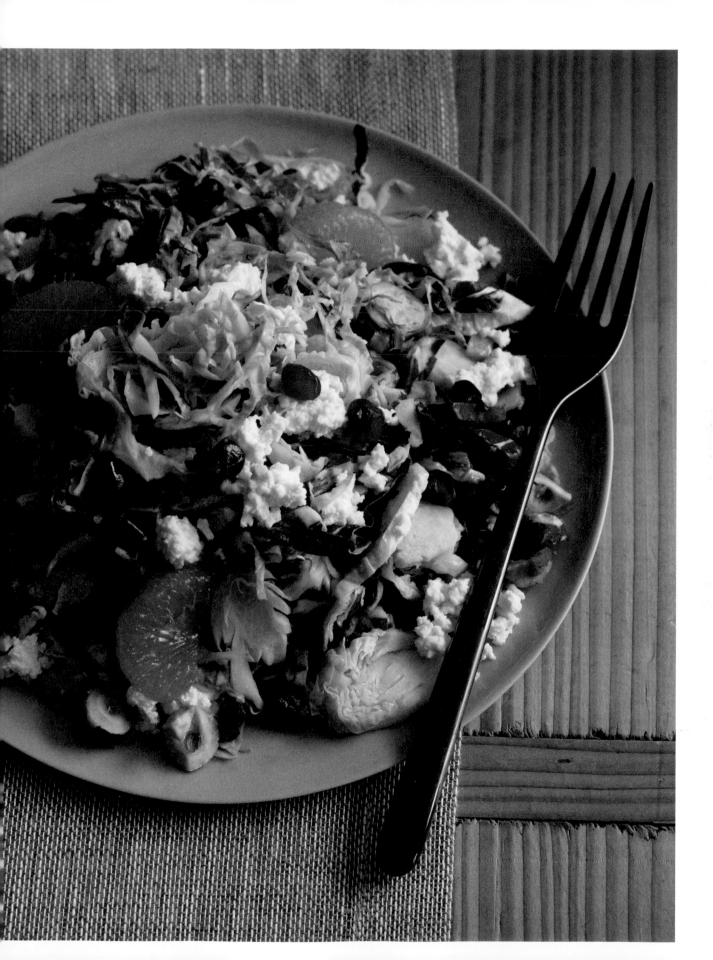

Vegan Antipasto

My own twist on traditional antipasto salad tossed with a balsamic vinaigrette. It's light and delicious with warm baguette slices.

MAKES 4 SERVINGS

⅓ cup (75 ml) balsamic vinegar

⅓ cup (75 ml) grapeseed oil

1 lemon, zested and juiced

1 clove garlic, minced

1 tablespoon dried oregano

1 teaspoon dried thyme

½ teaspoon red pepper flakes

Salt and pepper, to taste

1 cup (150 g) black olives

1 cup (150 g) green olives

1 (15-ounce/430 g) can artichoke hearts in water, drained and quartered

1 cup (140 g) julienned roasted red bell pepper

In a small bowl, whisk together the vinegar, oil, lemon zest and juice, garlic, oregano, thyme, and red pepper flakes. Season with salt and pepper and set aside.

In a large bowl, combine the olives, artichoke hearts, and bell pepper. Add the vinegar marinade and gently toss until thoroughly combined. Cover and chill for at least an hour or up to 2 days.

Srv: 242 g | Cal: 430 | Fat: 38 g | Sat Fat: 6 g | Col: 0 mg | Carb: 16 g | Fib: 3 g | Pro: 1 g

Miso Crunch Salad

A simple miso salad always has me at hello. The salad itself is fresh and nutritious, but the dressing is remarkable. On page 136, you will find a recipe for the crunchy wonton strips, which are optional since the eggless versions are only available at traditional Asian markets. If you have an Asian market in your 'hood, they do add some filling texture. (Just don't overdo it.)

MAKES 6 SERVINGS

2 tablespoons light yellow miso

¼ cup (60 ml) plain soy yogurt

¼ teaspoon soy sauce

1 tablespoon dark brown sugar

1 teaspoon toasted sesame oil

1 tablespoon rice wine vinegar

¾ teaspoon mirin

½ teaspoon grated fresh ginger

1 small garlic clove, minced

½ cup (120 ml) soybean oil

Salt and pepper, to taste

2 cups (145 g) shredded iceberg lettuce

1 cup (90 g) shredded Napa cabbage

1 cup (90 g) shredded red cabbage

2 Persian cucumbers, julienned

1 cup (150 g) shelled and cooked edamame

1 small bunch of cilantro, finely chopped and large stems removed

3 green onions, thinly sliced, white and pale green parts only

¼ cup (30 g) sliced almonds, toasted

1 cup (130 g) julienned jicama

1 cup (100 g) julienned snow peas

½ cup (65 g) shredded carrots

2 cups (115 g) Deep Fried Wonton Strips (see recipe on page 136)

1 ripe avocado, peeled, pitted, and cut into ½-inch (12 mm) cubes

2 tablespoons black sesame seeds, for garnish

In a blender or food processor, combine the miso, yogurt, soy sauce, brown sugar, sesame oil, vinegar, mirin, ginger, garlic, oil, and salt and pepper, and blend until creamy.

In a large bowl, combine the lettuce, cabbage, cucumbers, edamame, cilantro, onions, almonds, jicama, snow peas, and carrots. Pour the dressing on the salad and toss well. Add the wonton strips and avocado. Garnish with the sesame seeds.

Srv: 288 g | Cal: 200 | Fat: 10 g | Sat Fat: 1 g | Col: 0 mg | Carb: 21 g | Fib: 6 g | Pro: 10 g

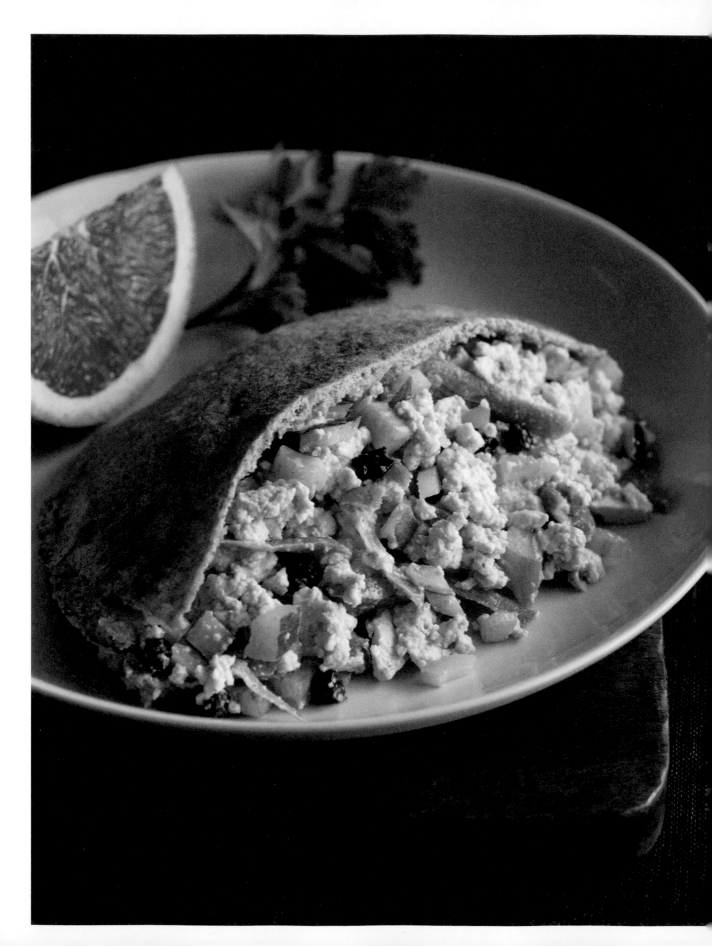

Curried Tofu Egg-Less Salad

Prior to going vegan, I couldn't eat my morning eggs without a side of ketchup. The two might as well have been sold as a boxed set in the grocery store. Tofu replaces eggs in this recipe, and the anti-inflammatory properties of curry make it a healthy alternative to processed ketchup. Truly an unconventional meal for lunch or dinner, and a cinch to prepare.

MAKES 6 SERVINGS

1 (14-ounce/400 g) package extra-firm tofu, drained, and crumbled

½ cup (80 g) diced red onion

1 carrot, grated

1 celery stalk, finely diced

¼ cup (45 g) currants

2 tablespoons sliced almonds (optional)

1 tablespoon curry powder

½ cup (120 ml) vegan mayonnaise

1 lemon, zested and juiced

2 tablespoons Dijon mustard

1 tablespoon agave nectar

Salt and pepper, to taste

2 pita breads, cut into quarters and toasted

In a steamer basket over 1 inch (2.5 cm) of boiling water, steam the tofu 10 minutes. Remove from the heat and place in a towel-lined bowl to remove excess water. In a large bowl, mix together the tofu, onion, carrot, celery, currants, and almonds. In a small bowl, whisk together the curry powder, mayonnaise, lemon juice, lemon zest, mustard, agave nectar, salt, and pepper for the dressing. Add the dressing to the tofu and salad mixture, and toss well. Chill in the refrigerator 15 to 30 minutes. Serve on toasted pita breads.

Srv: 166 g | Cal: 230 | Fat: 16 g | Sat Fat: 2 g | Col: 0 mg | Carb: 17 g | Fib: 3 g | Pro: 6 g

Wonton Wrappers

....

MAKES 24 WRAPPERS

2 cups (255 g) all-purpose flour, plus more for dusting

½ teaspoon salt

½ cup (120 ml) warm water

Whisk together the flour and salt in a medium bowl. Slowly stir in the warm water with a fork until the dough turns stiff. Place the dough on a floured surface and knead the until smooth, about 12 minutes. Cover with a clean kitchen towel. Let stand for 20 minutes. Divide the dough in half and roll out to $\frac{1}{16}$-inch (2 mm) thick, re-flouring the surface as needed to prevent dough from sticking. Cut the dough into 3-inch squares if using for ravioli, and ¼-inch (6 mm) strips for salad toppings; toss to separate pieces. Store unused wrappers in a zip-top plastic bag. They can be refrigerated for 1 day or frozen for up to 2 weeks.

....

Srv: 1 Wrapper | Cal: 40 | Fat: 0 g | Sat Fat: 0 g | Col: 0 mg | Carb: 8 g | Fib: 0 g;

Deep-Fried Wonton Strips

....

1 cup (240 ml) grapeseed oil

1 recipe wonton wrappers

Heat the oil to 400° F (200° C) in a large, deep pot. While the oil is heating, cut the wonton wrappers into ¼-inch (6 mm) strips and toss to separate pieces. When the oil is hot, fry the wonton strips about 30 seconds, or until golden. Remove immediately with a wire skimmer, and drain on several layers of paper towels. Allow the wonton strips to cool. Store at room temperature in an airtight container for up to 3 days.

Artichoke Heart Avocado Salad with Garlic "Parmesan" Dressing

I am a big believer that artichokes just make everything taste better. Aside from taste, they are a diuretic that helps to rid your body of excess water and toxins and improves skin luminosity. Add a dash of garlic powder and croutons for one interesting salad. By interesting, I mean, *Someone please take the fork out of my hand.*

MAKES 4 SERVINGS

2 tablespoons red wine vinegar

⅓ cup (75 ml) olive oil

1½ teaspoons vegan Parmesan cheese

1 teaspoon Dijon mustard

¼ teaspoon garlic powder

Pinch of salt and pepper, to taste

1 (9-ounce/255 g) jar marinated artichoke hearts, drained, leaves or spikes removed

3 cups (140 g) chopped romaine lettuce

2 Persian cucumbers, thinly sliced (can substitute with regular cucumbers, peeled)

1 large avocado, cut into slices or chunks

3 green onions, minced

½ cup (40 g) garlic croutons, crushed

In a medium saucepan, prepare the dressing by combining the vinegar, oil, cheese, mustard, garlic powder, salt, and pepper. Cut the artichoke hearts into quarters. In a large bowl, add the lettuce, cucumbers, artichokes, and avocado. Sprinkle with the green onions. Toss with the dressing. Sprinkle with the crouton crumbs.

Srv: 328 g | Cal: 400 | Fat: 35 g | Sat Fat: 5 g | Col: 0 mg | Carb: 18 g | Fib: 4 g | Pro: 4 g

THE SKINNY: PERSIAN CUCUMBERS

VERY SIMILAR TO THE JAPANESE CUCUMBER, PERSIAN CUCUMBERS ARE CRUNCHY WITH FEW SEEDS, AND HAVE A WATERY, FRESH FLAVOR. THEY ARE AWESOME FOR COOKING BECAUSE THEY DON'T NEED TO BE PEELED OR SEEDED WHEN USED IN DISHES (UNLESS NOTED IN THE RECIPE). LOOK FOR ONES THAT ARE FIRM WITH A RICH GREEN COLOR AND NO SOFT SPOTS.

BBQ Seitan Chopped Salad

This salad is a spin-off of one of my favorite salads at Real Food Daily in Los Angeles, California. The combination of barbecue sauce with a creamy dressing instantly makes the salad into a cookbook front-runner. Not for the faint of heart.

MAKES 6 SERVINGS

2 (8-ounce/225 g) packages seitan, chopped

⅔ cup (165 ml) barbecue sauce (for homemade recipe see page 147)

1 (14-ounce/400 g) package silken tofu

1 lemon, zested and juiced

¼ cup (60 ml) unsweetened almond milk

½ cup (5 g) chopped dill

1 tablespoon apple cider vinegar

1 tablespoon agave nectar

2 tablespoons Dijon mustard

1 teaspoon celery seed

½ teaspoon salt, or more to taste

Pepper, to taste

5 cups (235 g) chopped romaine lettuce

2 celery stalks, diced

1 carrot, peeled and julienned

2 avocados, cubed

Dulse flakes, for garnish

In a medium-size sauté pan, sauté the seitan with the barbecue sauce until well combined and heated through. In a blender or food processor, add the tofu, lemon juice, lemon zest, almond milk, dill, vinegar, agave nectar, mustard, celery seed, salt, and pepper, and blend until creamy. In a large bowl, add the romaine, celery, carrot, and avocados. Toss the seitan with the salad ingredients. Drizzle the dressing on top and sprinkle with the Dulse flakes, to garnish.

Srv: 251 g | Cal: 170 | Fat: 6 g | Sat Fat: 0.5 g | Col: 0 mg | Carb: 19 g | Fib: 4 g | Pro: 12 g

> **BITCHIONARY: DULSE FLAKES**
> SOUNDS LIKE FISH FOOD, DOESN'T IT? FISH CAN ONLY WISH. DULSE IS A RED SEAWEED OR ALGAE THAT CAN BE BROKEN INTO SMALL FLAKES FOR COOKING. DRIED DULSE HAS A SALTY TASTE, CHEWY TEXTURE, AND CAN BE SPRINKLED ON SALADS, SOUPS, AND EVEN PIZZA FOR ADDED FLAVOR.

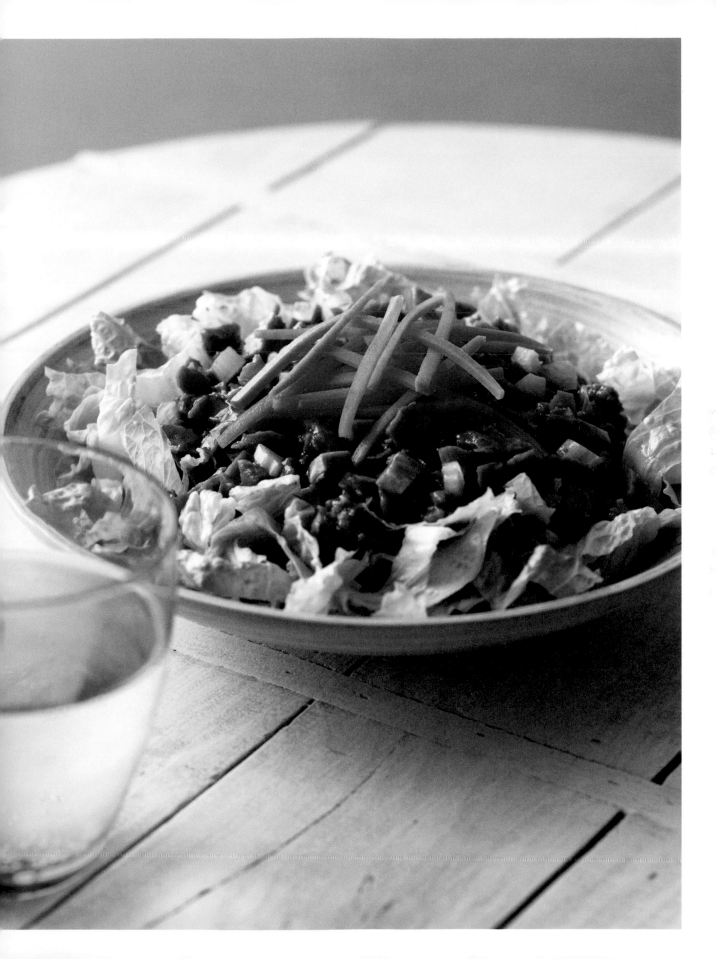

SAUCES &
DRESSINGS

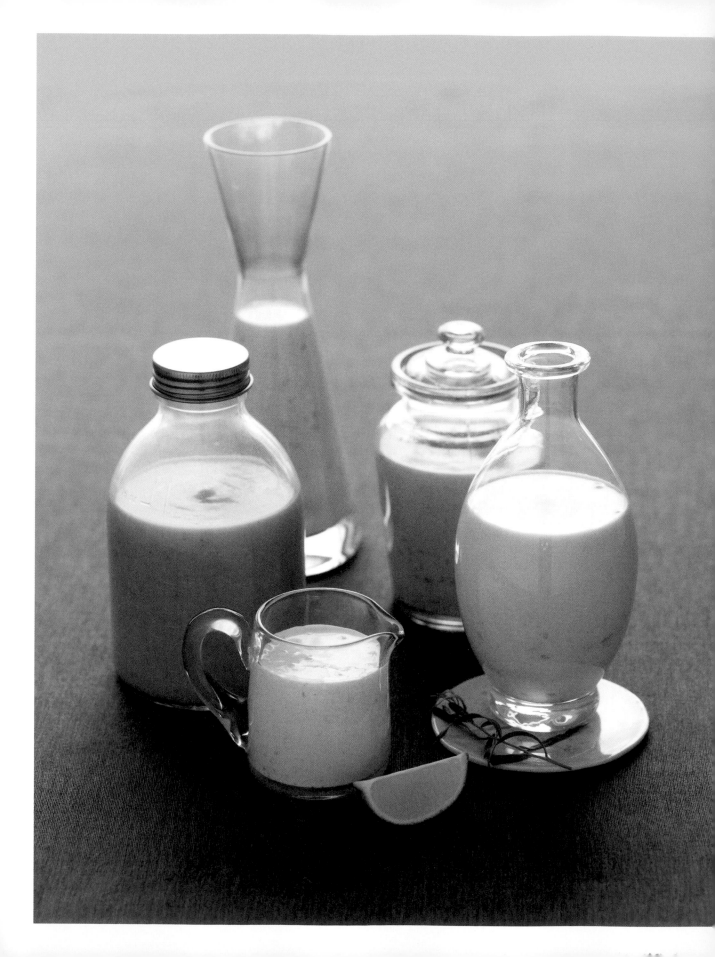

Tarragon Sauce

Tarragon sauce is great for all-purpose cooking. You can add this to pasta and steamed veggies for some unexpected flavor.

MAKES 2 ¼ CUPS (530 ML)

1½ cups (360 ml) white wine
¼ cup (40 g) finely chopped onion
2 sprigs fresh tarragon, plus 2 teaspoons chopped fresh
Salt and pepper, to taste
¼ cup (60 ml) vegetable broth
1 tablespoon unbleached all-purpose flour
1 cup (240 ml) soy creamer

In a large saucepan over medium-high heat, bring the wine, onion, 2 sprigs of the tarragon and a pinch of salt and pepper to a boil. Reduce the heat and simmer until the mixture is reduced by about two-thirds, 20 to 25 minutes.

In a small bowl, whisk together the broth and flour until smooth. Remove and discard the tarragon sprigs from the saucepan. Add the broth-flour mixture, soy creamer, and a pinch of salt and pepper to the wine mixture. Simmer gently until slightly thickened, about 15 minutes. Stir in the remaining 2 teaspoons chopped tarragon and remove from the heat. Serve warm.

Srv: 45 g | Cal: 35 | Fat: 1 g | Sat Fat: 0 g | Col: 0 mg | Carb: 3 g | Fib: 0 g | Pro: 0 g

> **BITCHWORTHY: VEGETABLE BROTH**
> VEGETABLE-BASED BROTH IS MY WINGMAN. I USE IT A LOT WHEN COOKING TO ENHANCE FLAVOR. HERE'S A TRICK: WHEN YOU'RE COOKING BARLEY, LENTILS, OR RICE, AND BARLEY, ADD VEGGIE STOCK TO THE WATER YOU'RE COOKING THEM IN AT A 1:1 RATIO (ONE PART STOCK, ONE PART WATER). THIS DOES WONDERS FOR THE FLAVOR.

Lime Cream

Top off the Black Bean and Tomato Soup (see page 99 for the recipe) with a citrus kick. This also works well on a baked potato with a scoop of Earth Balance.

MAKES ¾ CUP (180 ML)

½ cup (120 ml) vegan sour cream
2 tablespoons almond milk
2 tablespoons lime juice
¼ teaspoon salt
Pepper, to taste
1 teaspoon chopped fresh cilantro

In a blender or food processor, combine the sour cream, milk, and lime juice. Blend until thoroughly mixed and creamy. Add the salt, pepper, and cilantro. Blend until well combined. Use immediately or refrigerate in an airtight container.

Srv: 30 g | Cal: 35 | Fat: 3.5 g | Sat Fat: 0.5 g | Col: 0 mg | Carb: 3 g | Fib: 1 g | Pro: 0 g

Creamy Dill Sauce

This is the perfect dip to take to work. Bring a container of some raw mixed vegetables, such as carrots, celery, broccoli, and cherry tomatoes, to satisfy the midday munchies. The Creamy Dill Sauce is also a great topping for red potatoes.

MAKES 1 ¼ CUPS (300 ML)

½ cup (120 ml) vegan sour cream
½ cup (120 ml) vegan mayonnaise
3 tablespoons almond milk
1 tablespoon lemon juice
1 tablespoon chopped fresh dill
¼ teaspoon celery salt

In a blender or food processor, combine all of the ingredients. Blend until well combined. Use immediately or refrigerate in an airtight container.

Srv: 37 g | Cal: 80 | Fat: 7 g | Sat Fat: 1 g | Col: 0 mg | Carb: 2 g | Fib: 1 g | Pro: 1 g

Lemon Mayo

Add some tart to your veggie burger or work this mayo into a homemade potato salad. The bright lemon flavor changes a dish in a dash.

MAKES ½ CUP (120 ML)

½ cup (120 ml) vegan mayonnaise
2 tablespoons lemon juice
¼ teaspoon grated lemon zest
1 teaspoon fresh chives, chopped

In a small mixing bowl, combine all of the ingredients. Whisk together until well combined. Use immediately or refrigerate in an airtight container.

Srv: 25 g | Cal: 70 | Fat: 6 g | Sat Fat: 0.5 g | Col: 0 mg | Carb: 1 g | Fib: 0 g | Pro: 1 g

Rich and Creamy Squash Sauce

I like to change it up with the Marinated Tempeh and Veggie Skewers (see page 194 for the recipe) and switch out my homemade barbecue sauce for this dee-lish sauce. Add some jasmine rice, which soaks up the rich sauce, and it's to die for. The kids will love this too, but you may need to leave out the ginger.

MAKES 1½ CUPS (360 ML)

2 cups (280 g) peeled and cubed butternut squash
1 teaspoon salt, plus a pinch
¼ cup (60 ml) unsweetened applesauce
1 tablespoon tahini
1 teaspoon ground ginger

Bring a large pot of water to boil. Add the squash and a pinch of the salt. Reduce the heat to medium and gently boil until tender. Drain well. In a blender or food processor, add the squash, applesauce, tahini, ginger, and the remaining teaspoon of salt. Blend until creamy. Serve warm.

Srv: 61 g | Cal: 40 | Fat: 1.5 g | Sat Fat: 0 g | Col: 0 mg | Carb: 7 g | Fib: 1 g | Pro: 1 g

Savory Gravy

This gravy almost feels like it's bad for you because it's so rich and creamy. One scoop over holiday mashed potatoes or breakfast biscuits and you'll fool any relative. Since it's so good to have on hand for a handful of recipes, I upped the measurements for a bigger serving of gravy. Just freeze half and dig it out for another day.

MAKES 4 CUPS (960 ML)

2 tablespoons grapeseed oil

½ yellow onion, diced

Pinch of salt

1 teaspoon dried sage

1 teaspoon dried thyme

1 teaspoon pepper

4 cups (960 ml) vegetable stock, divided

1 tablespoon balsamic vinegar

½ cup (65 g) unbleached all-purpose flour, or more as needed

½ cup (145 g) nutritional yeast

2 tablespoons white miso paste

Pinch of salt

Chopped fresh parsley for garnish

Heat the oil in a medium saucepan, and add the onion and a pinch of salt. Sauté over medium-high heat until translucent, about 2 minutes. Add the sage, thyme, and pepper and sauté 2 minutes.

Add 2 cups (480 ml) of the stock and the vinegar. Slowly add in the flour and nutritional yeast, stirring constantly with a whisk to prevent lumping. Dissolve the miso in ½ cup (120 ml) of the stock. Add the remaining stock and the stock with the miso to the saucepan while continuing to cook. Reduce heat and simmer until the gravy thickens. Season with a pinch of salt, as needed. Add more flour gradually, if needed, to get the desired thickness. Stir in the parsley just before serving. Serve warm with Skinny Stuffing (see page 180) or Root Veggie Mash (see page 185).

Srv: 75 g | Cal: 60 | Fat: 2 g | Sat Fat: 0 g | Col: 0 mg | Carb: 7 g | Fib: 1 g | Pro: 3 g

Barbecue Sauce

This do-it-yourself barbecue sauce from scratch is a fun summer recipe. It keeps well in an airtight container in the refrigerator and has a special tang that you won't find on any grocery shelf.

MAKES 2 CUPS (480 ML)

1 (15-ounce/430 g) can tomato purée
½ cup (120 ml) water
1 tablespoon apple cider vinegar
1 tablespoon balsamic vinegar
1½ teaspoons Dijon mustard
1½ teaspoons soy sauce
2 tablespoons maple syrup
2 tablespoons molasses
1 teaspoon vegan Worcestershire sauce
1 teaspoon chili powder
Salt and pepper, to taste

In a large saucepan, add the tomato purée and the water. Combine the vinegars in a small bowl and add the mustard. Stir until the mustard dissolves and then pour into the saucepan. Add the remaining ingredients and whisk together over medium heat until well combined. Serve immediately or refrigerate in an airtight container.

Srv: 37 g | Cal: 20 | Fat: 0 g | Sat Fat: 0 g | Col: 0 mg | Carb: 5 g | Fib: 0 g | Pro: 0 g

Sesame Dipping Sauce

A perfect dipping sauce for Vegetable Tempura (see page 217 for the recipe).

(see page 217 for the recipe)

MAKES ⅔ CUP (165 ML)

½ cup (120 ml) tahini
1 tablespoon soy sauce
1 tablespoon mirin
½ teaspoon minced garlic
½ teaspoon minced fresh ginger
Pinch of salt and pepper
¼ cup (60 ml) olive oil

In a blender or food processor, add the tahini, soy sauce, mirin, garlic, ginger, salt, and pepper. Blend until well combined. With the motor running, add the oil in a slow, steady stream until the mixture is creamy. Use immediately or refrigerate in an airtight container.

Srv: 35 g | Cal: 210 | Fat: 20 g | Sat Fat: 3 g | Col: 0 mg |
Carb: 5 g | Fib: 1 g | Pro: 4 g

Avocado and Jicama Salsa

I'm a bit obsessed with whole-wheat tortillas. One of my favorite snacks is to roll up a tortilla with some shredded vegan cheddar and heat over the stovetop on all sides. Serve with this salsa and you'll feel like you just invented electricity.

MAKES 2 CUPS (400 G)

2 medium-size firm avocados, diced into small cubes
1 cup (130 g) peeled and finely diced jicama
1 red bell pepper, seeded and chopped
½ small red onion, finely diced
Freshly squeezed lime juice, to taste
¼ cup (4 g) finely chopped cilantro
Salt, to taste
Red chili powder, to taste (optional)

In a large mixing bowl, combine the avocado, jicama, bell pepper, onion, and lime juice. Toss in the cilantro, and season with the salt and chili powder (if using).

Marinate 10 to 15 minutes in the refrigerator. Serve cold.

Srv: 60 g | Cal: 45 | Fat: 3 g | Sat Fat: 0 g | Col: 0 mg |
Carb: 5 g | Fib: 3 g | Pro: 1 g

Champagne Vinaigrette

A friend once told me she had a few half-full bottles of bubbly leftover from her 30th birthday bash, and instead of chugging it down, she made a dressing with it. Now that's what I call an inventive mixologist! Her story inspired me to mess around with ingredients in the kitchen to develop a vinaigrette with a twist—*sans* the bubbly. This Champagne Vinaigrette dresses up almost any salad, and is also a great dipping sauce for fresh fruit. Cheers!

MAKES ¾ CUP (180 ML)

¼ cup (60 ml) Champagne vinegar
2 tablespoons agave nectar
1 tablespoon freshly squeezed lemon juice
½ teaspoon Dijon mustard
½ cup (120 ml) olive oil
Salt and pepper, to taste

Place the vinegar, agave nectar, lemon juice, and mustard in a blender or food processor and pulse to combine. With the motor running, add the oil in a slow, steady stream. Continue blending until the mixture is creamy. Use immediately or refrigerate in an airtight container.

Srv: 29 g | Cal: 140 | Fat: 14 g | Sat Fat: 2 g | Col: 0 mg | Carb: 5 g | Fib: 0 g | Pro: 0 g

Blue Cheese Dressing

Blue Cheese has always worked against me. I could eat an entire wedge of the stinky cheese in one bite back in my non-vegan days. But, it's not what we Skinny Bitches call "healthy." This dressing is dairy-free and better on the bod.

MAKES 1 ¼ CUPS (300 ML)

⅓ cup (75 ml) vegan mayonnaise
⅓ cup (75 ml) vegan sour cream
¼ cup (60 ml) almond milk
¼ teaspoon apple cider vinegar
½ teaspoon vegan Worcestershire sauce
½ teaspoon dry mustard
¼ teaspoon garlic powder
¼ cup (35 g) plus 1 tablespoon vegan blue cheese
1 tablespoon chopped parsley
Pinch of salt and pepper

In a blender or food processor, add the mayonnaise, sour cream, almond milk, vinegar, Worcestershire sauce, dry mustard, garlic powder, and 1 tablespoon of the blue cheese and blend until creamy and well combined. Transfer to a bowl and stir in the blue cheese, parsley, salt, and pepper. Use immediately or refrigerate in an airtight container.

Srv: 30 g | Cal: 45 | Fat: 4 g | Sat Fat: 0.5 g | Col: 0 mg | Carb: 1 g | Fib: 1 g | Pro: 1 g

White Miso Dressing

When you only have spinach leaves or some lettuce in your fridge, top naked greens with this White Miso dressing for an instant pick-me-up. You can also use it as a dip for a roll-up quesadilla or veggie wrap. Just my style.

MAKES ⅔ CUP (165 ML)

1 (1-inch/2.5 cm) knob fresh ginger, peeled
1 garlic clove
2 tablespoons white miso paste
1 tablespoon agave nectar
2 teaspoons mirin
1 teaspoon soy sauce
½ teaspoon sesame oil
½ cup (120 ml) olive oil

Place the ginger, garlic, miso, agave nectar, mirin, and soy sauce in a blender or food processor and pulse to combine. With the motor running, add both oils in a slow, steady stream. Continue blending until the mixture is creamy. Use immediately or refrigerate in an airtight container.

Srv: 31 g | Cal: 200 | Fat: 19 g | Sat Fat: 2.5 g | Col: 0 mg | Carb: 5 g | Fib: 0 g | Pro: 1 g

---

THE SKINNY: MIRIN
A POPULAR JAPANESE RICE WINE, MIRIN HAS A SWEET TASTE AND LOW ALCOHOL CONTENT, LIKE VERY SWEET SAKE. IT'S MOSTLY USED IN COOKING, THOUGH SOMETIMES DRUNK CEREMONIALLY AT THE BEGINNING OF THE NEW YEAR. IN DISHES, IT COMPLEMENTS AND BALANCES THE FLAVOR OF NATURAL SOY SAUCE, AND IS GREAT FOR SAUTÉING, STIR-FRYING, AND SIMMERING. RING IN THE NEW YEAR EVERY DAY AND SWEETEN ANY JAPANESE-STYLE DISH THAT CALLS FOR IT.

Citrus Mint Vinaigrette

Wowsers! This baby's got a citrusy punch that's perfect for any salad. A summertime favorite, it gets me excited to pass off my son to the babysitter, and enjoy a salad and some much-needed R&R on my front porch. A mom has to have her vices.

MAKES 1 CUP (240 ML)

1 lemon, zested and juiced

1 lime, zested and juiced

1 orange, zested and juiced

2 tablespoons agave nectar

½ cup (45 g) fresh mint leaves, loosely packed

⅓ cup (6 g) cilantro, loosely packed

½ cup (120 ml) olive oil

Salt, to taste

Place the juice and zests of the lemon, lime, orange, the agave nectar, mint leaves, and cilantro in a blender or food processor and pulse to combine. With the motor running, add the oil in a slow, steady stream. Continue blending until the mixture is creamy. Use immediately or refrigerate in an airtight container.

Srv: 31 g | Cal: 130 | Fat: 11 g | Sat Fat: 1.5 g | Col: 0 mg | Carb: 6 g | Fib: 1 g | Pro: 1 g

Raspberry-Walnut Vinaigrette

Whenever I visit a restaurant, raspberry vinaigrette is usually one of the first dressings I look for on the menu. I don't care if I'm ordering a Caesar or Greek salad. It makes me happy, and I'm not sorry. This dressing is inspired by raspberry vinaigrette, but I went and threw everyone for a loop and threw in some walnuts. If you're feeling really wild, use pecans instead.

MAKES 1½ CUPS (360 ML)

1 cup (125 g) fresh raspberries
¼ cup (60 ml) white balsamic vinegar
1 tablespoon evaporated cane sugar
1 lemon, zested and juiced
½ cup (120 ml) olive oil
½ cup (55 g) walnuts, finely chopped

Place the raspberries, vinegar, evaporated cane sugar, and lemon juice and zest into a blender or food processor and pulse to combine. With the motor running, add the oil in a slow, steady stream. Continue blending until the mixture is creamy. Stir in the walnuts. Use immediately or refrigerate in an airtight container.

Srv: 32 g | Cal: 110 | Fat: 11 g | Sat Fat: 1.5 g | Col: 0 mg | Carb: 4 g | Fib: 0 g | Pro: 1 g

Julie's Balsamic Dressing

My friend Julie C. May developed this recipe after an exhausting taste test that went on for months. But it was worth it. It was this fusion that encouraged her to think about starting her own dressing line. She just had to promise me that this recipe was mine, all mine.

MAKES ¾ CUP (180 ML)

½ cup (120 ml) olive oil

¼ cup (60 ml) balsamic vinegar

1 garlic clove, minced

1 teaspoon Dijon mustard

1 teaspoon agave nectar

1 teaspoon strawberry jam

1 teaspoon salt, plus pinch, to taste

¼ teaspoon pepper, plus pinch, to taste

1 teaspoon herbes de Provence

¼ teaspoon dried thyme

½ teaspoon ground mustard

¼ teaspoon ground ginger

¼ teaspoon dried sage

¼ teaspoon ground nutmeg

In a medium bowl, pour in the oil and vinegar. Add the garlic, Dijon mustard, agave nectar, and jam. Whisk in 1 teaspoon of the salt, ¼ teaspoon of the pepper, the herbes de Provence, thyme, mustard, ginger, sage, and nutmeg. Add pinches of salt and pepper, to taste. Cover and chill. Let stand at room temperature for 15 minutes after removing from the refrigerator. Always whisk to blend before serving.

Srv: 26 g | Cal: 140 | Fat: 14 g | Sat Fat: 2 g | Col: 0 mg | Carb: 3 g | Fib: 0 g | Pro: 0 g

Ranch Dressing

Ah, the ever-so-popular ranch dressing. I had to include this for my girlfriend who would have dabbled in veganism years ago had she owned a recipe for a dairy-free ranch dressing. The girl dips everything in it.

MAKES 1½ CUPS (360 ML)

½ cup (120 ml) almond milk
1 tablespoon freshly squeezed lemon juice
½ package (7 ounces/200 g) silken tofu
½ cup (120 ml) almond milk
1 teaspoon minced garlic
1 teaspoon chopped fresh parsley
1 teaspoon chopped fresh dill
1 teaspoon chopped chives
¼ teaspoon onion powder
¼ teaspoon salt
Pinch of pepper

In a blender or food processor, add the almond milk and lemon juice and let set 2 minutes. Add the remaining ingredients and blend until smooth and creamy. Use immediately or refrigerate in an airtight container.

Srv: 34 g | Cal: 15 g | Fat: 0.5 g | Sat Fat: 0 g | Col: 0 mg | Carb: 1 g | Fib: 0 g | Pro: 1 g

Caesar Dressing

A creamy Caesar dressing is just good to have on hand for a quick-fix salad. This recipe also doubles as a dipping sauce for raw or cooked vegetables.

MAKES 1⅓ CUPS (315 ML)

½ cup (115 g) silken tofu
¼ cup (60 ml) freshly squeezed lemon juice
4 garlic cloves, lightly chopped
1 tablespoon Dijon mustard
1 tablespoon vegan Worcestershire sauce
½ teaspoon salt
1 tablespoon capers
½ cup (120 ml) olive oil

In a blender or food processor, add the tofu, lemon juice, garlic, mustard, Worcestershire sauce, salt, and capers and pulse until blended. With the motor running, add the oil in a slow, steady stream until the mixture is smooth and creamy. Use immediately or refrigerate in an airtight container.

Srv: 29 g | Cal: 90 | Fat: 10 g | Sat Fat: 1.5 g | Col: 0 mg | Carb: 1 g | Fib: 0 g | Pro: 1 g

Herbed Croutons

These are a savvy substitute in any recipe that calls for breadcrumbs. Just blend them in a food processor to break into smaller crumbs.

MAKES 3 CUPS (120 G)

¼ cup (60 ml) cold-pressed olive oil

2 teaspoons dried sage

2 teaspoons dried marjoram

2 teaspoons dried thyme

½ teaspoon salt

¼ teaspoon pepper

3 cups (430 g) chopped whole grain bread

Preheat the oven to 250° F (120° C).

In a small bowl, whisk the oil, sage, marjoram, thyme, salt, and pepper together. Place the bread in a large mixing bowl. Slowly drizzle the herb oil over the breadcrumbs, mixing the oil evenly into the bread with your hands. Spread evenly on a baking sheet. Bake 20 minutes, or until dry and crispy, stirring occasionally. Use for Skinny Stuffing (see page 180). You could also use it to top a vegan green bean casserole.

Srv: 79 g | Cal: 190 | Fat: 8 g | Sat Fat: 1 g | Col: 0 mg | Carb: 29 g | Fib: 11 g | Pro: 4 g

THE SKINNY: COLD-PRESSED OLIVE OIL
COLD-PRESSED OIL IS NOT A TYPE, BUT ACTUALLY HOW AN OLIVE IS PROCESSED. PREMIUM OLIVE OIL IS COLD-PRESSED IN THE WINTER, MEANING DESCRIBES THE OLIVE PASTE IS GENTLY WARMED JUST TO ROOM TEMPERATURE TO RETAIN THE DELICATE FLAVORS, ANTIOXIDANTS, AND HEALTH BENEFITS.[110]

Spicy Mango Chutney

I like it hot. Plain and simple, I want something that sets my mouth ablaze. With that said, I have become an avid fan of chutney for the sweet-yet-sour flavor it brings to an Indian dish. This chutney is a fine balance between what I love and what my family can handle. Family cooking is all about compromise.

MAKES 2 CUPS (640 G)

1 tablespoon grapeseed oil
½ jalapeño chile, seeded and diced
⅓ cup (55 g) diced red onion
3 ripe mangoes, peeled, pitted, and diced
1 cup (240 ml) vegetable broth
1 tablespoon agave nectar
½ teaspoon ground cinnamon
¼ teaspoon ground nutmeg

In a large sauté pan, heat the oil over medium heat. Add the jalapeño and onion and sauté 5 minutes, stirring frequently. Add the mangoes, broth, and agave nectar, stirring to combine. Cover, reduce heat to low, and let cook 20 minutes. Stir in the cinnamon and nutmeg. Gently mash the mango with the back of a wooden spoon. Simmer 5 minutes. Use immediately or refrigerate in an airtight container.

Srv: 60 g | Cal: 40 | Fat: 1 g | Sat Fat: 0 g | Col: 0 mg | Carb: 8 g | Fib: 1 g | Pro: 0 g

BITCHWORTHY: Is your chutney done cooking? Place a scoop of cooked chutney on a plate. Take a fork or thin utensil and draw a line through the middle. If the chutney doesn't bleed liquid into the clear line you just drew, it's ready to serve.

SIDES

Masoor Daal (Split Red Lentils)

Adopting their mothers' traditions and reinventing them to tell the story of the modern-day woman, Naveen Kahn and her girlfriends have built a traveling cooking club that hosts fifteen to thirty-person dinner parties as a means of exploring worldly cuisine. They've taken conventional Pakistani cuisine and added a western flair, creating new flavors for time-honored dishes. Here's one of Naveen's favorites:

MAKES 4 SERVINGS

3 cups (720 ml) water

1 cup (170 g) dried red lentils

½ teaspoon salt

¼ teaspoon evaporated cane sugar

1 teaspoon garam masala, divided

½ teaspoon turmeric powder

1 teaspoon fresh ginger, chopped

1 garlic clove, chopped

2 fresh green chiles, chopped

2 dried red chiles

2 tablespoons grapeseed oil

1 small onion, finely diced

2 bay leaves

1 tablespoon chopped fresh cilantro

2 whole pita breads, cut into quarters

In a large saucepan, bring the water to a boil. Add the lentils and cook for about 10 to 15 minutes. Stir in the salt, sugar, ½ teaspoon of the garam masala, and turmeric. Continue to cook uncovered until the lentils are soft. Stir in the ginger, garlic, and both chiles. Remove from heat. Heat oil in a separate large saucepan and add the onion and the remaining garam masala, and sauté until onion is dark yellow to light brown. Pour in the lentils, add the bay leaves and simmer on low for 5 minutes. Remove from heat. Serve hot with rice and garnish with cilantro. Serve with pita bread.

Srv: 268g | Cal: 240 | Fat: 8g | Sat Fat: 0.5g | Col: 0mg | Carb: 31 g | Fib: 8 g | Pro: 13 g

---

THE SKINNY: GARAM MASALA

GARAM MASALA AIN'T YOUR MAMA'S AVERAGE SPICE MIX. A COMMON BLEND OF GROUND SPICES POPULAR IN INDIA AND OTHER SOUTH ASIAN CUISINES, GARAM MASALA IS NOW A COMMERCIALIZED SEASONING AVAILABLE AT MANY MAJOR GROCERY STORES NATIONWIDE. WHILE BLENDS WILL DIFFER FROM BRAND TO BRAND, TYPICAL INGREDIENTS INCLUDE BLACK AND WHITE PEPPERCORNS, CLOVES, BAY LEAVES, BLACK CUMIN, CUMIN SEEDS, CINNAMON, BLACK, BROWN, AND GREEN CARDAMOM, NUTMEG, STAR ANISE, AND CORIANDER SEEDS.

"Buttery" Green Beans with Toasted Almonds

If you ask me, Earth Balance is all that and a bag of chips. Vegans have been able to reinvent so many traditional recipes with the "butter" by our sides. But this one may just take the prize. While it's a satiating side dish, I've been known to serve it as the main course. You won't ever find anyone at my dinner table complaining.

MAKES 4 SERVINGS

1 pound (455 g) green beans
2 tablespoons Earth Balance
1 shallot, minced
1 clove garlic, minced
Salt and pepper, to taste
½ cup (55 g) sliced almonds, toasted

Fill a large pot with water and bring to a boil over high heat. Add the green beans and let cook until barely tender, 3 to 5 minutes. Place the Earth Balance in a large skillet over medium-high heat. Add the shallot and garlic, and sauté for 2 minutes. Drain the green beans and add to the skillet. Add a pinch of salt and pepper and cook 6 to 8 minutes, or until the green beans have cooked through. Stir frequently. Add the almonds and stir to combine.

Srv: 136 g | Cal: 180 | Fat: 11 g | Sat Fat: 2.5 g | Col: 0 mg | Carb: 18 g | Fib: 6 g | Pro: 5 g

Warm Spring Rolls with Spicy Sesame Sauce

My healthy version of traditional spring rolls. These aren't fried so they are a dozen times fresher, but the great flavor is not sacrificed.

SERVES 4

1 (6-ounce/170 g) package cellophane (glass) noodles

¼ cup (60 ml) sesame oil, divided

2 garlic cloves, minced

2 teaspoons minced fresh ginger, divided

¼ cup (60 ml) soy sauce, divided

1 tablespoon hoisin sauce

⅔ cup (60 g) shiitake mushrooms

¼ cup (35 g) thinly sliced carrot

¼ cup (25 g) bean sprouts

2 tablespoons potato starch mixed with 3 tablespoons water

Salt and pepper, to taste

½ teaspoon red pepper flakes

4 rice paper wrappers

Put the noodles in a large bowl and add hot water to cover completely; soak until soft, 20 to 30 minutes. Drain and set aside. In a medium-size frying pan, heat 2 tablespoons of the sesame oil and then add half the minced garlic, 1 teaspoon of the ginger, 2 tablespoons of the soy sauce, and the hoisin sauce and sauté 1 minute. Add the mushrooms, carrot, and beans sprouts and sauté about 3 minutes, or until the vegetables are soft. Add the noodles and toss to combine. Add the potato starch mixture and mix well. Turn off heat. Let cool. Add salt and pepper, to taste.

In a small bowl, whisk together the remaining garlic, soy sauce, sesame oil, ginger, and the red pepper flakes. Lay the spring roll wrappers out and put an even row of filling down the middle. Fold one side over to cover the filling. Fold both edges in to hold in the filling, roll tightly to the other end. Serve fresh with sauce.

Srv: 1 Spring Roll | Cal: 320 | Fat: 15 g | Sat Fat: 2 g | Col: 0 mg | Carb: 41 g | Fib: 2 g | Pro: 8 g

> **BITCHWORTHY:** IF YOU CAN'T FIND POTATO STARCH AT YOUR LOCAL GROCER, YOU CAN SUBSTITUTE WITH CORNSTARCH. POTATO STARCH IS A BIT MILDER AND SWEETER WHICH IS WHY I USE IT IN RECIPES, BUT CORNSTARCH IS A COMPETENT ALTERNATIVE.

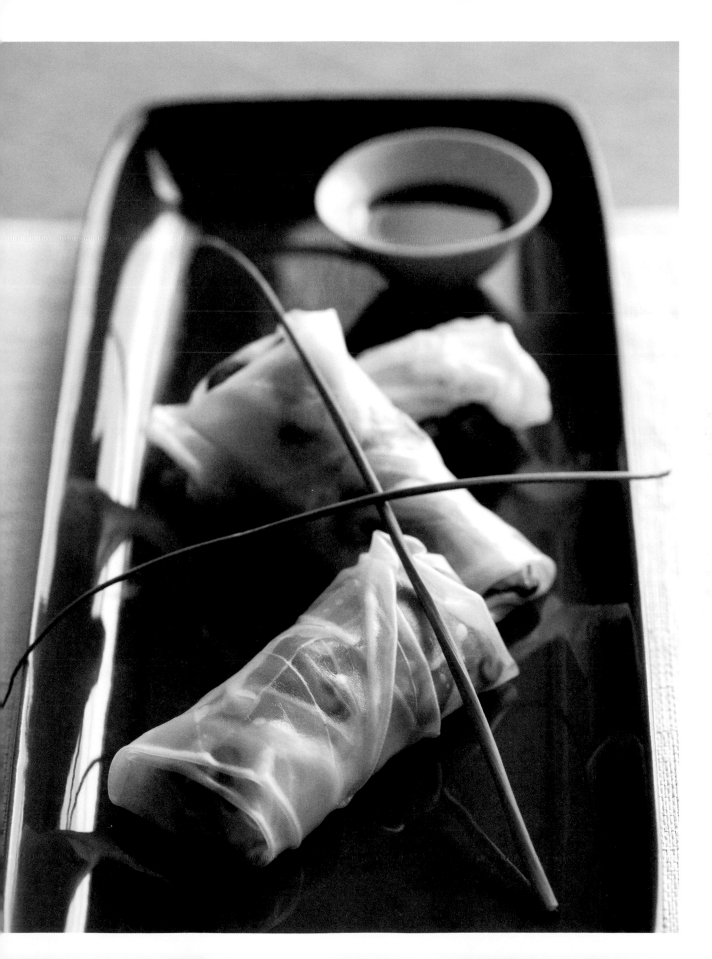

Roasted Carrots & Parsnips with Cumin Vinaigrette

There are so many different culinary influences in this one side dish. The slightly warm flavor of cumin just gives these backyard vegetables a fresh new twist. Pair it with a simple main course, since it is overpowering in flavor and texture.

MAKES 4 SERVINGS

1½ cups (180 g) baby carrots, peeled

1½ cups (200) 2-inch parsnip strips, peeled

¼ cup (60 ml) olive oil, divided

Salt and pepper, to taste

1 teaspoon cumin seeds or ½ teaspoon ground cumin

⅓ cup (75 ml) sherry vinegar

1 garlic clove, chopped

1 tablespoon Dijon mustard

⅓ cup (75 ml) mirin

1 avocado, sliced

2 cups (40 g) arugula

1 tablespoon chopped fresh parsley

Preheat the oven to 375° F (190° C).

In a large mixing bowl, add the carrots, parsnips, 1 tablespoon of the olive oil, and toss to coat the vegetables. Add a pinch of salt and pepper. Place the carrots and parsnips in a large baking pan and bake 20 to 25 minutes, or until soft.

Toast the cumin seeds in a small sauté pan over medium heat until the seeds turn dark brown like espresso beans, 1 to 2 minutes (if using ground cumin, skip the toasting step). In a medium-size bowl, add the toasted cumin seeds, the remaining oil, the vinegar, garlic, mustard, and mirin, for the sauce. Remove the vegetables from the oven and place in a large serving bowl. Add the avocado, arugula, and parsley. Add the sauce and lightly toss together.

Srv: 136 g | Cal: 190 | Fat: 13 g | Sat Fat: 2 g | Col: 0 mg | Carb: 17 g | Fib: 5 g | Pro: 2 g

Sautéed Broccolini with Garlic-Infused Soy Sauce

Broccolini is one of the best veggies you can give your body. It is chock-full of calcium, folate, and iron, with a well-established reputation for reducing the risk of breast and cervical cancer. Eat up, girls.

MAKES 4 SERVINGS

2 ½ cups (100 g) broccolini

1 teaspoon salt

2 tablespoons grapeseed oil, divided

2 garlic cloves, chopped

3 tablespoons soy sauce

2 tablespoons mirin

2 tablespoons sliced almonds

2 teaspoons chopped fresh parsley

Preheat the oven to 350° F (180° C). Bring a large pot of water to a boil. Add the broccolini and salt, and cook about 2 minutes. Turn off heat and let the water cool while making the sauce.

In a medium saucepan, heat 1 tablespoon of the grapeseed oil over medium heat, about 30 seconds. Add the garlic, soy sauce, and mirin, and cook about 1 minute. Pour the sauce into a bowl and set aside. Drain the broccolini and set aside.

Place the almonds on a cookie sheet and roast in the oven 10 to 12 minutes.

In a medium sauté pan, heat the remaining grapeseed oil over medium-high heat and sauté the broccolini about 1 minute. Add the sauce, parsley, and almonds to the pan and mix to coat. Serve warm.

Srv: 175 g | Cal: 150 | Fat: 7 g | Sat Fat: 1 g | Col: 0 mg | Carb: 15 g | Fib: 2 g | Pro: 7 g

THE SKINNY: BROCCOLINI

YOU'RE NOT CRAZY. YOU DID SEE BROCCOLINI IN THIS RECIPE. FOR THOSE NOT FAMILIAR WITH THE LEAFY GREEN, BROCCOLINI IS KNOWN AS THE "BABY BROCCOLI" IN AMERICA. IT IS A CROSS BETWEEN BROCCOLI AND CHINESE KALE WITH LONG, THIN STALKS TOPPED BY DELICATE BUDS. THE BABY IS SWEET AND TENDER WITH A BROCCOLI-LIKE FLAVOR, AND VERY RICH IN VITAMINS A AND C, POTASSIUM, IRON, AND FIBER. [111]

Quinoa-Stuffed Poblano Peppers with Tomatillo Sauce

Quinoa should be stocked in every pantry. High in protein, it is great at absorbing flavor. Hence the reason it works so well in this dish. The quinoa just takes on the spice of the poblano peppers and tomatillo sauce for a distinctively flavored side or main course.

SERVES 4

4 poblano peppers
2 tablespoons grapeseed oil
¼ cup (40 g) chopped onion
2 garlic cloves, minced
½ cup (70 g) corn, fresh or frozen
½ cup (45 g) cubed portobello mushrooms
½ cup (95 g) quinoa, cooked
½ cup (55 g) cubed tofu
Salt and pepper, to taste
10 medium tomatillos, husks removed
¼ cup (60 ml) lime juice
2 tablespoons chopped fresh cilantro
1 avocado, sliced
1 jalapeño pepper, seeded and chopped
3 tablespoons olive oil

If you are using a gas stove, use metal tongs to place the poblano peppers, one at a time, over the direct flame on the stovetop, rotating often until the skin is black and the pepper is soft, about 5 minutes. If you have an electric stove, preheat the oven to broil. Line a cookie sheet with foil and place poblano peppers on the sheet. Place in the broiler, turning several times to evenly roast. Broil for 5 to 10 minutes, or until blackened and soft. Remove from the broiler. Place the peppers in a large plastic zip-top bag and seal closed to keep the steam inside for about 20 minutes. Cool in the refrigerator 15 to 30 minutes. Once cooled, carefully peel off the skin. Halve the peppers lengthwise and remove the stems and seeds. Set aside.

In a medium frying pan, heat the grapeseed oil over medium heat. Add the onion and half of the garlic and sauté 1 minute. Add the corn, mushrooms, and quinoa and sauté 5 minutes. Add the tofu and salt and pepper to taste. Remove from the heat.

Remove the husks from the tomatillos, rinse, and place in a baking dish. Broil, turning over halfway through cooking, until softened and slightly charred, 7 to 10 minutes. Remove from the broiler and set aside.

Change the oven setting to 350° F (180° C). Prepare the sauce by combining the tomatillos, the remaining garlic, the lime juice, cilantro, avocado, jalapeño, olive oil, and a pinch of salt in the blender. Blend until smooth.

Stuff each poblano with the quinoa filling. Place in a large baking dish and bake 15 to 20 minutes. Serve with the tomatillo sauce.

Srv: 366 g | Cal: 340 | Fat: 26 g | Sat Fat: 3 g | Col: 0 mg | Carb: 25 g | Fib: 6 g | Pro: 8 g

THE SKINNY: QUINOA

THIS SNEAKY LITTLE BASTARD IS NOT CONSIDERED A TRUE GRAIN. QUINOA (PRONOUNCED "KEEN-WAH,") IS ACTUALLY A SEED FROM THE GOOSEFOOT PLANT, OR MORE COMMONLY KNOWN AS THE CHENOPODIUM PLANT. QUINOA COMES IN A VARIETY OF DIFFERENT COLORS TO DRESS UP YOUR DISH: IVORY, PINKISH HUES, BROWNS, VIBRANT REDS, AND DEEP BLACK. HOWEVER, NORMALLY THREE KINDS ARE IN ROTATION: THE WHITE OR SWEET QUINOA, THE RED-FRUITED VARIETY, AND BLACK QUINOA. WHEN COOKED, QUINOA IS LIGHT AND FLUFFY LIKE RICE, BUT ITS MILD, NUTTY FLAVOR MAKES IT A TASTY ALTERNATIVE.

Cholay and Āaloo
(Chickpeas and Potatoes)

When I lived in South Beach, one of my closest friends was French-Moroccan. She was a remarkable cook and would open her front door for everyone until her house was full. This dish reminds me of her. She made something very similar, and it never fails to bring me back to her apartment, sitting on big, bright pillows, eating, and drinking mint tea. Hafida, thank you for the great memories.

MAKES 6 SERVINGS

2 cups (480 ml) water

1 bay leaf

1 (15.5-ounce/445 g) can garbanzo beans, drained, divided

2 tablespoons grapeseed oil, divided

1 teaspoon ground coriander

1 teaspoon cumin seeds

1 teaspoon grated fresh ginger

1 teaspoon minced garlic

1 teaspoon ground turmeric

½ cup (80 g) finely chopped onion, plus ½ cup (60 g) sliced onion

3 potatoes, peeled and cubed

2 cups (315 g) chopped tomatoes, divided

Cayenne pepper, to taste

Salt, to taste

¼ cup (4 g) fresh cilantro leaves, divided

In a medium saucepan, bring the water and bay leaf to a boil. Add 1½ cups (360 ml) of the garbanzo beans to the boiling water. Let boil for 5 minutes, then discard the bay leaf and drain the beans, reserving the leftover water. Set aside.

In a skillet, heat 1 tablespoon of the oil over medium heat. Add the coriander, cumin seeds, ginger, and garlic. Cook and stir 15 to 20 seconds, or until lightly browned. Mix in the turmeric. Add the ½ cup (80 g) chopped onion, and cook until tender. Add the potatoes and 1½ cups (240 g) of the tomatoes. Season with the cayenne pepper and the salt. Bring to a boil and cook about 15 minutes.

In a separate large skillet, heat the remaining oil over medium heat and caramelize the sliced onion until tender. Add the remaining garbanzo beans, the remaining tomato, and 2 tablespoons of the cilantro leaves. Add the first bean and tomato mixture and add ¼ cup (60 ml) of the reserved bean water at a time to attain a thick, gravy-like consistency. Continue to cook and stir 5 minutes. Garnish with the remaining cilantro leaves.

Srv: 305 g | Cal: 170 | Fat: 6 g | Sat Fat: 0.5 g | Col: 0 mg | Carb: 28 g | Fib: 5 g | Pro: 6 g

Baigan Aaloo
(Eggplant and Potatoes)

This Indian dish makes such good use of the harmonizing flavors of fresh herbs and ground spices. I always found eggplant a bit plain, but everything in this dish works together to give it some love. Eggplant is also a great source of phytonutrients and fiber.

MAKES 6 SERVINGS

1 teaspoon cumin seeds
1 large onion, puréed
2 to 3 garlic cloves, puréed
1 teaspoon ground turmeric
1 teaspoon red chili powder
Salt, to taste
4 red potatoes, cubed
1 large eggplant, cubed
1½ tablespoons chopped fresh dill
1½ tablespoons chopped fresh cilantro
1 to 2 fresh green chiles, chopped
3 whole pita breads, cut into quarters

In a large sauté pan or pot, add the cumin seeds and heat over medium heat for 1 minute, or until dark brown. Stir with a wooden spoon to ensure the cumin seeds do not overcook. Add the onion and garlic purée, ground turmeric, chili powder, and salt. Cook this over medium heat 5 to 7 minutes, or until it forms a thick paste. Add the potatoes and cook until they are slightly tender, about 5 minutes. Add the eggplant and cook until the eggplant and potatoes are completely tender, about 15 minutes. Right before serving, mix in the dill, cilantro, and green chiles. Serve hot with pita bread.

Srv: 228 g | Cal: 140 | Fat: 0 g | Sat Fat: 0g | Col: 0 mg | Carb: 30 mg | Fib: 6 g | Pro: 4 g

Antioxidants | The Body's Crime Fighters

Chow Down on a Diet of Natural Disease-Fighters

Oxygen can be so two-faced. Sure, it walks around like a superhero taking down bad guys and saving babies, but behind closed cell walls, it's on a deadly mission to produce villains called free radicals that hunt down and damage our proteins, fats, and DNA. What'd we ever do to you, oxygen? Breathe?! Real cool, oxygen. Real cool.

Free radicals could give a shit. They are mad because they were born with only one electron. So rather than grow up and accept it like a big kid, they prey on innocent healthy cells to steal their missing part.

But all is not lost. Say hello to your neighborhood crime fighters—antioxidants. Your body's friendly

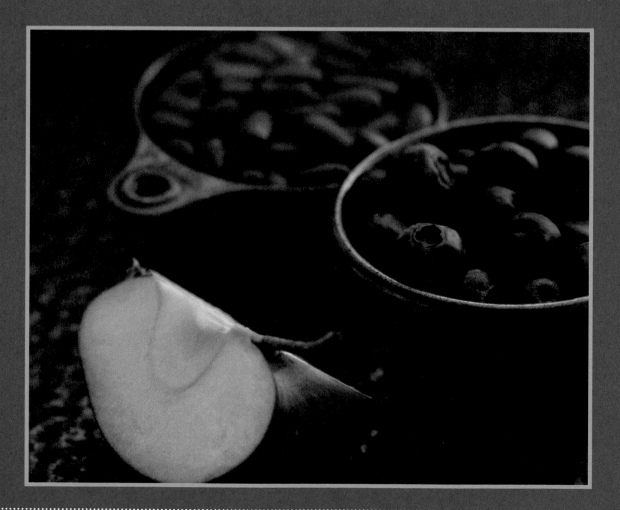

protestors, antioxidants won't take any of this cellular unrest lying down. They take a non-violent approach, surrounding these free radicals, giving them their damn electron, and ending the disruption. Though antioxidants are now short one electron, they do it with pride. It's a small price to pay to protect your cells' freedom.

This system has a happy ending when there are enough antioxidants to fight the good fight. When there are not, the free radicals run around like menaces to society pillaging your healthy cells. The result? The development of chronic diseases like cancer, heart disease, stroke, Alzheimer's disease, rheumatoid arthritis and cataracts. [112] Your body naturally produces a force of nutrients and enzymes that make up antioxidants, but it's not enough. It's up to you to keep the peace.

Luckily, it's simpler than you think. Your body needs food. Not just any food, but healthy, antioxidant-packed foods. Eat up. Your body has diseases to fight.

Rebels with a Cause: The Best Antioxidant-Rich Foods

HERBS AND SPICES: Seasonings like cloves, parsley, coriander, allspice, cinnamon, rosemary, and oregano are among the most antioxidant-rich sources of all.[113]

WHOLE GRAINS: Eat your Wheaties, kiddo. The polyphenols in whole grains have been shown to reduce the risk of coronary heart disease and cancer.[114] Indulge in the healthy stuff like 100 percent whole wheat, brown rice, corn, buckwheat, and oatmeal.

DARK CHOCOLATE: This would have been great to know when I was five. I would have had a valid argument for mom and pops. A small dose of antioxidants derived from chocolate has shown to help lower blood pressure.

BRIGHT FRUITS AND VEGGIES: Go ahead, judge these veggies by their color. Brighter fruits and vegetables pack more useful vitamins and are the antioxidant leaders. Think blueberries (which have the highest concentration by weight), cranberries, strawberries, kale, and carrots. These puppies neutralize the damage caused by free radicals. [115]

NUTS AND SEEDS: Pecans are a hot source for vitamin E, and Brazil nuts are pumped with selenium. Both are powerful antioxidant nutrients. Walnuts carry the most antioxidants by weight.[116]

GREEN TEA: Go figure. There is nothing a cup of green tea can't fix. Green tea is a lofty source of flavonoids, which prevent blood clots, lower LDL ("bad") cholesterol, and reduce inflammation. [117]

RED WINE AND GRAPE JUICE: The grape skins are the silent hero here. In the fermentation of white wine, these skins are removed, hence the reason red wine makes the cut. The skins are bursting with flavonoids and resveratrol, the latter of which is responsible for lowering cholesterol and fighting cancer cells. With grape juice, you want the all-natural, unprocessed stuff or you're just triggering other problems.[118]

> **THE SKINNY: FOUR MOST POWERFUL ANTIOXIDANTS**
> WORK A GOOD AMOUNT OF FOODS HIGH IN BETA-CAROTENE, VITAMIN C, VITAMIN E, AND SELENIUM INTO YOUR DIET, AND TELL FREE RADICALS TO SUCK IT.

Red Potato Salad with Black Niçoise Olives

....

One of my favorite things about potato salad is that you can use any leftover veggies as added ingredients. Though you can use any type of black olives, my son and I are slightly obsessed with black niçoise olives, and we love to throw them into a potato salad for unique flavor. My mother-in-law sends them in bulk from France a few times a year. It's like Christmas every time.

MAKES 4 SERVINGS

2 cups (300 g) large-cubed small red potatoes

½ cup (65 g) peeled, seeded, and cubed cucumber

½ cup (75 g) black niçoise olives (or black olives)

½ cup (75 g) cherry tomatoes, halved

⅓ cup (55 g) diced red onion

2 tablespoons capers

2 tablespoons chopped fresh parsley

⅓ cup (75 ml) Julie's Balsamic Dressing (recipe on page 153)

½ cup (75 g) faux feta, crumbled

Fill a large saucepan with water and bring to a boil. Add the potatoes, return to a boil, reduce the heat, and gently boil until the potatoes are tender but firm, about 10 minutes. Drain and set aside to cool.

In a large mixing bowl, add the cucumber, olives, cherry tomatoes, red onions and capers. Once the potatoes are cool, add to the cucumber mix. Mix in the parsley. Toss all of the ingredients together. Drizzle with Julie's Balsamic Dressing. Sprinkle with feta.

....

Srv: 185 g | Cal: 230 | Fat: 13 g | Sat Fat: 2 g | Col: 0 mg | Carb: 20 g | Fib: 4 g | Pro: 5 g

Barley and Red Bean Bowl

Barley is so underrated in my opinion, both for its health benefits and sweet, nutlike flavor. The Barley and Red Bean Bowl is my updated version of a traditional Southern dish, red beans and rice. When I make this, my son won't leave for school unless I pack leftovers in his lunch.

MAKES 6 SERVINGS

3 cups (720 ml) vegetable broth

1 cup (200 g) uncooked pearl barley

1 (14-ounce/400 g) can red kidney beans, drained and rinsed

½ cup (75 g) chopped yellow bell pepper

½ cup (75 g) chopped green bell pepper

2 tablespoons vegan Worcestershire sauce

¼ cup (60 ml) olive oil

1 garlic clove, minced

2 tablespoons chopped fresh parsley

Salt and pepper, to taste

In a medium saucepan, bring the broth to a boil. Add the barley and stir. Cover tightly and reduce the heat to low. Simmer 35 to 40 minutes, or until barley is tender and the liquid is absorbed.

In a large bowl, combine the beans and bell peppers. In a small bowl, prepare the dressing by whisking together the Worcestershire sauce, oil, garlic, and parsley. Add the barley to the bean mixture and mix well. Drizzle with the dressing and add salt and pepper, to taste.

Srv: 244 g | Cal: 380 | Fat: 3.5 g | Sat Fat: 0 g | Col: 0 mg | Carb: 69 g | Fib: 22 g | Pro: 20 g

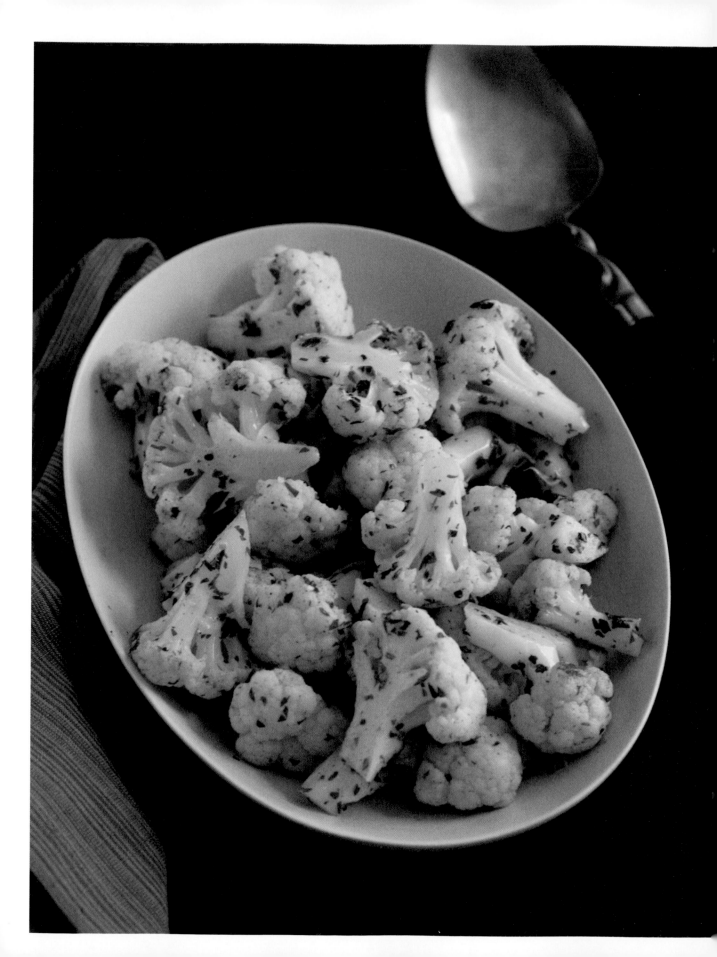

Roasted Curried Cauliflower

Cauliflower can be so underappreciated—but it's really one of the most versatile vegetables. Sometimes I cook it as a side dish, other times I put it in a spinach salad, and every so often, I add it to my morning tofu scramble. Here's a simple recipe that will show you that cauliflower can have a spicy side.

MAKES 4 SERVINGS

¼ cup (60 ml) olive oil

2 garlic cloves, minced

2 teaspoons curry powder

¼ teaspoon chili powder

¼ teaspoon red pepper flakes

Pinch of salt and pepper

1 head cauliflower, cut into florets

1 tablespoon minced fresh parsley

Preheat the oven to 350°F (180°C).

In a large bowl, whisk together the oil, garlic, curry powder, chili powder, red pepper flakes, salt, and pepper. Add the cauliflower and toss until well coated. Pour into a 13 x 9-inch (33 x 23 cm) baking dish and bake until tender, 25 to 30 minutes.

Srv: 158 g | Cal: 80 | Fat: 5 g | Sat Fat: 0 g | Col: 0 mg | Carb: 9 g | Fib: 4 g | Pro: 3 g

THE SKINNY: CAULIFLOWER—THE ANTI-DEPRESSANT

It seems America is down in the dumps. More than 15 million people suffer from depression per year in the United States. But remember: *You are what you eat.* Vegetables like cauliflower work to stabilize blood sugar, which can help in overcoming signs of depression.

Wild Rice Pilaf with Pine Nuts, Currants, and Caramelized Onions

Every household needs a good recipe for rice pilaf. It can be paired with almost any dish and is easily revamped by switching out a few ingredients to complement the main dish. This country recipe just feels inviting.

MAKES 8 SERVINGS

½ cup (80 g) uncooked wild rice

3 cups (720 ml) vegetable broth, divided

½ cup (95 g) uncooked basmati rice

⅓ cup (55 g) dried currants

2 tablespoons grapeseed oil

1 small onion, diced

2 cloves garlic, crushed

⅓ cup (55 g) pine nuts, toasted

2 tablespoons chopped fresh parsley

Rinse the wild rice in a large sieve under cold water and drain. In a medium saucepan, bring 2 cups (480 ml) of the broth to a boil. Add the wild rice and return to a boil. Turn down the heat to low, cover the saucepan, and simmer 40 minutes, or until tender.

Rinse the basmati rice in a large sieve under cold water and drain. In a separate saucepan, bring the remaining 1 cup (240 ml) of the broth to a boil. Add the basmati rice and the currants and return to a boil. Turn down the heat to low, cover the saucepan, and simmer 20 to 25 minutes, or until tender. Remove from the heat and fluff with a fork to release the steam.

Heat the oil in a medium sauté pan over medium-high heat. Add the onion and sauté, stirring frequently, about 5 minutes. Turn down the heat to medium. Add the garlic and sauté. Place in a bowl and set aside.

In a large bowl combine the cooked basmati rice, the wild rice, onions and garlic. Add the pine nuts and parsley and stir. Serve hot.

Srv: 135 g | Cal: 170 | Fat: 6 g | Sat Fat: 0.5 g | Col: 0 mg | Carb: 28 g | Fib: 4 g | Pro: 4 g

BITCHWORTHY: If you stepped away for a primetime reality TV moment and overcooked your rice, you can often "save" it by spreading it out on a cookie sheet in a thin layer to dry out. If you have some space, put it in your freezer immediately to stop the cooking.

Caramelized Eggplant with Red Miso

The minute I tasted this dish, I almost didn't know how to respond. There is truly nothing like it. The eggplant is so tender, and the caramelized miso tastes like a thick, fruity coating. It is close to perfection.

MAKES 6 SERVINGS

1 large eggplant

½ cup (120 ml) grapeseed oil, divided

⅓ cup (90 g) red miso paste

¼ cup (60 ml) mirin

2 tablespoons sake

Pinch of sanshou pepper powder

¼ teaspoon red pepper flakes

1½ tablespoons dark brown sugar

1 tablespoon chopped green onion, both white and light green parts

BITCHWORTHY: SANSHOU PEPPER IS NOT ACTUALLY A PEPPER, IT IS A DRIED BERRY FROM THE PRICKLY ASH TREE. IT IS TYPICALLY SOLD AS A GROUND SPICE FOR ASIAN CUISINE. FLAVOR IS EARTHY AND TANGY WITH A HINT OF LEMON.

Preheat the oven to broil.

Slice the eggplant into 1½-inch (4 cm) disks. Make ½-inch (12 mm) deep cuts on both sides of each disk to make a checker pattern. Heat ¼ cup (60 ml) of the oil in a large frying pan over medium-high heat. Add the eggplant in batches and fry on each side about 1 to 2 minutes, or until soft and brown. Remove from the oil and set on paper towel-lined plate. Continue frying remaining eggplant, adding additional ¼ cup (60 ml) of oil as needed. Set aside.

In a medium-size saucepan, whisk together the miso, mirin, sake, sanshou powder, red pepper flakes, and brown sugar. Cook slowly over low heat stirring often, about 3 minutes. Place the eggplant in baking dish, and coat with sauce. Broil in the oven for 30 seconds to 1 minute. Garnish with green onion.

Srv: 138 g | Cal: 170 | Fat: 9 g | Sat Fat: 1 g | Col: 0 mg | Carb: 17 g | Fib: 6 g | Pro: 1 g

Quinoa Lettuce Cups

Whenever I dine out for Chinese food, I always start with the vegetable lettuce wraps. Most of the time, they fill me up and I have to take my dinner to go. But it never stops me from ordering them. In this version, the quinoa has a delicate texture that pairs well with the crisp lettuce.

MAKES 4 SERVINGS

2 tablespoons sesame oil

⅔ cup (70 g) bean sprouts

½ cup (115 g) peeled and diced jicama

1 cup (185 g) quinoa, cooked

2 tablespoons chopped red onion

½ cup (55 g) green beans, cut in thirds

1 carrot, peeled and julienned

2 teaspoons soy sauce

Salt and pepper, to taste

¼ cup (60 ml) grapeseed oil

½ cup (60 g) rice vermicelli

4 large iceberg or romaine lettuce leaves

2 tablespoons hoisin sauce

2 teaspoons chopped fresh cilantro, for garnish

2 tablespoons thinly sliced green onion, both white and light green parts, for garnish

In a medium-size frying pan, heat sesame oil over medium heat. Add the bean sprouts, jicama, quinoa, onion, green beans, and carrot. Sauté for about 5 minutes. Add the soy sauce, and salt and pepper to taste.

In a medium-size sauce pan, heat the grapeseed oil on medium-high heat. Deep fry the vermicelli until it rises to the surface of the oil and expands in size. Remove from the oil and place on a plate covered with a paper towel. Add salt and pepper, to taste. Spoon the filling into lettuce leaves and top with hoisin sauce and vermicelli. Garnish with the cilantro and green onion.

Srv: 161 g | Cal: 240 | Fat: 9 g | Sat Fat: 9 g | Col: 0 mg | Carb: 35 g | Fib: 6 g | Pro: 8 g

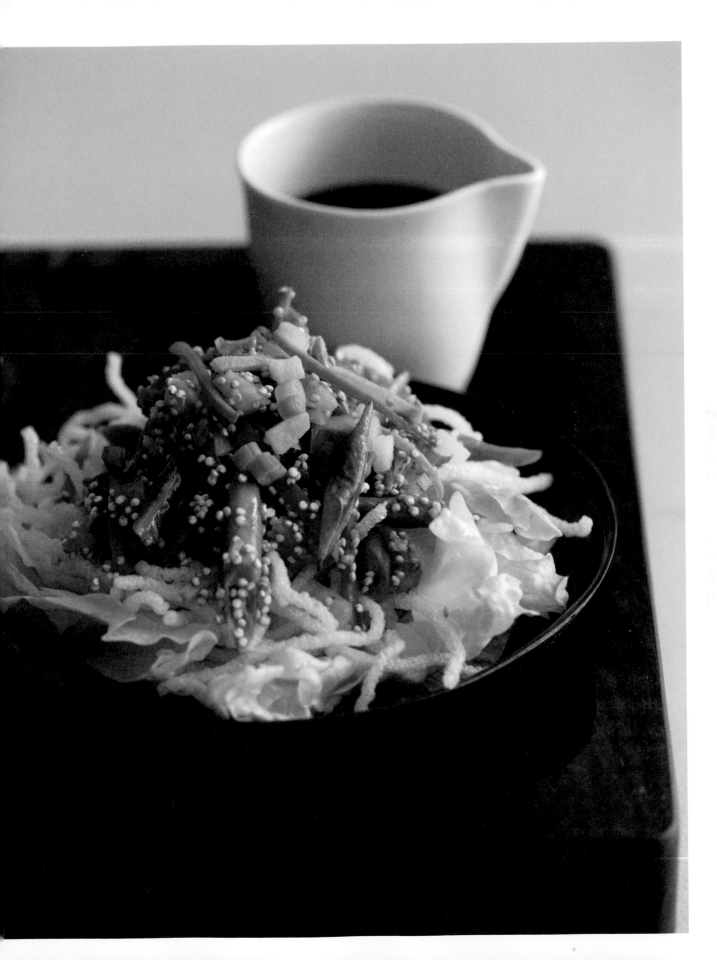

Skinny Stuffing

I am one of those people who makes Thanksgiving dinner a handful of times in late fall, early winter. And a home-cooked holiday dinner would not be complete without a filling vegan stuffing. It adds such a nice touch to Tofurkey and gravy.

MAKES 8 SERVINGS

2 tablespoons grapeseed oil

1 small onion, chopped

2 celery stalks, chopped

Pinch of salt

1 teaspoon dried thyme

1 teaspoon dried marjoram

4 cups (160 g) Herbed Croutons
   (see recipe on page 156)

2 tablespoons chopped fresh parsley

⅓ cup (40 g) walnuts, chopped

1 to 2 cups (240-480 ml) vegetable stock

Preheat the oven to 350° F (180° C).

In a medium saucepan, heat the oil. Sauté the onion and celery with a pinch of salt over medium heat 2 minutes. Add the thyme and marjoram, and sauté another 2 minutes. Set aside to cool slightly. In a large bowl, mix the croutons, vegetable mixture, parsley, and nuts. Add the stock, 1 cup (240 ml) at a time, while mixing with your hands. You want the mixture to be damp but not soaking wet. Press evenly into a 13 x 9-inch (33 x 23 cm) casserole dish. Bake, uncovered, 30 minutes.

Srv: 97 g | Cal: 170 | Fat: 10 g | Sat Fat: 2 g | Col: 0 mg | Carb: 16 g | Fib: 2 g | Pro: 3 g

> ## THE SKINNY: PLAY WITH YOUR STUFFING
> IF YOU WANT TO CHANGE THINGS UP, ADD RAISINS OR CHOPPED APPLES TO STUFFING FOR A DIFFERENT VARIATION. THEY BLEND INTO THE RECIPE WITHOUT A HITCH AND CAN BE ADDED WITHOUT REMOVING ANY OTHER INGREDIENTS.

Mexicali Roasted Vegetables

Roasting is typically a great cooking method for colder months. However, this quick dish uses summer vegetables for warmer times of year, as well. A vegetable medley goes well with any course and holds well for leftovers, too!

MAKES 6 SERVINGS

1 yellow squash, cut into ½-inch (12 mm) strips

1 zucchini squash, cut into ½-inch (12 mm) strips

2 cups (270 g) cauliflower florets

1 cup (70 g) sliced mushrooms

2 tablespoons olive oil

1 teaspoon ground cumin

1 teaspoon dried oregano

Pinch of chili powder

Pinch of ground cinnamon

Salt and pepper, to taste

Preheat the oven to 350° F (180° C).

In a medium-size bowl, toss together the squash, cauliflower, mushrooms, olive oil, cumin, oregano, chili powder, cinnamon, salt, and pepper. Mix well to coat all the vegetables with the oil and spices.

In a large baking pan, spread out the vegetables evenly. Bake 30 minutes, tossing once halfway through cooking.

Srv: 161 g | Cal: 70 | Fat: 5 g | Sat Fat: 0.5 g | Col: 0 mg | Carb: 7 g | Fib: 3 g | Pro: 2g

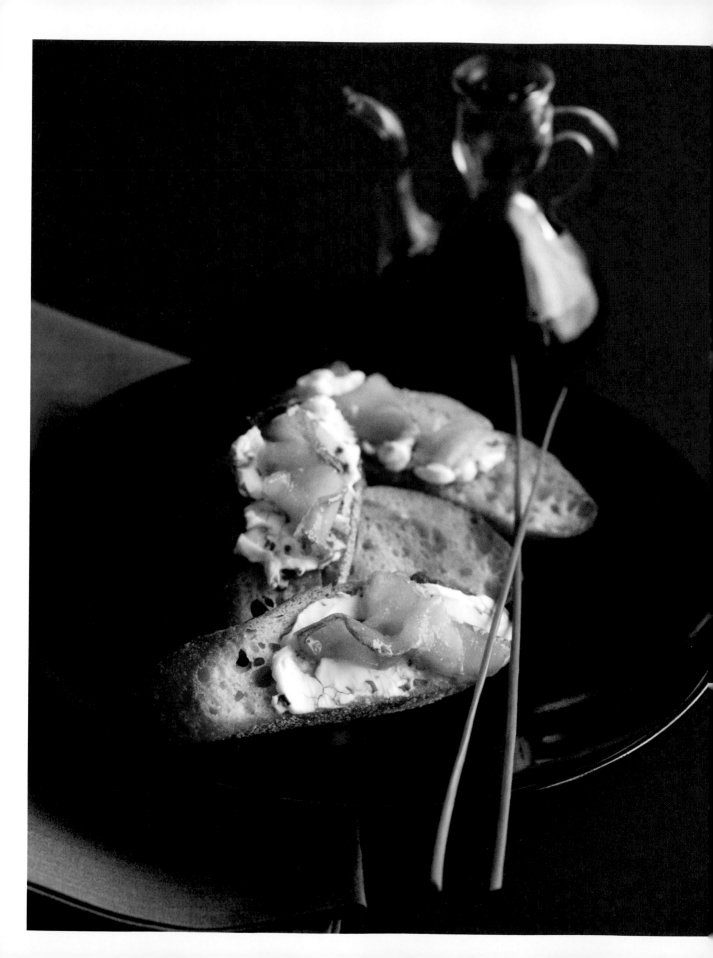

Caramelized Pear and "Cheese" Crostini with Balsamic Reduction

Oh, Caramelized Pear and Cheese Crostinis, you complete me. This fancy tapas dish takes a little patience and some time. After all, caramel can be temperamental and tricky. But the end result is almost too good to be true. This is one I recommend saving for a special occasion or romantic rendezvous, when you want to show off your skills in the kitchen.

MAKES 16 MINI APPETIZERS

1 cup (480 ml) balsamic vinegar

½ cup (100 g) evaporated cane sugar plus 2 tablespoons

¼ cup (60 ml) olive oil

2 teaspoons garlic powder, divided

½ French baguette sliced into ¼-inch (6 mm) slices (about 16 to 20 slices)

4 ripe pears, peeled and cored

3 tablespoons brown rice syrup

½ cup (120 m) hot water

1 (8-ounce/225 g) container of vegan cream cheese

1 tablespoon chives, minced

Preheat the oven to 350° F (180° C).

In a medium saucepan, add the vinegar and 2 tablespoons of the sugar. Cook over medium-low heat until reduced by 75 percent, stirring frequently. You will have a thick syrup.

In a small bowl, whisk together the olive oil and 1 teaspoon of the garlic powder. Lay the bread slices out on a baking sheet. Brush both sides with the olive oil mixture. Bake about 5 minutes, or until the bread is crisp but not too dark. Transfer to a large plate.

Cut the pears into thin slices lengthwise. Heat a large sauté pan and add the remaining ½ cup (100 g) sugar, the brown rice syrup, and the water. Simmer over medium-high heat, stirring occasionally, about 5 minutes. Add the pears and stir with a wooden spoon. Continue to cook another 5 minutes. Remove from the heat and set aside.

In a small bowl, mix the cream cheese with the remaining 1 teaspoon of garlic powder. Spread the garlic cream cheese mixture on each of the crostini slices, top with a pear slice and then drizzle with the balsamic reduction. Add a sprinkle of chives, for garnish. Repeat with each bread slice.

Srv: 2 Crostinis (114 g) | Cal: 130 | Fat: 5 g | Sat Fat: 0 g |
Chol: 0 mg | Carb: 20 g | Fib: 3 g | Pro: 3 g

Boston Baked Beans

This is one of my all-time favorite comfort foods, but the canned version usually contains boatloads of sugar and salt. Try this homemade version for a nice treat. To bulk it up for a meal, throw in some veggie or tofu hotdogs for franks and beans.

MAKES 8 SERVINGS

2 tablespoons grapeseed oil

1 small onion, diced

2 (15-ounce/430 g) cans of navy beans, drained and rinsed

⅔ cup (165 ml) Barbecue Sauce (recipe on page 147)

⅓ cup (55 g) barley malt

Salt and pepper, to taste

5 soy hot dogs, chopped (optional)

Preheat the oven to 350° F (180° C).

In a medium-size saucepan, heat the oil over medium-high heat. Add the onion and sauté until translucent, about 5 minutes. Add the beans and cook 2 minutes. Transfer to a medium-size baking dish and add the barbecue sauce and barley malt. Add salt and pepper, to taste. Mix well, cover with foil, and bake 20 minutes. Stir in the soy hot dogs (if using) and bake an additional 5 minutes.

Srv: 141 g | Cal: 410 | Fat: 3.5 g | Sat Fat: 0 g | Col: 0 mg | Carb: 73 g | Fib: 27 g | Pro: 25 g

Root Veggie Mash

Though mashed potatoes are yummy, they have little nutritional value. This Root Mash is a delicious alternative to traditional mashed potatoes and is high in fiber and vitamins. Add a generous serving of savory gravy (see recipe on page 146) and you've got something to smile about.

MAKES 8 SERVINGS

2 rutabagas, peeled and cubed
2 parsnips, peeled and cut into chunks
1 potato, peeled and cut into chunks
Pinch of salt
3 tablespoons Earth Balance
⅓ cup (75 ml) almond milk
½ teaspoon salt
Pepper, to taste
1 tablespoon chives, for garnish

Bring a large pot of water to a boil. Add the rutabagas, parsnips, potato, and a pinch of salt. Cook the vegetables until tender, about 15 minutes. Drain and place in large bowl. Add the Earth Balance, almond milk, salt, and pepper. Beat with an electric mixer and whip until fluffy. Garnish with the chives. Serve immediately.

Srv: 170 g | Cal: 120 | Fat: 4.5 g | Sat Fat: 1 g | Col: 0 mg | Carb: 18 g | Fib: 4 g | Pro: 2 g

Kale with Peanut Dressing

This is a fresh take on one of my favorite salads at M Café in Venice, California. Kale is the perfect match for a rich peanut dressing. If you have a peanut allergy, you can substitute almond butter.

MAKES 4 SERVINGS

1 large bunch of kale with hard spine removed, chopped

1 carrot, julienned

½ cup (130 g) peanut butter

¼ cup (60 ml) water

2 tablespoons tamari

2 tablespoons rice vinegar

1 tablespoon agave nectar

Red pepper flakes, for garnish

Sesame seeds, for garnish

Fill a steamer basket with the kale and carrot and steam over an inch of boiling water in a medium saucepan until the vegetables soften, about 5 minutes. Remove from the pan and transfer to a large bowl.

In a small bowl whisk together the peanut butter, water, tamari, rice vinegar, and agave nectar. Toss the vegetables with the dressing until well combined. Garnish with red pepper flakes and sesame seeds.

Srv: 135 g | Cal: 250 | Fat: 17 g | Sat Fat: 3.5 g | Col: 0 mg | Carb: 18 g | Fib: 3 g | Pro: 11 g

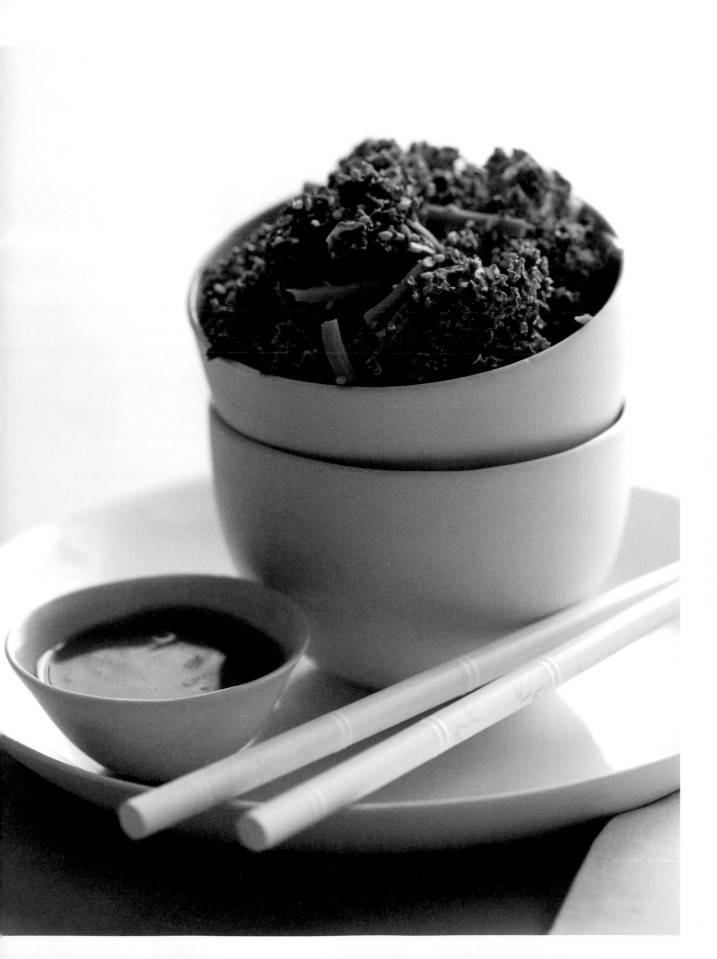

Summer Squash Fritters

Every now and then, you need to indulge. You need to eat something that if you ate it every day, you'd look like the Pillsbury Doughboy. What better way to cheat on your diet than to slip something extra healthy in, as well? These breaded fritters may make you feel guilty on the outside, but on the inside, you're getting your veggies, girl. For an extra treat, drizzle fritters with Citrus Mint Vinaigrette (see recipe on page 151).

MAKES 4 SERVINGS

½ cup (120 ml) grapeseed oil

3 zucchini, cut in half and julienned

2 yellow squash, cut in half and julienned

2 cups (255 g) unbleached all-purpose flour

2 tablespoons garlic powder

½ teaspoon salt, plus a pinch, to taste

¼ teaspoon pepper, plus a pinch, to taste

2 tablespoons light coconut milk

¾ cup (180 ml) sparkling water

Place the oil in a heavy-bottomed skillet over medium-high heat. Monitor the oil heat carefully. If the surface begins to ripple, reduce the heat. Place several layers of paper towels on a baking sheet and set aside.

Place the zucchini and yellow squash in a medium bowl and toss together. Set aside. In another medium bowl, combine the flour, garlic powder, ½ teaspoon of the salt, and ¼ teaspoon of the pepper. Whisk the coconut milk and sparkling water into the flour mixture until smooth. Pick up a small amount of the squash mixture with a pair of tongs and dip it in the batter, shaking off any excess. Carefully place into the hot oil. Allow to cook about 2½ minutes on each side or until golden brown. Drain on paper towels. Season with the remaining salt and pepper, to taste. Serve hot.

Srv: 167 g | Cal: 130 | Fat: 10 g | Sat Fat: 0.5 | Col: 0 mg | Carb: 10 g | Fib: 2 g | Pro: 3 g

Coconut-Saffron Rice

Saffron is used in Mediterranean and Middle Eastern kitchens to add an avant-garde flavor to a dish. This one is no different. It's a perfect partner for the Coconut- and Almond-Crusted Tofu (see recipe on page 203), since one can never have too much coconut in a dish. (Well, if you're me.) I always make extra rice because it's good to have on hand for a last-minute meal or lunch the next day.

see recipe on page 203

MAKES 8 SERVINGS

Pinch of saffron

3 tablespoons light coconut milk, plus ½ cup (120 ml)

2 tablespoons grapeseed oil

8 green cardamom pods

¼-inch (6 mm) cinnamon stick

1½ cups (360 ml) water

½ teaspoon salt

1 cup (215 g) uncooked jasmine rice

In a small pan, quickly toast the pinch of saffron on low heat, about 20 seconds. Remove from the pan and crumble into a small bowl. Warm 3 tablespoons of the coconut milk and pour into a bowl with the saffron. Let sit to infuse.

In a large pot, heat the oil over medium-high heat. Add the cardamom and cinnamon. Stir a few times to infuse the flavor into the oil. Add the water, the remaining ½ cup (120 ml) of the coconut milk, and the salt. Bring to a boil and stir in the rice. Cover and reduce the heat to low. Simmer about 20 minutes. Remove the pan from the heat and stir in the saffron-infused coconut milk. Replace the lid and let sit for 5 minutes. Remove the lid and fluff with a fork.

Srv: 191 g | Cal: 90 | Fat: 3.5 g | Sat Fat: 0 g | Col: 0 mg | Carb: 9 g | Fib: 0 g | Pro: 1 g

---

THE SKINNY: CARDAMOM PODS

THESE LITTLE GREEN PODS USUALLY CONTAIN ABOUT 12 CARDAMOM SEEDS FOR YOUR COOKING PLEASURE. (TEN PODS YIELD ABOUT 1 TEASPOON OF GROUND CARDAMOM SPICE.) THEIR ABILITY TO RETAIN FLAVOR AND AROMA MAKES THEM A SUPERIOR CHOICE TO PRE-GROUND SPICE IN ITS NATIVE COUNTRY OF INDIA. YOU CAN BUY THEM AT SELECT HEALTH FOOD STORES AND ONLINE AT WWW.CARDAMOMSPICE.COM.

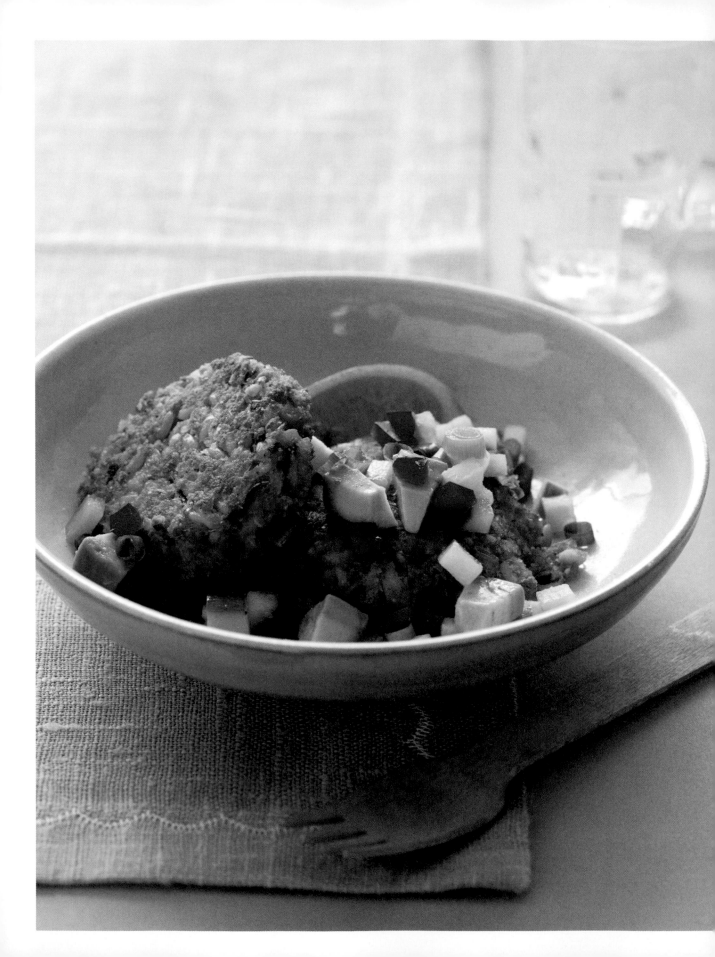

Curried Chickpea Cakes

One of my girlfriends, TV chef personality and cookbook author Candice Kumai, came over to make these with me, and she couldn't make them fast enough. I was eating them one by one as she set them on the plate. They are that good. The Curried Chickpea Cakes can be eaten as a side dish with some mango salsa, or on a bed of butter lettuce with Citrus Mint Vinaigrette (recipe page 151).

MAKES 10 SERVINGS

1 (15-ounce/430 g) can chickpeas, drained and rinsed

⅓ cup (20 g) sliced green onions, both white and light green parts

⅓ cup (75 ml) light coconut milk

2 teaspoons evaporated cane sugar

⅔ cup (75 g) breadcrumbs, plus ¼ cup (30 g) for coating

1 teaspoon curry powder

½ teaspoon ground nutmeg

½ teaspoon ground cumin

⅔ cup (130 g) brown rice, cooked

½ teaspoon salt

¼ cup (60 ml) grapeseed oil or toasted sesame oil, for pan searing

In a large food processor, combine the chickpeas and green onions. Pulse until combined. Transfer to a large mixing bowl. Add the coconut milk, sugar, ⅔ cup (75 g) of the breadcrumbs, curry powder, nutmeg, and cumin. Stir together with a wooden spoon until well combined. Stir in the brown rice and the salt. Mold into 10 mini patties.

In a large sauté pan, heat the oil over medium heat. Add the chickpea cakes to the pan in batches and sauté until there's a nice golden sear on the bottom. Flip and sear the other side as well. Continue with the remaining cakes. Transfer to a paper-towel-lined plate to drain.

Srv: 123 g | Cal: 170 | Fat: 7 g | Sat Fat: 1 g | Col: 0 mg | Carb: 23 g | Fib: 3 g | Pro: 4 g

DINNERS

Marinated Tempeh and Veggie Skewers

I grew rather tired of stomping my feet at cocktail parties when the tray of skewers came around, and I had to look the other way. Chicken and beef. Just peachy. I decided to take matters into my own hands and create my own little version of skewers, perfect as a main course for dinner parties, backyard barbecues, picnics at the beach, and of course, cocktail parties.

MAKES 6 SERVINGS

8 to 12 wooden skewers

2 (6-ounce/170 g) packages tempeh, cut into
   ½-inch (12 mm) cubes

2 zucchini, cut into ½-inch (12 mm) rounds

1 yellow onion, cut into ½-inch (12 mm) pieces

1 cup (150 g) cherry tomatoes

1 recipe Barbecue Sauce, divided
   (see recipe on page 147)

Place the skewers in a shallow dish and cover with water. Allow to soak for at least 30 minutes (this prevents burning). In a large bowl, add the tempeh, zucchini, onion, and tomatoes. Add to the tempeh mixture half of the barbecue sauce. Cover and refrigerate at least 1 hour, or up to 4 hours. Skewer the tempeh and vegetables onto 6 bamboo skewers, alternating ingredients, until all ingredients have been used.

Heat a grill or grill pan on medium-high heat. Place the skewers onto the grill and cook about 12 minutes, turning every 3 minutes. Serve with the remaining barbecue sauce.

Srv: 210 g | Cal: 140 g | Fat: 6 g | Sat Fat: 1.5 g | Col: 0 mg | Carb: 12 g | Fib: 2 g | Pro: 12 g

> ### RECIPE VARIATION: FRUIT SKEWERS
> IN THE HEAT OF SUMMER, STICK SOME FRESH, SEASONAL FRUIT ON THOSE SKEWERS FOR A REFRESHING SNACK. TO MAKE THEM PRETTY, PICK FRUITS WITH BRIGHT, CONTRASTING COLORS AND SCOOP OR CUT INTO DIFFERENT SHAPES BUT SIMILAR SIZES. SLIDE THEM ON EACH SKEWER, ALTERNATING COLORS AND FLAVORS. NOW, THAT'S A FRUIT SALAD.

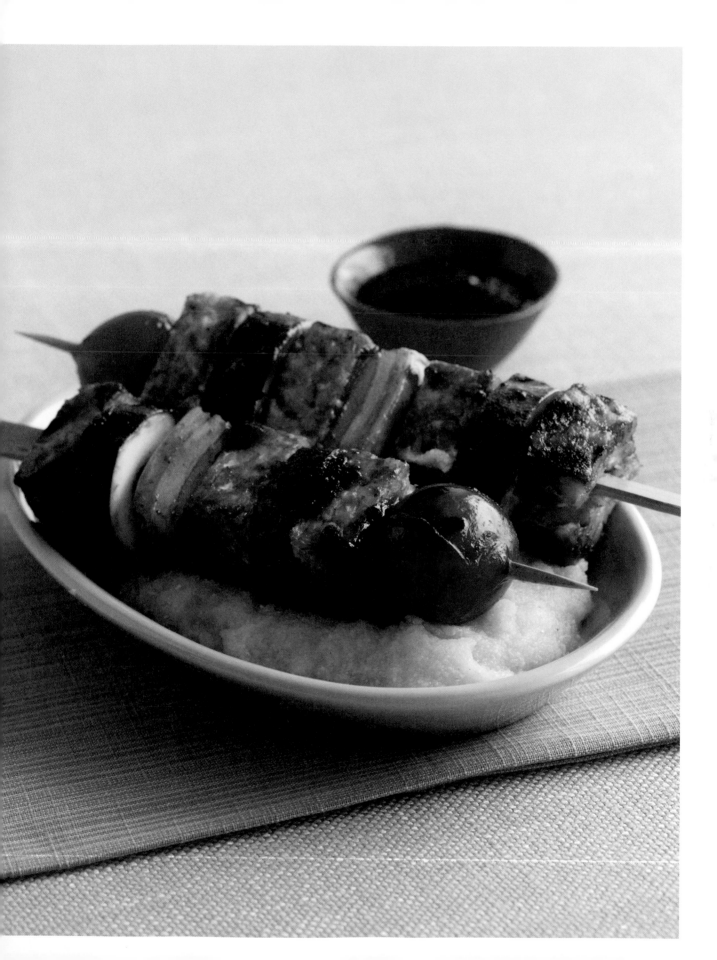

Match Vegan Chicken Marsala

I can feel my mouth watering already. The thick and robust wine sauce reminiscent of chicken marsala is what does it for me. And you don't lose that with this dish.

MAKES 4 SERVINGS

2½ tablespoons grapeseed oil, divided

1 pound (455 g) Match chicken, divided and shaped into 4 patties

Salt and pepper, to taste

¼ cup (30 g) whole wheat flour, plus 1 tablespoon for breading

3 medium portabella mushrooms, sliced ¼ inch (6 mm) thick

¼ cup (15 g) coarsely chopped green onions

1 teaspoon minced garlic

¾ cup (180 ml) vegetable stock

½ cup (120 ml) Marsala wine

In a large nonstick skillet, heat 2 tablespoons of the oil over medium heat. Lightly salt and pepper both sides of the Match chicken patties. Pour ¼ cup (30 g) of the flour in a small bowl, and dredge each of the patties, shaking off any excess. Place all 4 of the patties in the skillet. Brown both sides of the patties about 4 minutes on each side. Transfer to a plate, cover, and keep warm.

Return the same skillet to medium heat and add the remaining oil. Add the mushrooms, green onions, and garlic. Sauté 3 minutes and sprinkle with the remaining flour. Toss until the flour coats the mushroom mixture and cook about 1 more minute. Add the stock and wine and bring to a low simmer, letting it reduce until the alcohol cooks out and it becomes a sauce consistency, about 5 minutes. Adjust the seasoning, if needed, and add the reserved Match chicken medallions. Heat through about 1 minute more. Serve hot.

Srv: 254 g | Cal: 280 | Fat: 13.5 g | Sat Fat: 1 g | Col: 0 mg | Carb: 20 g | Fib: 6 g | Pro: 19 g

BITCHWORTHY: MATCH PREMIUM MEATS

What looks like meat and feels like meat, but isn't *quite* meat? Ooohhh, this could get fun. But, let's keep the star quarterback from high school out of this, honey . . . he's not here to defend himself.

Match **"Guiltless"** premium meat alternatives are just what the vegetarian ordered. A gourmet, vegan match for animal meat, Match premium meat alternatives are changing the way people chow down with tons o' flavor packed into meatless supplements made from natural plant proteins.

With Match, you get the taste, texture, and nutrition that meat lovers want, without the saturated fats, cholesterol, hormones, or antibiotics. The meatless varieties are high in fiber, protein, iron, calcium, and vitamin C, with such natural flavoring ingredients as wheat, soy, and vegetable protein. Choose from a handful of Match products—ground beef, ground chicken, ground pork, crab, breakfast sausage and Italian sausage—and even get recipe suggestions from the culinary masterminds on their website.

Our buddies at Match meats, President Allison Burgess and Executive Chef Freddie Holland, worked with me to create a few of these dee-lish Match meat recipes exclusively for this cookbook. Put a fork in it.

Purchase Match premium meats online at www.matchmeats.com. The website also offers a library of vegan recipes and a list of stores that currently carry their products.

Noodles with Match Vegan Pork and Hot Bean Sauce

After a little discussion with Allison at Match premium meats, we decided this recipe was a must to include in the cookbook. Not only because it is a spicy and super-flavorful stir-fry that will open your sinuses in a matter of seconds, but also because we're suckers for the piggies. They probably see the worst of the goddamn factory farms. The more we indulge in this dish, the less pork we'll consume. It makes a world of difference, bitches. Because the serving size here is bigger, this is best prepared for a family get-together or cozy dinner party.

MAKES 6 TO 8 SERVINGS

1 pound (455 g) dried soba noodles

5 tablespoons (75 ml) Chinese hot bean sauce or Korean gochujang paste

2 teaspoons evaporated cane sugar

3 tablespoons grapeseed oil

¼ cup (25 g) finely chopped fresh ginger

1 pound (455 g) Match vegan pork

½ cup (30 g) sliced green onions

1 teaspoon sesame oil

KIM'S NOTE: BECAUSE OF THE HIGH TEMPERATURE, MAKE SURE THAT ALL OF YOUR INGREDIENTS ARE READY BEFORE YOU BEGIN, AS THE STEPS WILL GO RATHER QUICKLY. USE THIS RECIPE AS A BASE BUT BE BRAVE AND ADD ANY OTHER INGREDIENTS THAT YOUR LITTLE HEART DESIRES. TRY PEANUTS, TOASTED SESAME SEEDS, OR VEGETABLES!

Boil the noodles according to package instructions. Drain well. Lightly oil and set aside. Meanwhile, combine the hot bean sauce and sugar in a small bowl.

Heat a wok or a 12-inch (30.5 cm) nonstick skillet over high heat until a drop of water evaporates immediately. Add the oil while swirling the wok to coat. Add the ginger and stir-fry for 30 seconds. Add the Match vegan pork and stir-fry about 3 minutes, breaking up into bite-size pieces as it browns (cook longer if you like a crispier texture). Add the hot bean sauce mixture and cook, stirring constantly, for 3 minutes. Stir in the noodles, green onions, and sesame oil. Cook about 2 more minutes, or until the noodles are hot. Remove from the heat and serve.

Srv: 210 g | Cal: 480 | Fat: 13.5 g | Sat Fat: 1 g | Col: 0 mg | Carb: 70 g | Fib: 4 g | Pro: 27 g

BITCHWORTHY: IF YOU DON'T LIKE IT HOT AND SPICY, USE LESS OF THE HOT BEAN PASTE. ALSO, TRY TO PURCHASE A HOT BEAN PASTE WITH GARLIC. YOU CAN USUALLY FIND THIS AT GROCERY STORES AS SOYBEAN PASTE WITH CHILI. FOR THOSE WHO NEED SOME MORE SPICE IN THEIR LIFE, TRY KOREAN GOCHUJANG PASTE, AVAILABLE AT SPECIALTY KOREAN MARKETS.

Match Vegan Ginger Chicken Stuffed with Dried Cherries and Fennel

This is my dressed-up version of a typical holiday meal, cranberry chicken. I traded out the cranberries for dried cherries, which gave it a sweeter and less bitter taste. I try to roll out this recipe when we have the in-laws or relatives in town, because it looks like a lot of work went into it. Little do they know, it took about 20 minutes to prepare.

MAKES 4 SERVINGS

1 tablespoon grapeseed oil

½ cup (40 g) finely sliced fennel bulb

¼ cup (40 g) medium-dice onion

¼ cup (45 g) coarsely chopped dried cherries

½ teaspoon orange zest

¼ teaspoon ground ginger or ½ teaspoon fresh, grated

1 clove garlic, minced

1 tablespoon chopped roasted red bell pepper

½ teaspoon soy sauce

1 teaspoon sesame oil, plus 2 tablespoons

½ cup (120 g) panko breadcrumbs

1 tablespoon vegetable stock

1 pound (455 g) Match vegan chicken, divided into 8 (2-ounce/60 g) portions

Salt and pepper, to taste

2 teaspoons sesame seeds

3 tablespoons teriyaki sauce

In a medium saucepan, heat the grapeseed oil over medium heat. Add the fennel and onion and sauté just until tender. Add the cherries, orange zest, ginger, and garlic. Sauté for 1 minute and then remove from the heat. Add the peppers, soy sauce, 1 teaspoon of the sesame oil, the breadcrumbs, and the stock. Combine all of the ingredients to form stuffing and set aside.

Roll each of the 8 Match chicken portions into balls. Place the portions on a sheet of plastic wrap, side-by-side, with 4 inches (10 cm) of space in between each piece. Place a second sheet of plastic wrap on top of the portions and flatten with palm of hand until about ½ inch (12 mm) thick. Divide the stuffing filling into 4 equal portions and place on 4 of the flattened portions, spreading the filling almost to the edge. Place the remaining flattened portions on top of the filling and cover with the previous piece of plastic wrap. Apply pressure around the edge to secure the filling and shape the portions into ovals. Season each stuffed portion with salt and pepper and sprinkle each side with the sesame seeds.

Pour the remaining 2 tablespoons of sesame oil into a sauté pan and cook each stuffed chicken portion over medium-high heat 5 minutes on each side. Glaze with teriyaki sauce and serve.

Srv: 193 g | Cal: 350 | Fat: 17.5 g | Sat Fat: 1.5 g | Col: 0 mg | Carb: 31 g | Fib: 6 g | Pro: 20 g

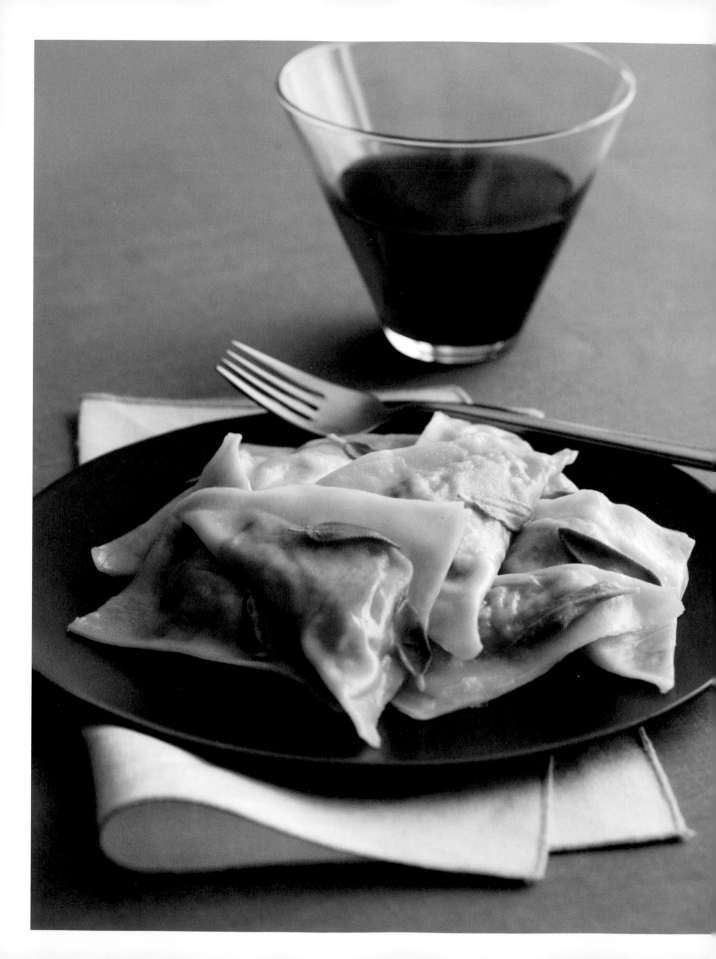

Butternut Squash Ravioli with Sage Sauce

Got a hot date with the guy you met in the elevator? (You little tramp [wink, wink].) Suggest dinner at your place. If you're looking to impress him with more than just your ridiculously good looks and charisma, this gourmet ravioli dish dolled up with a savory sage sauce is your golden ticket to Pleasureville. How do you like me now, stud?

MAKES 24 RAVIOLI

2 cups (455 g) frozen butternut squash, thawed
1½ sticks (170 g) Earth Balance, divided
½ cup (120 g) panko breadcrumbs
½ cup (40 g) vegan Parmesan cheese, grated
Salt and pepper, to taste
1 recipe Wonton Wrappers (see recipe on page 136)
1 bunch fresh sage, stems removed

Place the squash and ½ stick (55 g) of the Earth Balance in a blender or food processor and process until smooth. Transfer to a medium bowl and stir in the breadcrumbs, vegan cheese, and salt and pepper to taste. Place 1 tablespoon of the squash mixture into the center of each wonton wrapper. Brush the edges of the wrapper with water and fold one corner over to create a triangle. Press on edges to seal tightly. Bring a large pot of water to a boil over high heat. Add the ravioli and cook 5 to 6 minutes. Remove with a slotted spoon.

Meanwhile, melt the remaining Earth Balance in a large skillet over medium heat. Add the sage and cook 3 minutes. Remove from the heat and toss with the ravioli before serving.

Srv: 1 Ravioli (48 g) | Cal: 130 | Fat: 7 g | Sat Fat: 3 g | Col: 0 mg | Carb: 13 g | Fib: 0 g | Pro: 3 g

---

THE SKINNY: PANKO BREADCRUMBS VS. WESTERN BREADCRUMBS
FOR HEALTH NUTS, THERE IS NO COMPETITION. JAPANESE PANKO CRUMBS ARE TYPICALLY MADE FROM THE SOFT CENTERS OF BREAD AND ARE MUCH LIGHTER THAN THE PROCESSED WESTERNIZED VERSIONS. PANKO CRUMBS ABSORB LESS GREASE THAN THEIR POPULAR COUNTERPARTS, AND ARE EXCEPTIONALLY LOWER IN SODIUM AND CALORIES. BUT, WHO'S COUNTING? UMM. . . *ME*.

Celery Root and Fennel Gratin

Celery can be a bit bland without a scoop of peanut butter. But, the celery root and fennel gratin requires nothing of the sort. I love to make this comfort food to break up the midweek doldrums, and it's especially good in early fall when both veggies are in season.

MAKES 4 SERVINGS

3 small heads celery root, peeled, thinly sliced, and cut in half

1 cup (240 ml) almond milk, divided

Salt and pepper, to taste

½ cup (115 g) Earth Balance, divided

2 fennel bulbs, thinly sliced

½ yellow onion, thinly sliced

1 cup (120 g) panko breadcrumbs

Preheat the oven to 375° F (190° C).

Cover the bottom of a 13 x 9-inch (33 x 23 cm) baking dish with a layer of the celery root. Pour 2 tablespoons of the milk over the top. Season lightly with salt and pepper, and dot with 2 tablespoons of the Earth Balance. Place a layer of the fennel bulb on top of the celery root. Pour 2 tablespoons of the milk over the top. Season lightly with salt and pepper, and dot with 2 tablespoons of the Earth Balance. Place a layer of the onions on top of the fennel bulb. Pour 2 tablespoons of the milk over the top. Season lightly with salt and pepper, and dot with 2 tablespoons of the Earth Balance. Continue layering until all of the vegetables have been used. Pour the remaining milk over the gratin. Sprinkle with the breadcrumbs and remaining Earth Balance. Cover loosely with foil and bake 30 to 40 minutes, or until the vegetables are tender when pierced with a fork the gratin is bubbling. Remove the cover for the last 10 minutes of baking to allow the breadcrumbs to become golden brown. Serve hot.

Srv: 310 g | Cal: 400 | Fat: 25 g | Sat Fat: 10 g | Col: 0 mg | Carb: 39 g | Fib: 6 g | Pro: 7 g

Coconut- and Almond- Crusted Tofu

I've heard it before: *Tofu could never take the place of meat.* I dare you to crust these babies in coconut and almond, and then come talk to me. For those flirting with meatless recipes a few times a week, add this one to the weekly lineup. Top with Spicy Mango Chutney (see recipe on page 157).

MAKES 4 SERVINGS

1 cup (240 ml) grapeseed oil

1 cup (130 g) unbleached all-purpose flour

1 cup (240 ml) light coconut milk

1 cup (95 g) shredded unsweetened coconut

¼ cup (30 g) almond meal

¼ cup (60 g) panko breadcrumbs

1 (14-ounce/400 g) package extra-firm tofu, drained and cut into finger-size sticks

Salt and pepper, to taste

1 recipe Spicy Mango Chutney (see recipe on page 157)

Place the oil in a deep, heavy-bottomed large saucepan and place over medium heat. Place the flour in a shallow dish, and the milk in another shallow dish. In a third shallow dish, combine the coconut, almond meal, and breadcrumbs. Line a baking sheet with several layers of paper towels ready for draining. Dredge the tofu in flour, shaking off any excess. Dip the tofu in the coconut milk and then in the coconut mixture, shaking off any excess. When the surface of the oil begins to shimmer slightly (this means it's hot enough for frying) carefully drop in the tofu in several small batches, so as not to overcrowd. Fry until golden brown, about 4 minutes. Transfer to baking sheet to drain. Season with salt and pepper, to taste. Serve immediately with the Spicy Mango Chutney.

Srv: 174 g | Cal: 260 | Fat: 21 g | Sat Fat: 4 g | Col: 0 mg | Carb: 7 g | Fib: 2 g | Pro: 10 g

Seitan Sweet Potato and Onion Hash

This sweet potato hash is a wholesome, hearty meal for the entire family. Adults, kids, teenagers, and grandmas love it just the same. I usually save it for an evening when my husband and son can join me in the kitchen. Time spent with them just makes it taste that much better.

MAKES 4 SERVINGS

3 tablespoons grapeseed oil, divided

2 cups (330 g) seitan, chopped

½ sweet onion, diced

1 red bell pepper, seeded and diced

1 sweet potato, peeled and diced

Salt and pepper, to taste

½ cup (120 ml) vegetable broth

1 tablespoon minced fresh rosemary

1 tablespoon minced fresh thyme

1 tablespoon thinly sliced chives

Place 1 tablespoon of the oil in a large skillet over medium-high heat. Add the seitan to the skillet and sauté 5 minutes, stirring frequently. Remove the seitan from the pan and set aside. Add the remaining oil to the skillet. Add the onion and bell pepper and sauté 3 to 5 minutes, or until soft. Add the sweet potato and season with salt and pepper. Sauté 5 minutes, or until nearly tender. Reduce the heat to medium and stir in the broth. Return the seitan to the skillet. Stir in the rosemary, thyme, and chives, and cook for an additional 5 minutes, or until the potatoes are tender. Serve hot.

Srv: 224 g | Cal: 150 | Fat: 7 g | Sat Fat: 1 g | Col: 0 mg | Carb: 12 g | Fib: 3 g | Pro: 10 g

THE SKINNY: HOW TO CUT A BELL PEPPER

To start, rinse the pepper well and using a paring knife, cut around the stem to remove it. To chop or dice, cut the pepper in half lengthwise. Clean out the core and seeds. Place the pepper flat on a cutting surface, skin facing down. Then, chop into desired size.

Tofu Tortas

This is classic grub to ring in Cinco de Mayo. I fill these stacked tacos to the brim with the traditional Mexican works—beans, sweet corn, onions, tomatoes, and cheese (vegan, of course)—and add a few gourmet tricks of my own. I have two other recipes for tacos in the cookbook, because I decided they all deserved the ink.

MAKES 4 SERVINGS

1 (8-ounce/225 g) package silken tofu, drained and crumbled

½ cup (70 g) sweet corn, fresh or frozen

½ package vegan taco seasoning (or make your own with recipe below)

2 tablespoons vegetable broth

Salt and pepper, to taste

2 medium tomatoes, diced

¼ cup (40 g) diced onions

2 tablespoons minced fresh cilantro

2 teaspoons minced garlic

1 tablespoon freshly squeezed lime juice

1 (14.5-ounce/415 g) can refried beans

12 prepared fried corn tortillas (packaged flat for tostados)

1 cup (90 g) shredded vegan Cheddar cheese

Combine the tofu, corn, taco seasoning, and broth in a medium bowl and toss together. Season with salt and pepper and set aside. In a small bowl, combine the tomatoes, onions, cilantro, garlic, and lime juice. Gently toss together and set aside. Warm the beans in a saucepan over medium-low heat.

To prepare the tortas, spread the beans on four of the tortillas and then top each with another corn tortilla. Spoon the tofu mixture evenly onto the top tortilla and then top with the vegan cheese. Place a third tortilla on top and then spoon the tomato mixture on top. Serve immediately.

Srv: 422 g | Cal: 480 | Fat: 20 g | Sat Fat: 1.5 g | Col: 0 mg | Carb: 64 g | Fib: 11 g | Pro: 15 g

MAKE YOUR OWN TACO SEASONING

Sure, you can buy a packet of taco seasoning at the store, but isn't it better to know what the hell is in it? Unless you like hydrochloric acid in your tacos, make your own with a few simple steps:

In a small bowl, combine all of the ingredients. Store the mixture in a dry, cool place in an airtight container.

¼ cup (40 g) onion powder

1 tablespoon garlic powder

2 tablespoons chili powder

2 teaspoons dried paprika

2 teaspoons dried red pepper flakes, crushed

1½ teaspoons dried oregano

½ teaspoon dried marjoram

1 teaspoon ground cumin

1 tablespoon salt

½ teaspoon pepper

Cayenne pepper, to taste

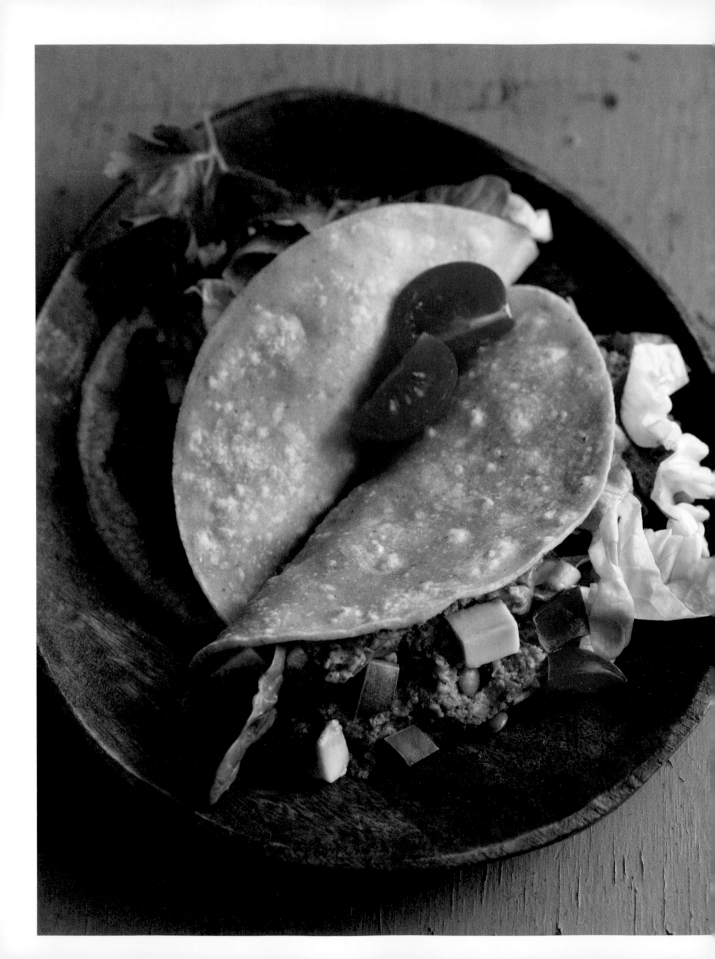

Lentil Tacos with Fresh Salsa

I didn't think it was possible to enjoy a taco without meat. But it is more than possible. The lentils in this dish have a texture and consistency that is similar to meat, and it tastes so much fresher! Lentils are an excellent source of protein, folate, fiber, iron, and tryptophan. It's a bite-size meal rolled up in your hand.

MAKES 4 SERVINGS

4 cups (960 ml) water
1 cup (170 g) dried green lentils
2 tablespoons diced white onion
2 tablespoons olive oil
Salt and pepper, to taste
2 tablespoons tomato paste
⅔ cup (100 g) diced cherry tomatoes
2 tablespoons finely sliced red onion
1 garlic clove, minced
¼ teaspoon diced jalapeño pepper
3 teaspoons lime or lemon juice
1 tablespoon finely chopped fresh cilantro
4 corn tortillas
1 avocado, sliced
½ cup (50 g) shredded lettuce

In a medium saucepan, bring the water to a boil over high heat. Add the lentils and white onion. Return to a boil and then reduce heat, cover, and simmer until soft, 30 to 40 minutes. Drain any remaining water, and place half of the lentils in a blender or food processor. Process while drizzling 1 tablespoon of the oil into the mixture. Season with salt and pepper, to taste. Add the tomato paste and purée until combined. Put the lentil mixture in a medium bowl and stir in the remaining lentils.

In a separate medium bowl, mix together the cherry tomatoes, red onion, garlic, jalapeño, lime or lemon juice, cilantro, and remaining oil, for the salsa. Add salt and pepper, to taste.

Heat a small frying pan over low heat, and quickly warm the corn tortillas on each side. Spread the lentil mixture on top. Top with the sliced avocado, salsa, and lettuce.

Srv: 169 g | Cal: 330 | Fat: 12 g | Sat Fat: 1 g | Col: 0 mg | Carb: 47 g | Fib: 11 g | Pro: 13 g

RECIPE VARIATION: MINI TACO BOWLS

Out with the fried taco shells, and in with the baked mini-taco bowls. This is a stylish and simple variation on the Lentil Taco recipe. Rather than warm the tortillas in a frying pan as instructed, get creative. Hint: You will need a muffin tin or muffin cups.

1: Heat the oven to 350° F (180° C).

2: Quickly microwave the tortillas on high for 30 seconds.

3: Press the middle of each tortilla into a muffin cup, leaving an opening in the center for filling. It should look like a cup.

4: Bake 10 minutes.

5: Now, follow the recipe for Lentil Tacos, filling each center with the lentil mixture and topping with avocado, salsa, and lettuce.

Tempeh Tomato and Tarragon Stew

There's no better way to feel at home than with a hearty tomato stew. Maybe it's those Campbell's soup commercials that pull at my heartstrings, but it reminds me of kids coming in from the snow and curling up next to the fire with mom and a steamy bowl of stew. This meatless version is packed with protein from tempeh soaked in a thick vegan gravy.

MAKES 4 SERVINGS

2 tablespoons grapeseed oil, divided

2 cups (165 g) 1-inch tempeh cubes

Salt and pepper, to taste

1 small yellow onion, diced

1 carrot, peeled and diced

1 celery stalk, diced

3 tablespoons minced tarragon

1 tablespoon minced thyme

1 bunch Swiss chard, thinly sliced

2½ cups (395 g) diced tomatoes

1 (15-ounce/430 g) can garbanzo beans, drained and rinsed

2 cups (480 ml) red wine

4 cups (960 ml) vegetable broth

Place 1 tablespoon of the oil into a large saucepan over medium-high heat. Add the tempeh and sauté 5 minutes, or until golden brown. Season with salt and pepper to taste. Remove the tempeh from the saucepan and set aside. Add the remaining oil, the onion, carrot, and celery to the saucepan. Sauté 3 to 4 minutes, or until the onions become slightly translucent. Season with salt and pepper. Add the tarragon and thyme, and sauté for 1 additional minute. Stir in the Swiss chard and cook 6 minutes. Return the tempeh to the saucepan. Stir in the tomatoes and garbanzo beans. Add the wine and simmer 8 minutes, or until liquid has reduced by half. Pour in the broth and bring to a boil over high heat. Reduce the heat to low and cover. Simmer 20 minutes longer. Serve hot.

Srv: 309 g | Cal: 220 | Fat: 9 g | Sat Fat: 1.5 g | Col: 0 mg | Carb: 19 g | Fib: 3 g | Pro: 11 g

> ### BITCHWORTHY: SWISS CHARD
> ONE CUP OF THIS COLORFUL LEAFY GREEN HAS ONLY THIRTY-FIVE CALORIES. WHILE THAT MIGHT SOUND PEACHY, GET THIS: YOU ALSO GET 110 PERCENT OF THE DAILY VALUE FOR VITAMIN A FROM BETA-CAROTENE, AND NINETEEN THOUSAND MCG OF *LUTEIN* AND *ZEAXANTHIN*. THE LATTER ARE POTENT CAROTENOIDS THAT ARE MAKING HEADLINES FOR PROTECTING THE EYES AND SHIELDING AGAINST VISION PROBLEMS. HOW'S THAT FOR EASY ON THE EYES?[119]

Veggie Calzones

Calzones make me feel young again. They bring me back to the days of heating up a Hot Pocket from the freezer or, as I reached my teens, begging the pizza guy to make one last delivery before they closed for the night. Filled with yellow squash, zucchini, onion, mushrooms, and bell pepper, these Veggie Calzones are a healthy take on every man's and woman's favorite guilty pleasure.

MAKES 6 SERVINGS

1/4 cup (60 ml) grapeseed oil, plus 1 tablespoon

1/3 cup (40 g) yellow onion, thinly sliced

1/2 zucchini, thinly sliced

1/2 yellow squash, thinly sliced

1 cup (70 g) button mushrooms, thinly sliced

Salt and pepper, to taste

2 cloves garlic, minced

1 tablespoon dried oregano

1 teaspoon dried thyme

1/3 cup (75 ml) red wine

1 cup (160 g) tomatoes, crushed

1 recipe Vegan Pizza Dough, divided into 4 equal balls (see page 234)

1 cup (90 g) shredded vegan mozzarella

Preheat the oven to 375° F (190° C).

Pour 1/4 cup (60 ml) of the oil into a large sauté pan over medium heat. Sauté the onion, zucchini, yellow squash, mushrooms and bell pepper 5 to 7 minutes, or until vegetables are just tender. Season with salt and pepper and set aside.

Place the remaining oil in a saucepan over medium heat. Add the garlic, oregano, and thyme and cook 2 minutes, stirring frequently. Add the wine and bring the mixture to a boil. Let the mixture cook at a slow boil until the liquid has reduced by half. Stir in the tomatoes and season with salt and pepper. Reduce the heat and partially cover the pan. Simmer about 20 minutes, stirring occasionally. Remove from the heat and stir in the vegetable mixture.

To assemble the pizzas, roll out the balls of dough to 8-inch (20 cm) circles. Place a quarter of the vegetable mixture on half of each crust. Top with the vegan mozzarella. Fold the dough over to cover the filling and pinch the edges to seal. Cut a small incision on the top of each calzone to allow steam to escape. Place each calzone onto a sheet pan lined with parchment paper, and dot the tops with remaining oil.

Bake 15 to 20 minutes, or until the crust is golden brown. Serve hot.

Serv: 1 Calzone | Cal: 590 | Fat: 20 g | Sat Fat: 2 g | Col: 0 mg | Carb. 09 g | Fib. 0 g | Pro. 13 g

Vegan Cassoulet

My husband has lived most of his life in a French kitchen. Whether he was helping his mother crush herbes de Provence for a comfort meal, or preparing dishes for a crowded French restaurant in Los Angeles, he has always appreciated a rich, slow-cooked *cassoulet* (French for casserole). Now that he has to cater to a veggie, it requires some creativity.

MAKES 6 SERVINGS

2 tablespoons grapeseed oil

6 tablespoons (85 g) Earth Balance, divided

2 leeks, thinly sliced

1 carrot, peeled and diced

1 stalk celery, diced

1 garlic clove, minced

3 tablespoons minced fresh tarragon

1 tablespoon minced fresh thyme

1 tablespoon thinly sliced chives

1 bay leaf

3 (15-ounce/430 g) cans white cannellini beans, rinsed and drained

1 cup (240 ml) vegetable broth

½ cup (120 g) panko breadcrumbs, divided

Salt and pepper, to taste

Preheat the oven to 350° F (180° C).

Place the oil and 2 tablespoons of the Earth Balance in a large pot over medium-high heat. Add the leeks, carrot, celery, and garlic, and cook 5 minutes, stirring occasionally. Add the tarragon, thyme, chives, and bay leaf, and cook another 4 minutes. Stir in the beans, broth, and ¼ cup (60 g) of the breadcrumbs. Reduce the heat and simmer 20 minutes, stirring occasionally. Season with salt and pepper.

Meanwhile, melt the remaining Earth Balance and toss with the remaining breadcrumbs in a small bowl until well combined. Set aside. Pour the bean mixture into a 13 x 9-inch (33 x 23 cm) baking dish, removing and discarding the bay leaf. Cover loosely with foil and bake about 25 minutes, or until bubbly. Remove the foil and sprinkle with the breadcrumb mixture. Continue cooking until the top is golden. Serve hot.

Srv: 330 g | Cal: 370 | Fat: 18 g | Sat Fat: 5 g | Col: 0 mg | Carb: 41 g | Fib: 10 g | Pro: 12 g

Veggie Pot Pies

Pot pies require a bit more handiwork in the kitchen. Which is why I can't think of a better time to get the kids involved. Give them the chance to pour the creamy batter into the pie tray and poke holes in the dough once baked. I even let my son roll the dough balls while I'm stirring on the stovetop. He feels like a hotshot being able to handle a big man's job and, in the end, eats those veggies like they're candy.

MAKES 6 SERVINGS

2 tablespoons grapeseed oil
½ yellow onion, diced
1 medium carrot, peeled and sliced
1 stalk celery, diced
Salt and pepper, to taste
1 cup (90 g) broccoli florets
1 cup (135 g) frozen sweet peas, thawed
½ stick (55 g) Earth Balance
¼ cup (30 g) unbleached all-purpose flour
2 cups (480 ml) almond milk
½ recipe vegan pie dough (see page 267)

Preheat the oven to 375° F (190° C).

Place the oil in a large skillet over medium-high heat. Add the onion, carrot, and celery and cook about 5 minutes. Season with salt and pepper. Add the broccoli and peas and cook 5 to 6 minutes. Remove from heat and set aside.

In a medium saucepan, melt the Earth Balance over medium heat. Sprinkle in the flour and whisk together until smooth. Cook 3 minutes, whisking constantly. Whisk in the milk, stirring constantly to prevent lumps. Simmer about 3 minutes, or until slightly thickened. Add the vegetable mixture to the sauce, stirring to combine. When done, spoon the mixture into a 9-inch (23 x 3.5 cm) glass pie pan. Roll the dough out a little bit larger than the pie pan and place on the top of the pie. Trim off the excess dough, crimping edges. Using a knife or fork, poke a couple of holes into the top of the pie to allow the steam to escape. Bake 35 to 40 minutes, or until the crust is golden brown. Serve hot.

Srv: 284 g | Cal: 545 | Fat: 42 g | Sat Fat: 14.5 |
Col: 0 mg | Carb: 35 g | Fib: 4.5 g | Pro: 6.5 g

Squash Linguini with Vegan Cream Sauce

Surprisingly, spaghetti squash can be used in place of pasta. The texture is a little crunchier than pasta but when paired with this light cream sauce, you won't believe you're eating a vegetable. It's a great occasional replacement for pasta, high in nutrients and low in calories.

MAKES 4 SERVINGS

1 medium-size spaghetti squash

1 tablespoon grapeseed oil

1 clove garlic, minced

½ yellow onion, diced

2 ripe tomatoes, diced

Salt and pepper, to taste

2 cups (480 ml) almond milk, divided

1 tablespoon cornstarch

4 cups (120 g) loosely packed baby spinach

½ cup (40 g) vegan Parmesan cheese

Preheat the oven to 350° F (180° C).

Pierce the shell of the squash several times with a small, sharp knife and place in a baking dish. Cook 1 hour. When done, remove from the oven and cut in half lengthwise. Scoop out the seeds from the shell. Be particularly careful to avoid burns when opening the squash, as the heat is trapped inside. Separate the strands with a fork, from a stem-to-stem direction. Do not cut too small or you will have short strands. Set spaghetti strands aside.

Place the oil in a large skillet over medium-high heat. Add the garlic and onion and sauté 5 minutes. Add the tomatoes and sauté 3 minutes. Season with salt and pepper. Add 1¾ cups (420 ml) of the milk to the garlic mixture. In a small bowl, whisk the remaining milk and cornstarch together. Pour into the skillet, stirring to combine. Let simmer for 5 minutes. Stir in the spinach and cook just until the spinach begins to wilt. Gently stir in 2 cups of the spaghetti squash strands and cook 3 minutes. Add the vegan cheese, for garnish.

Srv: 291 g | Cal: 160 | Fat: 7 g | Sat Fat: 0 g | Col: 0 mg | Carb: 19 g | Fib: 2 g | Pro: 8 g

Tofu Saag with Brown Rice

This recipe follows the traditional style of *saag paneer* (a northern Indian curry made with a spiced spinach purèe) but swaps out cheese for tofu.

MAKES 6 SERVINGS

2 tablespoons grapeseed oil

1 yellow onion, chopped

¼ cup (60 ml) vegetable broth

1 pound (455 g) spinach, stems removed

⅓ cup (75 ml) light coconut milk

2 teaspoons ground cumin

1 teaspoon ground cinnamon

1 (8-ounce/225 g) package firm tofu, cut into ½-inch (12 mm) cubes

Salt and pepper, to taste

2 cups (390 g) freshly cooked brown rice

Place the oil in a large skillet over medium-high heat. Add the onion and sauté until translucent, about 6 minutes. Add the broth and spinach, cooking until the spinach begins to wilt. Add the coconut milk, cumin, and cinnamon, and simmer 7 minutes. Pour the mixture into a blender or the work bowl of a food processor and process until smooth. Transfer the mixture to a large saucepan and place over medium heat. Gently add the tofu and cook 8 minutes. Season with salt and pepper. Serve over hot brown rice.

Srv: 291 g | Cal: 190 | Fat: 7 g | Sat Fat: 1 g | Col: 0 mg | Carb: 25 g | Fib: 6 g | Pro: 7 g

---

THE SKINNY: HOW TO COOK BROWN RICE

EVER NOTICE THAT BROWN RICE IS A BIT TRICKIER AND MORE TIME CONSUMING TO COOK THAN SAY, WHITE RICE? YOU WEREN'T TRIPPIN'. WITH BROWN RICE, THE NUTRITIOUS BRAN LAYER COVERING THE GRAIN IS STILL INTACT, CAUSING THE LONGER COOKING TIME. I USED TO HATE TO COOK BROWN RICE BECAUSE IT ALWAYS CAME OUT TOO TOUGH, BUT WHEN I MET MY HUSBAND HE TAUGHT ME HOW TO COOK RICE A SLIGHTLY DIFFERENT WAY. IT'S REALLY EASY, AND I NEVER MESS IT UP ANYMORE. (DIRECTIONS AT RIGHT)

AS FOR BUYING BROWN RICE, THERE ARE A FEW DIFFERENT VARIETIES TO CHOOSE FROM. THERE'S SHORT GRAIN, WHICH HAS A SLIGHTLY SWEETER TASTE BUT TENDS TO BE STICKIER THAN THE OTHERS. MEDIUM GRAIN IS MOIST AND TENDER, AND LONG GRAIN IS MORE CHEWY AND FIRM WITH A NUTTY FLAVOR. IF YOU HAVE THE TIME BEFORE STARTING TO COOK, SOAK YOUR BROWN RICE FOR THIRTY MINUTES TO ONE HOUR TO SOFTEN THE BRAN LAYER AND TO ENHANCE THE NUTRITIONAL VALUE.

1. [IF SOAKING] IN A LARGE BOWL, POUR IN 1 CUP OF BROWN RICE AND FILL THE BOWL HALF-FULL WITH WATER. LET SIT FOR THIRTY MINUTES TO ONE HOUR. STRAIN THE RICE AND RINSE.

2. BRING A LARGE POT OF WATER AND 1 TEASPOON OF SALT TO A BOIL.

3. ONCE BOILING, ADD IN 1 CUP OF BROWN RICE AND REDUCE HEAT TO MEDIUM-HIGH.

4. SIMMER FOR ABOUT 45 MINUTES, STIRRING FREQUENTLY. TEST THE RICE TO SEE IF IT IS DONE.

5. DRAIN THE RICE AND RETURN TO THE POT.

6. FLUFF THE RICE WITH A FORK.

Lentil Seitan Sloppy Joes

Sloppy Joes were my guilty little pleasure in my grade-school cafeteria days. They were so messy and yummy. This version is healthy and made with whole foods instead of fattening meat. But just because you're not a kid anymore doesn't mean you can't be messy. Use this dish to help you remember what it feels like.

MAKES 6 SERVINGS

1½ cups (360 ml) water
½ cup (170 g) dried lentils, rinsed
1 tablespoon safflower oil
⅓ cup (55 g) minced onion
1 red bell pepper, finely chopped
1 large carrot, peeled and finely chopped
½ cup (85 g) seitan, finely chopped
1 (6-ounce/170 g) can tomato paste
1 tablespoon Dijon mustard
1 tablespoon balsamic vinegar
2 tablespoons tamari
¼ cup (60 ml) ketchup
6 whole wheat burger buns
1 avocado, sliced
Pickles, sliced for garnish

In a medium saucepan, heat the water over high heat. Once the water is boiling, add the lentils. Reduce the heat, cover, and simmer until tender, about 30 minutes. In a separate sauté pan, heat the oil over medium-high heat and sauté the onion, bell pepper, and carrot until tender, about 10 minutes. Add in the seitan. Add the tomato paste to a blender or the work bowl of a food processor and purée.

In a medium bowl, mix together the tomato purée, mustard, vinegar, tamari, and ketchup. Then add the tomato mixture to the pan of vegetables. Combine thoroughly. Drain the lentils, but save the cooking liquid in case it's needed. Add the lentils to the pan of vegetables and simmer 5 minutes. If the mixture seems dry, add some of the lentil cooking liquid.

Toast the burger buns. Serve the mixture on the toasted buns with avocado slices and sliced pickles.

Srv: 1 sandwich (221 g) | Cal: 230 | Fat: 5 g | Sat Fat: 0.5 g | Col: 0 mg | Carb: 40 g | Fib: 7 g | Pro: 10 g

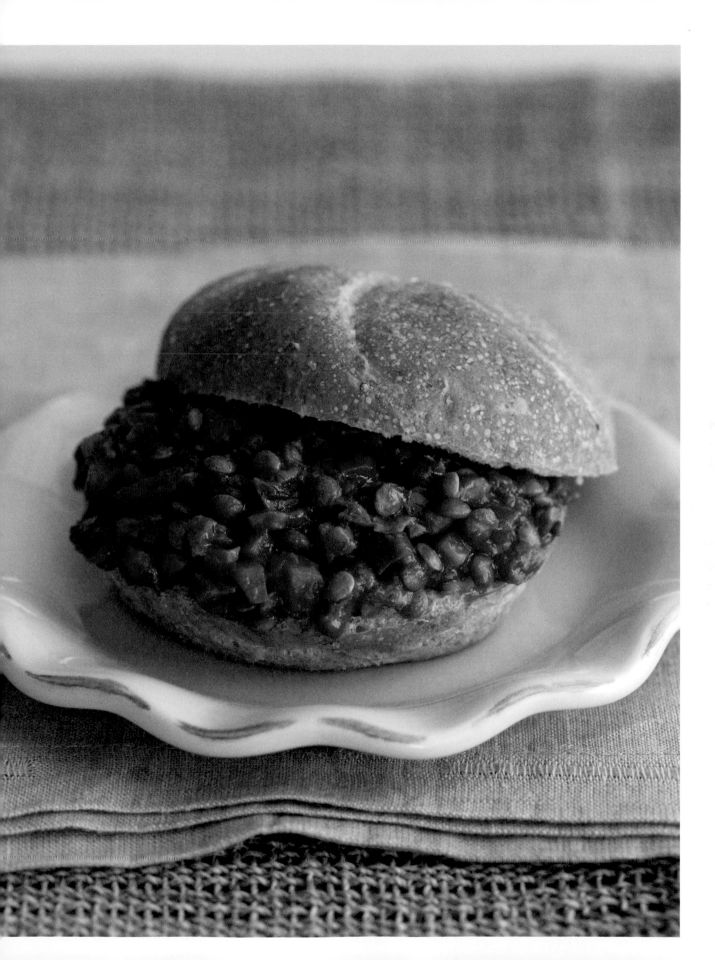

Potato Samosas

Samosas remind me of a steamy pot pie, but more convenient. Creamy, savory filling in a bubbly breaded pastry. Yum. These Indian street snacks are traditionally vegetarian, so they easily find their way into the vegan kitchen.

MAKES 14 MINI SAMOSAS

½ pound (225 g) red potatoes, peeled and quartered

Salt and pepper, to taste

¼ cup (60 ml) hot vegetable broth

½ cup (70 g) frozen peas, thawed

½ cup (70 g) diced frozen carrots, thawed

2 tablespoons curry powder

1 tablespoon ground cumin

1 teaspoon ground cinnamon

½ teaspoon ground nutmeg

1 recipe Vegan Pizza Dough (see page 234), divided into 12 equal balls

¼ cup (55 g) Earth Balance, melted

Preheat the oven to 375° F (190° C).

Bring a large pot of water to a boil, add the potatoes, and return to a boil. Reduce the heat, and gently simmer until soft, about 20 minutes. Drain, transfer to a large bowl and mash slightly with a fork. Season with salt and pepper. Add the broth, peas, carrots, curry, cumin, cinnamon, and nutmeg to bowl. Stir together to combine.

Roll out the dough to 2-inch (5 cm) squares. Place 1½ tablespoons of the potato mixture in the center of each square, folding the four corners up to the center and pinching the edges to seal. Brush the surface of a baking sheet lightly with melted Earth Balance. Place samosas on baking sheet and bake 20 minutes, or until the samosas are light golden brown. Serve hot.

Srv: 1 Samosa (93 g) | Cal: 230 | Fat: 6 g | Sat Fat: 1.5 g | Col: 0 mg | Carb: 39 g | Fib: 3 g | Pro: 5 g

Vegetable Tempura with Daikon Radish Soy Dip

I love eating out at the Asian restaurant down the street from my house, and ordering veggie tempura. But what I love even more is that an amazing chef friend of mine taught me how to make it at home! It's a fun, crunchy snack or main dish, and the original dip is a fiery take on miso dip. This is definitely one dish that will make you look like a pro in the kitchen!

MAKES 4 SERVINGS

⅔ cup (80 g) potato starch

3 tablespoons unbleached all-purpose flour

2 tablespoons baking soda

2 cups (480 ml) ice water

¼ cup (60 ml) soy sauce

¼ cup (60 ml) mirin

1 teaspoon evaporated cane sugar

2 tablespoons grated daikon radish

3 cups (720 ml) peanut oil

1 cup (80 g) 1-inch (2.5 cm) eggplant sticks

1 cup (100 g) okra

8 shiso leaves

1 cup (40 g) broccolini or broccoli

1 cup (140 g) ½-inch (12 mm) peeled kabocha squash or sweet potato strips

1 cup (225 g) firm tofu, drained and cut into 1-inch (2.5 cm) slices

In a medium bowl, blend the potato starch, flour, and baking soda. Add the ice water and slowly whisk until the batter is smooth, for the tempura.

In a separate medium bowl, whisk together the soy sauce, mirin, sugar, and daikon radish. Set aside.

Heat the oil in a large sauté pan or amall pot over medium-high heat. Dip the eggplant, okra, shiso leaves, broccolini, kabocha squash, and tofu in the tempura batter, one at a time. Deep-fry the vegetables and tofu, one at a time, until crispy. Remove each vegetable from the pan and place on paper towels to drain. Serve with Daikon Radish Soy Dip.

Srv: 208 g | Cal: 200 | Fat: 10 g | Sat Fat: 1.5 g | Col: 0 mg | Carb: 19 g | Fib: 4 g | Pro: 9 g

BITCHWORTHY: DAIKON RADISH

MEANING "REALLY BIG RADISH," A DAIKON RADISH LOOKS PRETTY MUCH LIKE A WHITE CARROT WITH SUPERSIZE ROOTS. IT IS SPICIER THAN YOUR AVERAGE RADISH, AND THE PICK OF THE LITTER FOR STIR-FRIES, SALADS, SOUPS, AND PICKLING. BUT YOU CAN EAT IT RAW, TOO! THOUGH THEY ARE HARVESTED IN TEXAS AND CALIFORNIA IN THE U.S., YOU CAN FIND THEM YEAR-ROUND AT FARMERS' MARKETS, LOCAL GROCERY STORES, OR ASIAN SPECIALTY MARKETS. THEY ALSO HAVE A SPECIAL SUPERPOWER: THE CHINESE RADISHES ARE POTENT ANTIOXIDANTS THAT HELP SLOW DOWN THE AGING PROCESS. DAIKONS ALSO CONTAIN DIGESTIVE ENZYMES THAT HAVE AWESOME DETOXIFYING POWERS.[120]

Asian Persuasion

Traditional Japanese Soy Sauces

One can only imagine the culture shock soy sauce experienced when East met West. In Japan, it was a symbol of tradition and authentic food enhancers. But when it landed on friendly soil, we adopted it as mini Chinese take-out packets in our kitchen drawers, and sodium-overkill bottles on the refrigerator shelves. The Chinese believe putting it on white rice is a sign of poverty, but we'll drench our rice in the brown sauce any given Sunday. For rich or for poor.

The point is, the soy sauce we've grown to love is not the stuff soybeans are made of. The cheaper brands on the market today are unfermented, synthesized from hydrolyzed vegetable protein (HVP), and then mixed with hydrochloric acid. Additives like caramel coloring, preservatives, salt, corn syrup, and other refined sugars are added to the HVP to get it all nice and tasty. Not so tasty anymore, eh?[121]

Here's the thing: Soy sauce can be a pretty healthful flavoring. Key words being *can be*. You just need to be conscious of what you are buying, and read your labels. I may sound like a goddamn broken record, but ask me if I care. It's important to follow some rules to protect your health.

Below are a few things you should look for when deciphering the back of the bottle. I also touch on two Japanese soy varieties that should be in every vegan pantry. Now, without further ado, let's put some oodle in that noodle.

THE SKINNY: SOY SAUCE ALTERNATIVES

BRAGG LIQUID AMINOS: BRAGGS IS MY RIGHT-HAND MAN IN THE KITCHEN. IT IS ALL-NATURAL, FLAVORFUL, VERSATILE, AND CONTAINS MUCH LESS SODIUM THAN COMMERCIAL SOY SAUCE. BRAGGS IS ALSO CERTIFIED NON-GMO AND CONTAINS MORE THAN SIXTEEN AMINO ACIDS! YOU CAN ALSO MAKE YOUR OWN SOY SAUCE WITH THREE SIMPLE INGREDIENTS.

DO-IT-YOURSELF SOY SAUCE

INGREDIENTS:
8 ounces (240 ml) molasses
3 ounces (90 ml) balsamic vinegar
Sugar, to taste

COMBINE ALL INGREDIENTS. STIR AND REFRIGERATE IN AN AIRTIGHT CONTAINER.

Soy Sauce: Label Language

NATURAL FERMENTATION: The highest quality sauces are made from naturally fermented or brewed soy products.

HVP: Make sure they do not contain HVP or any artificial coloring (i.e. caramel coloring).

LITE: You don't need to blow your whole daily sodium allotment on one spoonful of soy sauce. Keep in mind that the recommended daily allowance is fifteen hundred to twenty-four hundred milligrams a day. One tablespoon of the "regular" stuff has a whopping one-thousand milligrams![122] The "lite" version weighs in at five hundred.

NON-GMO AND ORGANIC: It is very important that you buy soy sauces made from non-genetically modified soybeans. Buying organic soy sauce is a safe way to avoid this. Genetically modified soybeans contain a harmful gene that make them resistant to pesticides and herbicides. In the U.S., 92 percent of soybeans are genetically modified, so be a smart skinny bitch and double-check the bottle. I cannot stress this enough.[123]

> **BITCHWORTHY:** According to the Food Channel, more people have soy sauce in their kitchen than tea, coffee, milk, or salsa.[124]

Traditional Japanese Soy Sauces: Tamari and Shoyu

Your rice bowl may never be the same. Many are discovering the value of natural, authentic, and traditional soy sauces that are brewed with traditional methods and used by the Japanese for thousands of years. Tamari and shoyu both cater to different styles of cooking and deliver the subtle flavor of quality soy sauce. *Tanoshimu.*

TAMARI: Made from whole soybeans, sea salt, and water, tamari was once a thick brown sauce considered more of a rare delicacy reserved for special occasions. Once the Japanese learned how to brew tamari as a liquid soy sauce, it became a common household product that is thought to bring strong, dominant flavor to a dish. Tamari is wheat-free for those with gluten allergies, and used in food processing for longer cooking, such as soups, stews, marinades, and baking.

SHOYU: Japanese for "soy sauce made of soybeans," shoyu is a mixture of wheat, sea salt, and soybeans. Shoyu is used to bring a soft, deep flavor to dishes, thus enhancing their flavor rather than overpowering it. Because shoyu is slowly fermented, it is easily broken down by our bodies and requires less energy to digest. It is more of an all-purpose cooking and condiment sauce best used in everyday dishes like stir-fries and or sauces, or for seasoning veggies.

Eggless Brown Fried Rice with Garlic Infusion

There's just something special about opening up your fridge and seeing that magical Chinese take-out carton filled with last night's brown rice leftovers. Somebody tell me why it tastes so much better the next day! Problem is, it can be like crap sitting in your stomach. This is a healthier, eggless rendition with a delicious garlic kick that you can prepare at home.

MAKES 4 SERVINGS

2 tablespoons sesame oil

2 garlic cloves, chopped

1 cup (225 g) firm tofu, drained and crumbled

2 tablespoons chopped green onions, both white and light green parts

1 cup (140 g) corn, fresh or frozen

1 cup (100 g) snow peas, cut in half

1 teaspoon minced fresh ginger

2 cups (390 g) cooked brown rice

Salt and pepper, to taste

2 teaspoons sesame seeds, for garnish

Teriyaki sauce or shoyu, for serving

Heat the oil in a frying pan over medium-high heat. Add the garlic and tofu and sauté for 30 seconds. Add the green onions, corn, snow peas, and ginger. Stir-fry about 3 minutes. Add the rice and cook an additional 5 minutes. Season with salt and pepper, to taste. Garnish with the sesame seeds. Serve with teriyaki sauce or shoyu.

Srv: 241 g | Cal: 250 | Fat: 8 g | Sat Fat: 1 g | Col: 0mg | Carb: 35 g | Fib: 5 g | Pro: 10 g

Kale Ravioli with Chili Vinaigrette

Raviolis were my favorite when I was a kid. It was like opening a birthday present every time, since I didn't know what was inside. I like to call this my "grown up" version of ravioli because wrapped inside is one of the best leafy vegetables you can put in your body—both taste-wise and health-wise. The chili vinaigrette dipping sauce just seals the deal.

MAKES 24 (4 SERVINGS)

4 tablespoons (60 ml) grapeseed oil, divided

2 cups (135 g) finely chopped kale, with hard spine removed

1 cup (90 g) chopped Napa cabbage

1 garlic clove, minced

2 tablespoons chopped green onions

1 tablespoon chopped shallots

1 teaspoon chopped fresh ginger

Salt and pepper, to taste

½ cup (100 g) brown rice, cooked

1 recipe Wonton Wrappers (see recipe on page 136)

½ cup (120 ml) water

¼ cup (60 ml) soy sauce

½ teaspoon red pepper flakes

½ jalapeño pepper, seeded and chopped

1½ teaspoons freshly squeezed lemon juice

1½ teaspoons rice wine vinegar

2 tablespoons olive oil

Heat 2 tablespoons of the grapeseed oil in a large sauté pan over medium heat. Add the kale, cabbage, garlic, green onionns, shallots, ginger, and salt and pepper. Cook about 5 minutes. Transfer the vegetable mixture to a medium bowl and mix in the cooked brown rice. Place a spoonful of the mixture in the center of each wonton wrapper. Fold and seal the wrapper in half over the filling. Fold the edges with moistened fingers. Heat the remaining grapeseed oil in a large frying pan over medium-high heat. Cook the ravioli in batches on both sides until light brown, 1 to 2 minutes. Add the water, cover, and steam until the water has evaporated, 2 to 4 minutes (check frequently). Repeat until all of the wontons have been cooked. Serve hot.

To make the dipping sauce, whisk together the soy sauce, red pepper flakes, jalapeño, lemon juice, vinegar, and olive oil in a small bowl.

Srv: 1 Ravioli (22 g) | Cal: 45 | Fat: 1 g | Sat Fat: 0 g | Col: 0 mg | Carb: 8 g | Fib: 0 g | Pro: 1 g

Sauce Srv: 49 g | Cal: 150 | Fat: 14 g | Sat Fat: 2 g | Col: 0 mg | Carb: 4 g | Fib: 0 g | Pro: 2 g

THE SKINNY: HAIL TO KALE

ARE YOU FAMILIAR WITH THE ORAC SCALE? YOU SHOULD BE. THIS IS A RANKING SYSTEM THAT CATEGORIZES VEGETABLES BY THEIR ANTIOXIDANT CAPACITY, AND HOW WELL THEIR CONCENTRATION OF ANTIOXIDANTS AND PHYTONUTRIENTS WORKS TOGETHER TO FIGHT FREE RADICALS. KALE RANKS NUMBER ONE, WITH AN ORAC RATING OF 1770. THE RUNNER UP: SPINACH WITH AN ORAC VALUE OF 1260.

Spicy Vegetable Curry

I am a sucker for Thai food delivery. Nothing beats having an exotic meal cooked for you and brought to your doorstep. Except making it yourself [Smile].

MAKES 4 SERVINGS

3 tablespoons grapeseed oil

1 teaspoon chopped fresh ginger

2 garlic cloves, chopped

1 (14-ounce/400 g) can light coconut milk

1½ cups (360 ml) water

2 teaspoons red curry paste

2 tablespoons white miso paste

1 teaspoon curry powder

½ cup (35 g) mushroom halves

½ cup (55 g) 1-inch (2.5 cm) zucchini slices, halved

½ cup (40 g) cubed eggplant

⅓ cup (35 g) sliced okra

Salt and pepper, to taste

1 teaspoon lime juice for garnish

½ teaspoon red pepper flakes for garnish

Freshly cooked jasmine rice, for serving

Heat 1 tablespoon of the oil in a large saucepan over medium heat. Add the ginger and garlic and sauté for 30 seconds. Add the coconut milk, water, red curry paste, miso, and curry powder, and stir until well combined. Reduce the heat to low and simmer 20 minutes.

In a medium frying pan, heat the remaining oil over medium-high heat. Add the mushrooms, zucchini, eggplant, and okra and sauté about 3 minutes. Add salt and pepper, to taste. Add the vegetable mixture to the curry sauce and cook an additional 10 minutes. Garnish with the lime juice and red pepper flakes. Serve with jasmine rice.

Srv: 255 g | Cal: 130 | Fat: 11 g | Sat Fat: 1 g | Col: 0 mg | Carb: 7 g | Fib: 7 g | Pro: 12 g

---

THE SKINNY: HOW TO COOK JASMINE RICE

Cooking rice can be a bit sticky (no pun intended). But, breathe a huge sigh of relief. Jasmine is much faster to cook than brown rice. Remember: 1 cup dry rice = 2 cups cooked.

1: Rinse the rice under cold water to improve the flavor and color and prevent it from getting too sticky.

2: Pour 2 cups (480 ml) water in a medium saucepan. Bring the water to a soft boil.

3: Add 1 cup Jasmine rice to the saucepan, along with 2 teaspoons salt. Stir 10 seconds, and then reduce the heat to medium heat. Cover tightly.

4: Cook 15 minutes and taste to make sure the rice is ready.

When done, serve with Spicy Vegetable Curry.

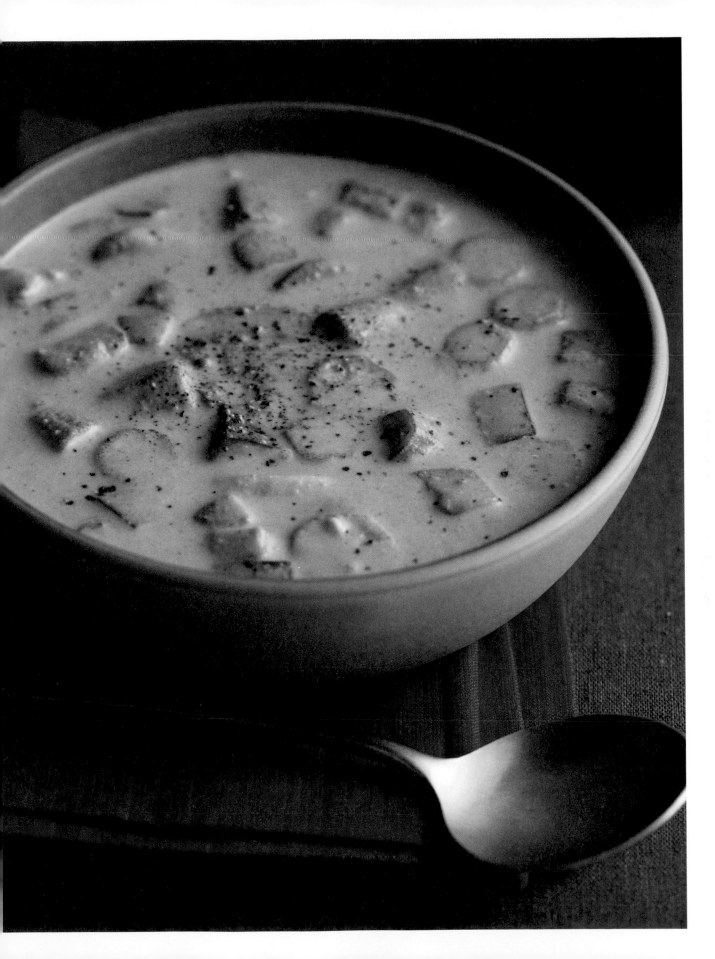

Asian Macaroni and Cheese

There are many recipes for vegan Mac 'n Cheese, but I have to boast that this one is un-freakin'-believable. You'll taste some signature Asian influences, but boy is it still rich and creamy.

MAKES 8 SERVINGS

2 cups (270 g) cauliflower, cut into small pieces and stems removed

1 cup (240 ml) light coconut milk

1 cup (240 ml) water

2 garlic cloves, chopped

¼ teaspoon ground nutmeg

1 teaspoon white miso paste

¼ teaspoon soy sauce

½ teaspoon Dijon mustard

½ teaspoon salt

Pinch of pepper

1 teaspoon potato starch

2 tablespoons grapeseed oil

½ cup (115 g) firm tofu, drained and cut into cubes

2½ cups (350 g) cooked elbow macaroni

½ cup (120 ml) panko breadcrumbs

¼ teaspoon garlic powder

Preheat the oven to 375° F (190° C).

In a medium saucepan, cook 1 cup (135 g) of the cauliflower with the coconut milk and 1 cup water over medium-high heat until soft. Add the garlic, nutmeg, miso, soy sauce, mustard, salt, and pepper. Cook about 3 minutes and add the potato starch to thicken. Pour the mixture into a blender or food processor and blend until smooth and creamy. Be careful when blending the hot liquids. It is best to divide the mixture in half when blending so it won't spill.

In a separate sauté pan, heat the oil and sauté the remaining 2 cups of cauliflower and the tofu over medium-high heat until lightly browned, about 3 minutes. Add salt and pepper, to taste. In a lasagna-style pan, add the macaroni, cauliflower, and tofu mixture. Mix in the cauliflower and coconut milk sauce. Sprinkle the breadcrumbs on top, and add the garlic powder over breadcrumbs. Bake 15 to 20 minutes, or until golden brown.

Srv: 287 g | Cal: 130 | Fat: 3 g | Sat Fat: 0 g | Col: 0 mg | Carb: 18 g | Fib: 2 g | Pro: 5 g

Tomato and Tofu Stew

This Tomato and Tofu Stew is easy enough for everyday cooking, and it doesn't need a lot of simmering time like traditional stews. Whip it up for a snack or pair it with a grilled vegan cheese sandwich for a more filling meal.

MAKES 4 SERVINGS

2 tablespoons grapeseed oil

1 tablespoon ginger-garlic paste, divided

1 package (14-ounce/400 g) firm tofu, drained and cubed

1 large onion, chopped

¼ teaspoon ground turmeric

1 teaspoon red chili powder

3 large tomatoes, seeds removed and cut into large chunks

1 Thai chile, cut in half lengthwise and seeds removed

Salt, to taste

One small bunch of cilantro, chopped

Freshly cooked rice or warm naan bread

In a medium frying pan, heat 1 tablespoon of the oil over medium heat. When the pan is hot, add ½ teaspoon of the garlic-ginger paste and let brown, about 30 seconds. Add the tofu and pan-fry until light brown, about 3 minutes. Set aside.

In a medium saucepan, add the remaining oil and heat over medium heat. Once heated, add the onions, turmeric, and chili powder and cook until translucent, 3 to 5 minutes. Add the tomatoes, Thai chiles, and salt and cook 3 to 5 minutes. Add the pan-fried tofu and cilantro to the tomato mixture. Cover and simmer until the tomatoes are completely cooked, 7 to 10 minutes. The skins will come off and roll up to the shape of a toothpick. Serve with rice or Indian naan bread.

Srv: 280 g | Cal: 130 | Fat: 4.5 g | Sat Fat: 1 g | Col: 0 mg | Carb: 12 g | Fib: 3 g | Pro: 10 g

---

THE SKINNY: HOW TO MAKE A GINGER-GARLIC PASTE

I JUST STARTED TAPPING INTO INDIAN COOKING IN THE LAST FEW YEARS. THE FIRST TIME I SAW A RECIPE THAT CALLED FOR GINGER-GARLIC PASTE, I ASSUMED IT WAS A TYPO. NEEDLESS TO SAY, I PROBABLY DIDN'T GET THE DESIRED FLAVOR. WHEN I SAW IT THE SECOND TIME, I KICKED MYSELF FOR MY LACK OF KNOWLEDGE OF SPICE TERMINOLOGY. GINGER-GARLIC PASTE IS VERY POPULAR IN INDIAN COOKING. YOU CAN BUY A JARRED PASTE FROM THE GROCERY STORE, BUT MAKING YOUR OWN IS EFFORTLESS. FOLLOW THESE STEPS FOR A DO-IT-YOURSELF GINGER-GARLIC PASTE:

INGREDIENTS:

7 TABLESPOONS (100 G) GARLIC, PEELED AND CHOPPED

½ CUP (120 ML) WATER

1 TABLESPOON VINEGAR

PLACE ALL OF THE INGREDIENTS IN THE BOWL OF A FOOD PROCESSOR, AND BLEND SMOOTH TO FORM A THICK PASTE. THE VINEGAR ACTS AS A PRESERVATIVE, BUT THE SMALL AMOUNT DOESN'T AFFECT THE FLAVOR OF THE PASTE. STORE IN AN AIRTIGHT CONTAINER IN THE REFRIGERATOR TO LAST ABOUT THREE TO FOUR MONTHS.

Vegetable Fondue

Nobody stopped me when I sold my fondue pot at a yard sale. I was sad but, as a new vegan cook, I couldn't really make any good use for it. Then I realized you didn't need cheese to make a kick-ass fondue. Damn it. This is a new spin on a classic dish. Healthy, yet creamy and good. The cheese might be missing, but not the taste.

MAKES 4 SERVINGS

1 cup (135 g) cauliflower florets

1½ cups (360 ml) light coconut milk

1 garlic clove, minced

¼ teaspoon ground nutmeg

1 teaspoon white miso paste

½ teaspoon Dijon mustard

¼ teaspoon soy sauce

1 teaspoon olive oil

2 tablespoons potato starch

Salt and pepper, to taste

½ cup (80 g) baby carrots, peeled

½ cup (45 g) broccoli florets

½ cup (65 g) asparagus halves

½ cup (75 g) fingerling potatoes (or small new potatoes)

French baguette, sliced

In a medium saucepan, add the cauliflower and coconut milk and cook over medium heat until the cauliflower is soft. Add the garlic, nutmeg, white miso, mustard, soy sauce, olive oil, potato starch, and salt and pepper, for the fondue sauce. Cook an additional 5 minutes. Let the fondue sauce cool, about 15 minutes. Then add to a blender or food processor and purée until smooth. Reheat the fondue sauce to serve. Steam the carrots, broccoli, asparagus, and potatoes until soft. Pour the fondue sauce in a bowl, and dip the vegetables and bread.

Srv: 193 g | Cal: 270 | Fat: 20 g | Sat Fat: 16 g | Col: 0 mg | Carb: 22 g | Fib: 2 g | Pro: 5 g

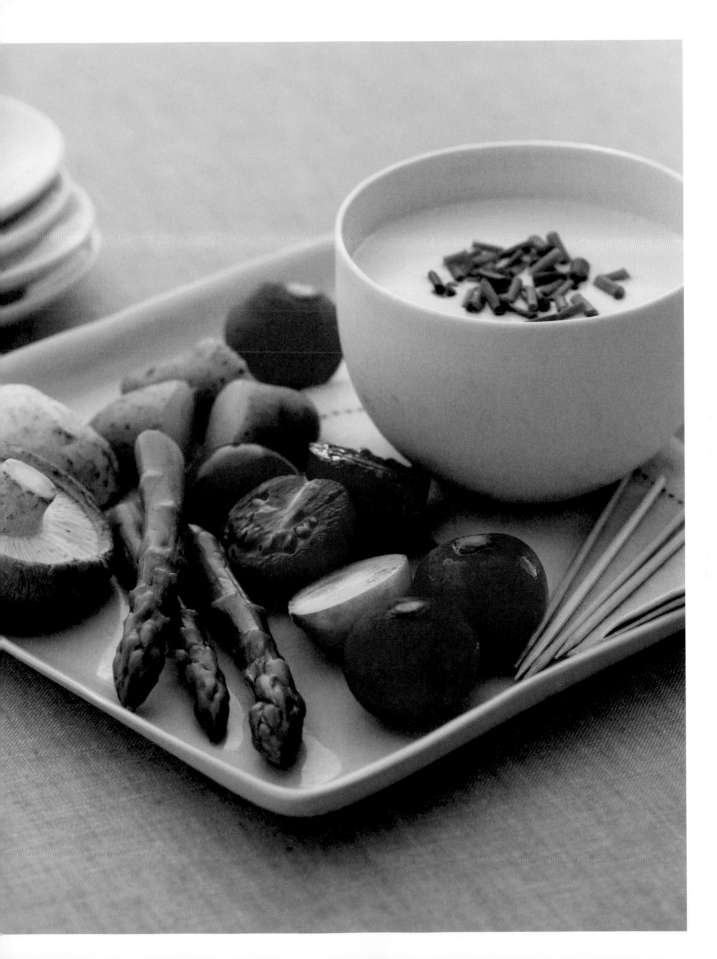

Spicy Black Bean Enchiladas

Put on some Mexican tunes and get ready to do some damage in the kitchen. These enchiladas are the perfect combination of saucy, spicy, and fresh. You can replace black beans with pinto beans to change up the recipe, but black beans bring this dish a more intense flavor.

MAKES 4 SERVINGS

2 tablespoons grapeseed oil

½ onion, chopped

1 red bell pepper, seeded and chopped

1 teaspoon chili powder

1 teaspoon ground cumin

¼ teaspoon red pepper flakes

2 (15-ounce/430 g) cans black beans, drained and rinsed

2 canned chipotle peppers

1 cup (150 g) diced tomato

Salt and pepper, to taste

12 corn tortillas

½ cup (120 g) shredded vegan cheese

2 tablespoons chopped fresh cilantro, for garnish

Fresh salsa, for serving

Preheat the oven to 350° F (180° C).

In a medium sauté pan, heat 1 tablespoon of the oil over medium-high heat. Add the onion and sauté about 5 minutes. Add the bell pepper and cook 6 to 8 minutes. Add the chili powder, cumin, and red pepper flakes and stir. Add the black beans and mix well. Pour a little less than half of the cooked bean mixture into a food processor or blender. Add the diced tomatoes and chipotle peppers and blend well, for the black bean sauce. Season with salt and pepper.

In a medium sauté pan, heat the remaining oil over medium-low heat. Place 1 tortilla at a time in the pan and flip to warm both sides.

In a 13 x 9-inch (33 x 23 cm) baking dish, spread just enough of the black bean sauce to cover the bottom of the pan. Fill each tortilla with about 3 tablespoons of the black bean sauce. Roll and fold the seam under and place seam-side down in the baking dish. When all of the tortillas have been filled and rolled tight, pour the rest of the black bean sauce on top. Sprinkle with vegan cheese and bake 40 to 45 minutes, or until it bubbles. Garnish with the cilantro. Serve with fresh salsa.

Srv: 1 Enchilada | Cal: 150 | Fat: 6 g | Sat Fat: 1 g | Col: 0 mg | Carb: 21 g | Fib: 5 g | Pro: 14 g

> **BITCHWORTHY:** Bell peppers know just how to ring my bell. One cup of bell peppers gives you 291 percent of your daily intake of vitamin C and 105 percent of vitamin A.[125]

Tempeh No-Meatloaf

It's tough to picture meatloaf without meat. But tempeh knows how to play the part. There is so much flavor in this hearty dish that it will appeal to any eater, not just veggies. Vegan cooking buddy and macrobiotic chef Christy Morgan helped put this meatless baby together. It pairs great with the Root Veggie Mash (see recipe on page 185).

MAKES 6 SERVINGS

2 tablespoons grapeseed oil

2 packages tempeh, crumbled

2 celery stalks, finely chopped

1 carrot, peeled and grated

1 teaspoon dried thyme

1 teaspoon dried basil

1 teaspoon dried oregano

Salt and pepper, to taste

¼ cup (60 g) panko breadcrumbs

¼ cup (20 g) rolled oats

3 tablespoons tahini

¼ cup (60 ml) soy sauce

⅓ cup (90 g) nutritional yeast

⅓ cup (75 ml) ketchup

Preheat the oven to 350° F (180° C). Lightly oil a large loaf pan.

In a large sauté pan, heat the oil over medium heat. Add the tempeh, celery, and carrot and sauté 5 minutes. Stir in the thyme, basil, oregano, and salt and pepper, to taste. Cook another 3 minutes and then remove from the heat. Pour the vegetable mixture into a large bowl and add the breadcrumbs, oats, tahini, soy sauce, yeast, and ketchup. Mash together until well combined. Press the mixture into the prepared loaf pan. Bake 45 minutes. Serve hot.

Srv: 224 g | Cal: 420 | Fat: 22g | Sat Fat: 4 g | Col: 0 mg | Carb: 30g | Fib: 4 g | Pro: 34 g

---

RECIPE VARIATION: MINI MEATLOAVES

PULL THAT STICK OUT OF YOUR ASS AND PLAY WITH YOUR FOOD! MAKE MINI MEATLOAVES IN A MUFFIN OR MINI PIE TIN. THIS WILL REDUCE THE BAKING TIME TO ABOUT 20-25 MINUTES. SERVE WITH MINI CARROTS WHILE YOU'RE SWEATING THE SMALL STUFF. SCREW DESSERT.

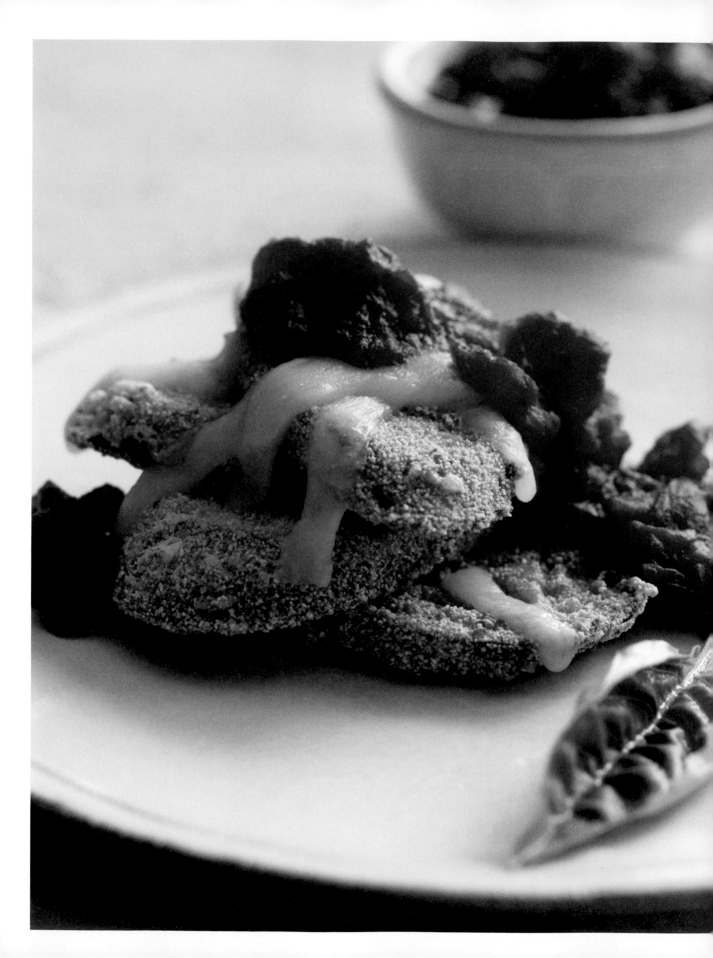

Polenta-Crusted Eggplant Parmesan

Yet another elegant dish for a special treat. The "Italian grits" make it a fun, comfort food, but eggplant Parmesan always breathes of class.

MAKES 6 SERVINGS

2½ cups (600 g) diced Italian-style tomatoes

⅔ packet vegan brown gravy mix

½ cup (70 g) dry, quick-cook polenta

¼ cup (20 g) vegan Parmesan cheese

2 tablespoons garlic powder

¼ teaspoon salt

White pepper, to taste

2 medium Japanese eggplants, sliced ¼-inch (6 mm) thick lengthwise

¼ cup (60 ml) vegan mayonnaise

3 tablespoons grapeseed oil

¾ cup (85 g) shredded vegan mozzarella cheese

2 tablespoons chopped fresh parsley

KIM'S NOTE: VEGAN BROWN GRAVY MIX IS AVAILABLE AT MOST SPECIALTY HEALTH RETAILERS, SUCH AS WHOLE FOODS. BRANDS LIKE HAIN PURE FOODS (WWW.HAINPUREFOODS.COM) AND SIMPLY ORGANIC (WWW.SIMPLYORGANICFOODS.COM) ARE BOTH HEALTHY OPTIONS.

Preheat the oven to broil.

In a small saucepan, simmer the tomatoes. Add the gravy mix and stir until blended. Cover and keep warm. In a small flat dish, combine the polenta, Parmesan cheese, garlic powder, salt, and white pepper. Spread both sides of each of the eggplant slices with about 1 teaspoon of the vegan mayo. Press the eggplant into the polenta mixture, making sure to cover both sides.

Heat a large sauté pan over medium-high heat and add the grapeseed oil. Place the coated eggplant slices into the hot oil, making sure that each piece is on top of oil, not just the hot, dry pan. Sauté until golden brown on each side. Remove the eggplant from the pan and top each one with 1 to 2 slices of the mozzarella cheese. Place on a cookie sheet and broil 2 to 3 minutes, or until the cheese melts. To serve, arrange on a plate and top with the tomato sauce. Garnish with fresh parsley.

Srv: 260 g | Cal: 310 | Fat: 19 g | Sat Fat: 2.5 g | Col: 0 mg | Carb: 26 g | Fib: 7 g | Pro: 7 g

---

BITCHWORTHY: EGGPLANT

ALWAYS THE FIRST TO MAKE EVERYONE ELSE LOOK BAD, EGGPLANT IS AN EXCELLENT SOURCE OF DIETARY FIBER, VITAMINS B1, B6, POTASSIUM, COPPER, MAGNESIUM, MANGANESE, PHOSPHORUS, NIACIN, AND FOLIC ACID. IS THAT ALL? NOPE. NASUNIN, AN ANTHOCYANIN FROM EGGPLANT PEELS, IS A POTENT ANTIOXIDANT AND FREE-RADICAL SCAVENGER. WHAT A SHOW OFF.[127]

Sweet Potato Leek Casserole

Sweet potatoes cater to all ages, so this is the perfect meal to replenish your family's appetite after a long, active day. Assemble it before hitting the gym, and pop it in the oven when you return. Voilà! Dinner is conveniently served right after you enjoy a steamy shower.

MAKES 4 SERVINGS

1 tablespoon olive oil

2 tablespoons grapeseed oil

3 medium leeks

1 garlic clove, minced

3 tablespoons chopped fresh rosemary

Salt and pepper, to taste

2 medium red-skinned sweet potatoes or garnet yams, peeled and sliced ⅛-inch (3 mm) thick

½ cup (60 g) panko breadcrumbs

⅓ cup (75 ml) vegetable broth

Preheat the oven to 400° F (200° C). Coat a medium casserole dish with the olive oil.

Heat a skillet with the grapeseed oil over medium heat. Cut the dark green tops off the leeks, and discard. Halve the leeks lengthwise. Make sure to thoroughly wash any dirt residue off the leeks. Chop the leeks and sauté with the garlic, rosemary, salt, and pepper until soft. Arrange one-third of the sweet potatoes across the bottom of the casserole dish. It is fine if they overlap and do not fit perfectly in the dish. Spread one-half of the leek mixture on top of the sweet potatoes. Then arrange another third of the sweet potatoes across the leeks. Repeat, ending with a layer of potatoes. Sprinkle breadcrumbs over the top. Pour the vegetable broth over the casserole. Cover and bake 30 minutes.

Srv: 205 g | Cal: 220 | Fat: 5 g | Sat Fat: 1 g | Col: 0 mg | Carb: 41 g | Fib: 5 g | Pro: 4 g

Black Bean and Yam Tacos

Sometimes, we just need a quick fix. These tacos are ideal for those nights. They are super-easy to prepare and come together in minutes. Beans and yams are also full of heart-friendly fiber.

MAKES 4 SERVINGS

2 tablespoons grapeseed oil

1 large garnet yam, peeled and cubed

1 green bell pepper, seeds removed and diced

1 garlic clove, minced

2 teaspoons ground cumin

1 teaspoon chili powder

1 teaspoon ground coriander

1 teaspoon dried Mexican oregano

1 (15-ounce/430 g) can black beans, drained and rinsed

1 large tomato, diced

Salt and pepper, to taste

4 whole wheat or sprouted tortillas

1 avocado, sliced, for garnish

In a large skillet, heat the oil over medium heat. Add the yam and sauté until almost soft. Add the green pepper, garlic, cumin, chili powder, coriander, and oregano. Sauté 3 minutes. Stir in the beans and tomato and cook 3 to 5 minutes, stirring frequently. Add salt and pepper, to taste. Warm the tortillas in a small skillet and then place on 4 plates. Spread the yam/bean mixture on the tortillas, and garnish with the avocado.

Srv: 1 Taco | Cal: 380 | Fat: 17 g | Sat Fat: 1.5 g | Col: 0 mg | Carb: 51 g | Fib: 11 g | Pro: 11 g

> **'TIS THE SEASON: GARNET YAM**
> NAMED FOR THEIR DARK REDDISH-BROWN SKINS, GARNET YAMS ARE ACUALLY SWEET POTATOES. THE POTATOES REACH THEIR PEAK SEASON FROM SEPTEMBER THROUGH MARCH.

Kale and Sweet Potato Pizza

Bravo to chef Noriyuki Sugie. Once again, you've outdone yourself. Chef Nori worked with me to create this unbelievable gourmet pizza. This is one of those dishes you make when Mom comes over to show her you're a big girl now. Wait until you see the look on her face. There are so many delectable flavors in this pie, it's difficult to pinpoint which one your taste buds appreciate the most.

VEGAN PIZZA DOUGH

Save this Vegan Pizza Dough recipe to use with the Veggie Calzones (page 209) and the Potato Samosas (page 216).

1 cup (240 ml) warm water

½ teaspoon dry yeast

½ teaspoon evaporated cane sugar

½ teaspoon sea salt

2 tablespoons olive oil, divided

2 cups (255 g) unbleached white pastry flour

1 cup (130 g) unbleached whole wheat flour

Preheat the oven to 250 F (120 C) for 10 minutes and turn off.

In a large mixing bowl, combine the water, yeast, and sugar and let sit until the mixture begins to bubble, typically about 5 minutes. Add the sea salt and 1 table-spoon of the olive oil to the yeast mixture. Slowly add the pastry flour. When the dough starts to thicken, use your hands to mix in the wheat flour and knead until smooth. Place the dough in a large oven-safe bowl that has been lightly oiled and cover with plastic. Set the dough in the oven until doubled in size, about an hour. When the dough has expanded, place on a floured cutting board or a flat surface, and roll out the dough.

PIZZA

MAKES 8 SLICES

2 tablespoons grapeseed oil

1 cup (160 g) chopped white onion

1 cup (90) thinly sliced leeks

2½ cups (170 g) medium-chop green kale

½ cup (65 g) peeled, small-cubed sweet potato

¼ teaspoon cumin seeds or ground cumin

¼ teaspoon salt, plus a pinch, to taste

½ cup (115 g) firm tofu, drained and cubed

2 garlic cloves, chopped

½ teaspoon dried oregano

⅛ teaspoon red pepper flakes

Preheat the oven to 400 F (200 C).

Transfer the dough to an oiled baking sheet. Heat the grapeseed oil in a large sauté pan over medium-high heat. Saute the onion and leeks until golden brown. Add the kale, sweet potato, cumin, and salt. Saute until the sweet potato starts to soften. Add the tofu and garlic and cook 2 minutes. Place the vegetables on the dough. Bake 10 to 12 minutes, or until the dough is golden brown on bottom. Top with the remaining olive oil, the oregano, red pepper flakes, and salt, to taste. Cut in slices to serve.

Srv: 1 slice (160 g) | Cal: 250 | Fat: 4.5 g | Sat Fat: 0.5 g | Col: 0 mg | Carb: 46 g | Fib: 3 g | Pro: 8 g

THE SKINNY: TRUE OR FALSE? SEA SALT IS HEALTHIER THAN TABLE SALT
LET'S CLEAR THE AIR. SEA SALT IS 98 PERCENT SODIUM CHLORIDE AND TABLE SALT IS 99.9 PERCENT SODIUM CHLORIDE WITH ADDED IODINE. SINCE ONLY 2 PERCENT OF SEA SALT IS MADE OF KEY MINERALS, IT REALLY ONLY ENHANCES THE FLAVOR, NOT YOUR HEALTH. THE DIFFERENCE IS IN THE TASTE, TEXTURE, AND PROCESSING, NOT THE NUTRITIONAL VALUE.[128] ANSWER: FALSE.

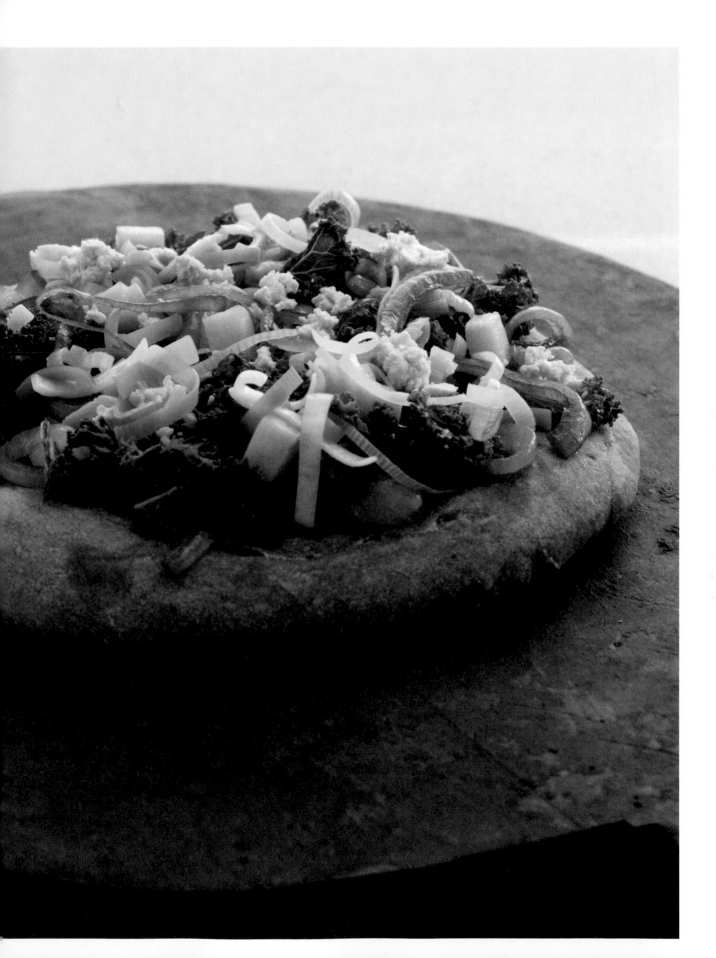

Orange-Battered Tempeh

Before I went vegan, my husband and I used to order orange chicken from our local hole-in-the-wall Chinese restaurant. I had too much determination to completely let it go. This is a much healthier version, but it IS deep-fried, so go easy.

MAKES 4 SERVINGS

1 cup (130 g) unbleached all-purpose flour

½ teaspoon baking powder

½ teaspoon salt

1 (12-ounce/340 g) can dark beer, cold (such as Newcastle)

2 oranges, zested and juiced

3 tablespoons tamari

4 tablespoons (60 ml) maple syrup

2 tablespoons rice vinegar

1 tablespoon arrowroot powder

½ cup (120 ml) safflower oil, plus 2 tablespoons or more for frying

2 green bell peppers, seeded and cubed

1 cup (165 g) pineapple chunks

2 packages tempeh, cut into 2-inch (5 cm) rectangles

½ cup (55 g) arrowroot powder for dredging (or substitute cornstarch)

In a medium bowl, mix together the flour, baking powder, and salt. Pour in the beer and whisk together until no clumps remain. Chill in the refrigerator 15 minutes.

Heat a small saucepan over medium heat, and add the orange juice and zest, the tamari, and maple syrup; whisk until well combined, for the orange glaze. In a small bowl, mix together the vinegar and arrowroot powder until smooth. Whisk the vinegar mixture into the orange juice mixture. It will begin to thicken after about 5 minutes. Do not boil. Remove the batter from the refrigerator. Heat 1 tablespoon of the oil in a skillet and stir-fry the peppers and pineapple about 3 minutes. Transfer to a bowl and set aside.

Add ¼ cup of the oil to the skillet and heat over medium-high heat. Dredge the tempeh in the arrowroot, shaking off any excess. Submerge the tempeh batter and cook in batches in the hot oil, flipping with metal tongs when one side turns golden brown. Remove the pieces and place on a paper-towel lined plate. Continue cooking the remaining tempeh pieces. (You will need to add an additional tablespoon of oil for each new batch of tempeh.) Toss the peppers, pineapple, and fried tempeh together in a bowl. Drizzle with the desired amount of orange glaze and serve immediately.

Srv: 290 g | Cal: 370 | Fat: 13 g | Sat Fat: 2 g | Col: 0 mg | Carb: 45 g | Fib: 3 g | Pro: 18 g

---

THE SKINNY: DARK BEER

DON'T PULL OUT THE BEER BONG JUST YET, BABE. WHILE YOU'LL NEVER CATCH ME ENCOURAGING YOU TO JOIN THE BOYS AT THE PUB EVERY SUNDAY, BEER ACTUALLY DOES HAVE A FEW HEALTH BENEFITS. EXPERTS HAVE FOUND BEER HELPS TO INCREASE HDL "GOOD" CHOLESTEROL IN THE BODY, PROTECT AGAINST HEART DISEASE, AND REDUCE BLOOD PRESSURE. KEEP IN MIND THAT DARK BEER CONTAINS MORE FLAVANOIDS THAN LIGHT BEER.[126] ENJOY ON OCCASION, BUT WATCH YOURSELF—SKINNY BITCHES DON'T HAVE BEER BELLIES.

Spaghetti with Spinach in a White Wine Garlic Sauce

Enjoy a big bowl of spaghetti in a traditional white wine garlic sauce, with the addition of a powerful veggie. Popeye would have loved this dish.

MAKES 6 SERVINGS

1 (1-pound/455 g) box thin spaghetti, uncooked
3 tablespoons grapeseed oil, divided
5 medium white or cremini mushrooms, thinly sliced
Salt and pepper, to taste
2 cups (480 ml) vegetable stock, divided
½ cup (80 g) finely chopped onion
3 garlic cloves, minced
8 ounces (225 g) fresh baby spinach
3 Roma tomatoes, chopped in large pieces
½ cup (120 ml) white wine
¼ cup (20 g) vegan Parmesan cheese

In a large pot, boil water over high heat and cook the spaghetti according to package directions until it is al dente. Drain and set aside.

Meanwhile, heat a large sauté pan over medium-high heat. Add 1 tablespoon of the oil and the mushrooms and sauté 5 to 8 minutes, or until they are slightly caramelized and golden. Add salt and pepper and cook 1 additional minute. Stir in 2 tablespoons of the stock and sauté until the stock is absorbed. Remove the mushrooms from the heat and transfer to a medium bowl. Add another tablespoon of the oil to the sauté pan and the onion. Sauté over medium heat for about 10 minutes, or until the onions are golden brown. Stir in the garlic and sauté 2 minutes, stirring constantly. Spoon the onion and garlic mixture into a small bowl.

Return the pan to the stove over medium-high heat and add the remaining oil. Add the spinach and sauté until the spinach is wilted, about 2 minutes. Add 2 tablespoons of the stock and cook until absorbed. Season with salt and pepper, to taste. Return the mushrooms, onions and garlic, and the tomatoes to the pan with the spinach, and cook over medium-high heat. Add the white wine and cook until reduced by two-thirds, stirring occasionally. Stir in the remaining stock and cook for 5 minutes until the sauce begins to reduce again and thicken (it should still be brothy). Add the Parmesan cheese. Top the pasta with the sauce and toss to coat.

Srv: 235 g | Cal: 210 | Fat: 1.5 g | Sat Fat: 0 g | Col: 0 mg | Carb: 45 g | Fib: 3 g | Pro: 18 g

THE SKINNY: ROMA TOMATOES— FINDING THE RIGHT ONE

GOLDILOCKS ISN'T AROUND TO HELP YOU FIND THE ROMA TOMATO THAT IS "JUST RIGHT." GOOD-QUALITY ROMA TOMATOES WILL BE FIRM, SMOOTH-SKINNED, AND SLIGHTLY PINK IN COLOR. IF THEY HAVE A GREEN BLUSH, PUT IN A PAPER BAG AND ALLOW THEM TO RIPEN AT ROOM TEMPERATURE ON THE KITCHEN COUNTER.

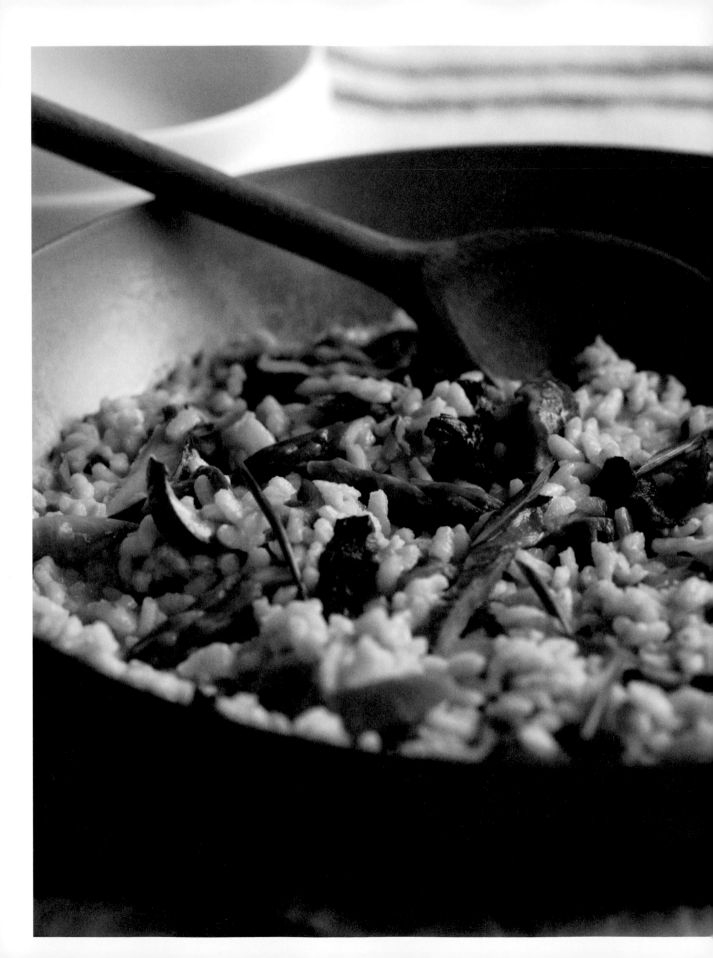

Wild Mushroom and Asparagus Risotto

I'm pretty sure that somewhere in my future there will be a cookbook devoted just to Italian cuisine. And no self-respecting Italian food lover would be caught dead without a special Risotto recipe on hand, so here is one for my mushroom lovers out there! This is creamy and delicious.

MAKES 6 SERVINGS

6 cups (1.41 ml) vegetable broth
¼ cup (10 g) dried wild mushrooms
½ cup (120 ml) hot water
3 tablespoons grapeseed oil
¼ cup (55 g) Earth Balance
¾ cup (70 g) coarsely chopped fresh mushrooms (such as porcini, chanterelles, crimini, portobello)
1½ cups (200 g) asparagus, cut into 1-inch pieces
Salt and pepper to taste
2 garlic cloves, minced
1 small onion, finely chopped
⅓ cup (55 g) shallots, finely chopped
1 cup (200 g) Arborio rice, uncooked
⅓ cup (75 ml) white wine
½ cup (40 g) vegan Parmesan cheese
1 teaspoon white truffle oil (optional)
1 teaspoon chopped chives, for garnish

In a large saucepan add the vegetable broth, cover and keep warm over low heat. Place hot water in a medium size bowl and add the 2 ounces of dried mushrooms. Allow to sit for about 20 minutes, or until the mushrooms are soft. Then add the mushrooms and the hot water to the vegetable broth.

In a large sauté pan over medium-high heat, add 1 tablespoon grapeseed oil and 1 tablespoon Earth Balance. Add the fresh mushrooms and asparagus, and sauté until lightly browned, about 10 minutes. Season with salt and pepper to taste, remove from heat and transfer to a medium size bowl. Using the same large saucepan, heat the remaining grapeseed oil over medium heat and add the onions and shallots, stirring, until soft, about 5 minutes. Add the garlic and remaining Earth Balance and sauté for 1 minute. Add the rice and stir until well combined. Add the wine and stir until the wine is absorbed. Add 1 cup of the warm broth and cook over medium heat, stirring constantly, until nearly absorbed. Continue adding the broth ½ cup (118 ml) at a time, stirring frequently and letting each additional broth be absorbed before adding more. Continue adding the broth until the rice is tender and creamy, about 30 to 40 minutes.

Stir in the sautéed mushrooms, asparagus, and parmesan cheese to the rice, and season with salt and pepper to taste. Garnish each serving with a sprinkle of chives, and the white truffle oil (if using).

Srv: 383 g | Cal: 320 | Fat: 0 g | Sat Fat: 3 g | Col: 0 mg | Carb: 47 g | Fib: 5 g | Pro: 11 g

DESSERTS

Mini Rustic Pear Tarts

Reinvent the classic tea party in your own home with these delectable pear tarts. You can use mini tart pie pans or mini pie pans to serve these sweet treats. Once baked, they are about four inches across, so count on a generous serving.

MAKES 6 SERVINGS

1 recipe pie dough, divided into 6 equal balls (see page 267)

4 Bosc pears, peeled, cored, and thinly sliced

1 tablespoon cornstarch

½ cup (120 ml) freshly squeezed lemon juice

½ cup (100 g) packed light brown sugar

1 teaspoon ground cinnamon

¼ teaspoon ground nutmeg

¼ teaspoon ground cloves

¼ cup (60 ml) plus 2 tablespoons agave nectar

1 tablespoon boiling water

½ cup (55 g) sliced almonds, toasted

Preheat the oven to 375° F (190° C).

Roll out the dough and cut into four 6-inch circles; place in the mini tart pans, trimming excess dough from the edges. Place the pans on a baking sheet and chill 15 minutes.

Leaving the tart shells on the baking sheet, place them in the oven for 7 minutes to partially bake. Meanwhile, place the pears, cornstarch, lemon juice, brown sugar, cinnamon, nutmeg, and cloves into a medium bowl and toss well to combine. Reduce the heat to 350° F (180° C). Remove the tart crusts from the oven and fill with the pear mixture. Return the tarts to the oven and bake 22 to 28 minutes, or until the crusts are golden brown and the pears have begun to caramelize.

Meanwhile, in a small bowl, make the glaze by whisking together the agave nectar and water. Once the tarts are baked and have cooled slightly, gently brush a thin layer of the glaze over the tops of each tart. Sprinkle with the toasted almonds.

Srv: 1 Tart (235 g) | Cal: 630 | Fat: 31 g | Sat Fat: 10 g | Col: 0 mg | Carb: 85 g | Fib: 6 g | Pro: 7 g

Blood Orange and Black Pepper Sorbet

Black pepper in sorbet . . . weird? Absolutely. Rest assured, the colorful presentation of blood orange and black pepper sorbet is utterly radiant. A lovely dessert to serve when you have company. Someone else has to play witness to your brilliance.

MAKES 4 SERVINGS

⅔ cup (130 g) evaporated cane sugar

⅔ cup (165 ml) water

6 whole black peppercorns, lightly crushed

2 cups (480 ml) freshly squeezed blood orange juice, chilled

In a medium saucepan, combine the sugar, water, and peppercorns over high heat. Bring to a boil, reduce the heat, and simmer until the sugar has dissolved, about 2 minutes, stirring frequently. Remove from heat. Stir in the blood orange juice and chill in the refrigerator for at least 1 hour.

Once chilled, remove from refrigerator and strain the mixture through a fine sieve to remove the peppercorns. Pour the liquid into an ice cream maker or a Vitamix, and follow the manufacturer's directions. Serve immediately, or store in a airtight container in the freezer.

Srv: 188 g | Cal: 130 | Fat: 0 g | Sat Fat: 0 g | Col: 0 mg | Carb: 37 g | Fib: 0 g | Pro: 1 g

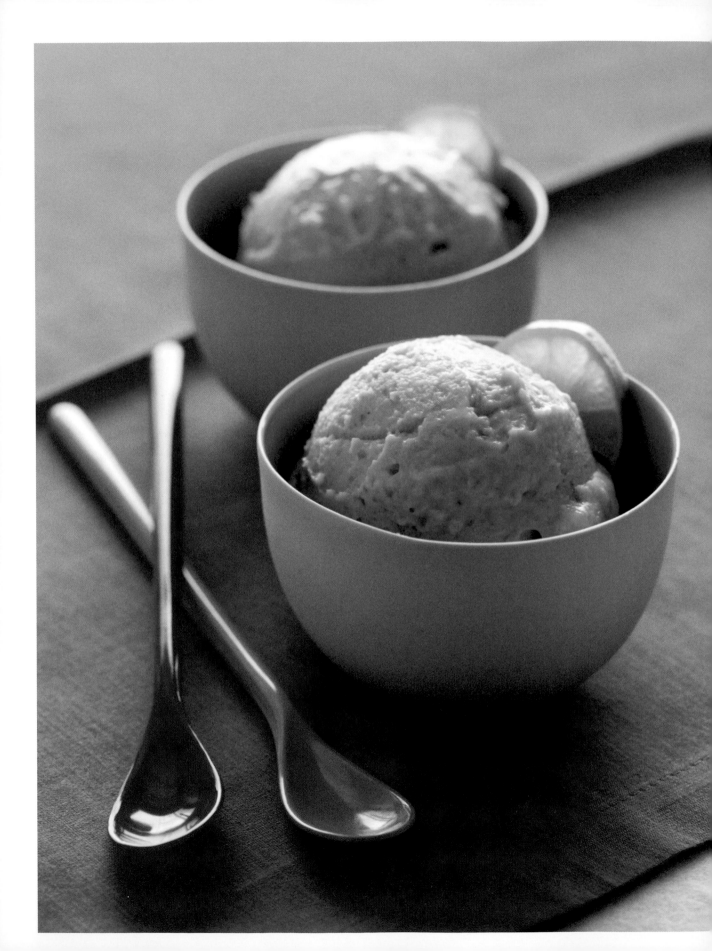

Avocado, Coconut, and Lime Sorbet

I know what you're thinking. Avocados in a sorbet? Oh, just you wait. The coconut and lime add a tropical panache, but the avocado gives it a very distinctive, smooth finish. I can't think of a more gratifying way to get a healthy scoop of monounsaturated fats.

MAKES 8 SERVINGS

1 cup (240 ml) water

1 cup (200 g) evaporated cane sugar

2 tablespoons lime zest

¾ cup (180 ml) freshly squeezed lime juice

3 avocados, peeled, seeded, and chopped

1 (8.5-ounce/240 g) can cream of coconut (like Coco Lopez)

1 teaspoon salt

In a medium saucepan, combine the water and sugar and cook over high heat. Bring to a boil, reduce the heat, and simmer until the sugar has dissolved, stirring frequently. Remove from the heat and set aside. Stir in the lime zest and chill in the refrigerator for at least an hour. Meanwhile, place the lime juice, avocados, and cream of coconut in a food processor and blend until smooth. Add the chilled lime syrup and pulse to combine. Pour into an ice cream maker or a Vitamix, and follow the manufacturer's directions. Serve immediately or store in an airtight container in the freezer.

Srv: 157 g | Cal: 270 | Fat: 6 g | Sat Fat: 0 g | Col: 0 mg | Carb: 42 g | Fib: 2 g | Pro: 2 g

Strawberry Shortcake

There is just something about strawberry shortcake that takes me to my happy place. Go to your local farmers' market during the summer and stock up on fresh organic strawberries. You can top this dessert with some vegan whipped cream or warm, melted chocolate sauce. Hey, go ahead, daredevil, top with both.

MAKES 8 SERVINGS

2 cups (330 g) sliced fresh strawberries

¼ cup (50 g) evaporated cane sugar plus 1 tablespoon

2 cups (255 g) unbleached all-purpose flour

1 tablespoon baking powder

½ teaspoon salt

⅔ cup (150g) Earth Balance, cold and cut in cubes

¾ cup (180 ml) almond milk

1½ teaspoons vanilla extract

Vegan whipped cream

Preheat the oven to 400° F (200° C).

In a large bowl, add the strawberries and 1 tablespoon of the sugar. Mix until the strawberries are coated well with sugar and then place in the refrigerator until the biscuits are done.

In a large bowl, mix together the flour, baking powder, the remaining ¼ cup sugar, and the salt. Add the Earth Balance and mix with a pastry cutter (or a fork if you don't have one). The batter will look crumbly. In a measuring cup, combine the almond milk and the vanilla extract. Add the milk mixture to the flour mixture and stir until just combined. Lightly flour a flat surface and knead the dough with your hands, adding more flour if necessary. Do not overknead the dough. Just knead until the dough is a good texture and not so sticky. Roll-out the dough, then use a round cookie cutter or a round drinking glass turned upside-down to cut out about 8 circles. Place them on a cookie sheet. You will need to re-mold the dough pieces back into another shape to cut the rest of it. Bake 10 minutes.

Allow the biscuits to cool for several minutes. Cut each biscuit in half horizontally so you have a bottom and top biscuit and place on plates. Add a desired amount of strawberries on the bottom half of the biscuit. Top the strawberries with a scoop of vegan whipped cream. Put the top half of the biscuit on the whipped cream, and top with another scoop of vegan whipped cream.

Srv: 1 Biscuit plus 57 g of Strawberries | Cal: 330 | Fat: 20 g | Sat Fat: 8 g | Col: 0 mg | Carb: 33 g | Fib: 2 g | Pro: 4 g

White Chocolate Chip Cookies

This is my new favorite cookie. They are a little crispy on the outside, but oh-so-soft on the inside. It will be harder to find the vegan white chocolate chips in a store, but you can order them online at *veganstore.com*. Trust me, you may find yourself waiting at the mailbox and flirting with the mailman.

MAKES 30 COOKIES

1¼ cups (150 g) unbleached all-purpose flour

½ cup (50 g) dark chocolate cocoa powder, unsweetened

½ teaspoon baking powder

½ teaspoon baking soda

½ teaspoon salt

2 tablespoons arrowroot (or cornstarch)

½ cup (120 ml) almond milk

½ cup (120 ml) canola oil

½ cup (100 g) packed light brown sugar

½ cup (100 g) evaporated cane sugar

2 teaspoons vanilla extract

⅔ cup (80 g) chopped walnuts

⅔ cup (115 g) vegan white chocolate chips

Preheat the oven to 350° F (180° C).

In a medium bowl, sift together the flour and cocoa powder. Add the baking powder, baking soda, salt, and arrowroot.

In a separate large bowl, combine the milk, oil, both sugars, and vanilla extract. Whisk together until well blended. Stir in the flour mixture until well combined. Add in the walnuts and chips. Let the dough sit for about 15 minutes to firm up a little.

Drop about 1 tablespoon of the dough at at time on an ungreased cookie sheet, leaving about 2 inches between each cookie (they will spread when baking). Bake 8 to 10 minutes. Let the cookies cool on the cookie sheet 5 minutes. Transfer to a wire rack to cool completely.

Srv: 1 Cookie (27 g) | Cal: 120 | Fat: 7 g | Sat Fat: 1.5 g | Col: 0 mg | Carb: 14 g | Fib: 1 g | Pro: 2 g

BITCH I LOVE:
ALICIA SILVERSTONE

There's just something about Alicia. There was a time when the blonde beauty was destined to go down in history as Steven Tyler's muse. Or as Cher, the spoiled prima donna with a heart, in the coming-of-age cult classic *Clueless*. Instead, Alicia's mark on VH1 music videos and the big screen will play as background music to her starring role as an animal activist. And now, a bestselling author. *As if.*

In her debut book, *The Kind Diet,* Alicia is showing people just how much better life can be when you say goodbye to your dirty vices in the kitchen. From enlightening us on food's ability to fight disease to encouraging us to "flirt" with a plant-based diet, Alicia is all about turning this planet around.

From the first day I met her, it would be wrong to say I didn't admire Alicia for her compassion for animals, and using her name to start a revolution. Because I did. But, what made me really fall for Alicia is that she is real. She is genuine and sweet, answers her own e-mail and cooks her own meals as much as humanely possible. There are no egos in Alicia's home. Just really good whole foods and a clan of rescue pups. Check out Alicia's blog at www.thekindlife.com.

Alicia's Crispy Peanut Butter Treats with Chocolate Chips

Alicia loves these Crispy Peanut Butter Treats with Chocolate Chips for a million reasons. They are a very delicious treat, but they are not all that bad for you. There is no crazy sugar, just nice, sweet, friendly brown rice syrup. They are versatile in that they can be chocolate peanut-butter or raisin-almond butter.They also like to travel. They have been to Egypt and London with her, and last forever in a big suitcase.

MAKES 12 SQUARES

1 (10-ounce/280 g) box brown rice crisps cereal

1¾ cups (420 ml) brown rice syrup

Salt, to taste

¾ cup (195 g) peanut butter or almond butter (preferably unsweetened and unsalted)

½ cup (85 g) grain-sweetened, nondairy chocolate or carob chips

Pour the rice cereal into a large bowl. In a small saucepan, heat the syrup with a pinch of salt over low heat. When the rice syrup liquefies, add the peanut butter and stir until well combined. Pour the mixture over the rice cereal, stirring well with a wooden spoon. When thoroughly mixed and cooled to room temperature, stir in the chocolate chips. Make sure the mixture is cool or you will end up with melted chocolate instead of chocolate chips in your treats. Spoon the mixture into an 8 x 8-inch (20 x 20 cm) or 13 x 9-inch (33 x 23 cm) baking dish. Wet the wooden spoon lightly and press the mixture evenly into the pan. Let cool for 1 hour, before cutting into squares or bars.

Srv: 1 square (101 g) | Cal: 400 | Fat: 12 g | Sat Fat: 3 g | Col: 0 mg | Carb: 71 g | Fib: 3 g | Pro: 7 g

RECIPE VARIATION: ALMOND RAISIN BARS
SUBSTITUTE ¾ CUP (195 G) OF THE ALMOND BUTTER FOR THE PEANUT BUTTER, AND ½ CUP (85 G) OF THE DARK OR GOLDEN RAISINS FOR THE CHOCOLATE CHIPS. GO CRAZY, AND USE BOTH!

Kabocha Squash Custard

Kabocha squash is amazingly sweet but not something you would expect in a dessert recipe. The combination of coconut milk, sugar, and vanilla adds a special touch to this fabulous after-dinner custard.

MAKES 8 SERVINGS

1 cup (140 g) cubed kabocha squash, with skin removed

4 cups (960 ml) light coconut milk, divided

2 tablespoons evaporated cane sugar

¼ teaspoon vanilla seeds scraped from vanilla bean (or 1 teaspoon pure vanilla extract)

¼ teaspoon agar agar flakes

2 tablespoons tapioca, uncooked

¼ cup (50 g) packed brown sugar

2 teaspoons brewed Earl Grey tea

1 tablespoon sliced almonds, for garnish

KIM'S NOTE: I chose Earl Grey tea because it gives the sauce an aromatic flavor, but if you must, you can swap out for black tea. Stubborn young lady, aren't you?

In a large saucepan, simmer the squash, 3 cups (720 ml) of the coconut milk, the sugar, and vanilla over medium heat, until soft. Remove the squash from the coconut milk and place in a bowl. Bring the coconut milk to a boil and then add the agar agar flakes. Whisk together until smooth. Put the squash and the coconut milk mixture in a blender or food processor, and blend or process until smooth. Pour into 8 custard cups or ramekins and refrigerate. Cook the tapioca according to package directions, and set aside.

In a small saucepan, cook the brown sugar over medium heat until sugar melts and browns. Add the remaining cup of coconut milk and whisk together. Add the Earl Grey tea and cook for 1 minute. Remove from the heat and let sit for 5 minutes. Pour into a mesh strainer and then pour into the tapioca. Bring the coconut milk custards to room temperature and pour the sauce over the top. Garnish with the almonds.

Srv: 413 g | Cal: 90 | Fat: 0.5 g | Sat Fat: 0 g | Col: 0 mg | Carb: 13 g | Fib: 0 g | Pro: 1 g

THE SKINNY: AGAR AGAR FLAKES

Agar agar may sound a bit funky, but it's a flavorless vegetarian gelatin substitute typically used as a stabilizing and thickening agent for baking. Made from a special variety of seaweed, agar agar flakes are available online and at most specialty health food stores like Whole Foods.

KABOCHA SQUASH

Known as the Japanese pumpkin, the kabocha squash is a cross between a sweet potato and a pumpkin. Its soft orange flesh is very nutty and sweet—sweeter than butternut squash—so it makes for a divine dessert. You will get the sweetest kabochas during late summer and early fall when they are in season. Look for them at specialty health retailers and some major grocers.

Vanilla Bean Cake

I love me some Vanilla Bean Cake. Vanilla has such an incredible aroma and flavor, and cooking it with the almond milk really brings out the taste. I also threw in some vegan pudding mix to help moisten the cake.

MAKES 8 SERVINGS

2 cups (255 g) unbleached all-purpose flour

1 teaspoon baking powder

½ teaspoon baking soda

½ teaspoon salt

3 tablespoons dry vanilla pudding mix

1 large vanilla bean

1 cup (240 ml) almond milk

1 cup (225 g) Earth Balance, at room temperature

1 cup (200 g) evaporated cane sugar

1 teaspoon almond extract

¼ cup (55 g) silken tofu, drained

Preheat the oven to 350° F (180° C). Lightly oil a round 8-inch (20 x 4 cm) or 9-inch (23 x 3.5 cm) cake pan and then lightly dust the pan with flour. Shake the pan to coat, discarding any remaining flour.

In a large bowl, sift the 2 cups flour. Add the baking powder, baking soda, salt, and dry pudding mix, and stir until well combined. Set aside. Lay the vanilla bean flat on a cutting board, and using a small, sharp knife make a cut through the top layer only of the bean, starting from the top and slicing downward. In a small saucepan over low heat, cook the almond milk and the vanilla bean about 10 minutes. Remove from the heat and, using a slotted spoon, remove the vanilla bean and set aside on a plate to cool. Pour the almond milk into a small bowl to cool as well.

In a separate large bowl, add the Earth Balance and beat with electric mixer until fluffy, about 30 seconds. Add the sugar and continue to beat until fluffy, 1 to 2

minutes. Add the almond extract and beat again just until combined. Once the vanilla bean has cooled, and using the same sharp knife, gently scrape out the black seeds from the vanilla bean and put them in the cooled of almond milk.

In a food processor or blender, add the tofu and pulse a couple of times. Add the almond milk and purée until well combined, just a few seconds.

In the bowl of the sugar mixture, add half of the flour mixture and beat on low. Continue to beat and add in half of the almond milk mixture. Combine briefly and then add the remaining flour and the remaining almond milk mixture. Beat until well combined. Pour the batter into the prepared pan and bake 35 minutes, or until golden brown on top and a toothpick inserted in the center of the cake comes out clean. Place on a wire rack to cool completely. When cooled, frost with Lemon Buttercream Frosting (see recipe on page 272).

Srv: 1 Slice | Cal: 410 | Fat: 23 g | Sat Fat: 9 g | Col: 0 m g | Carb: 48g | Fib: 1 g | Pro: 4 g

BITCHWORTHY: VEGAN PUDDING!

THOUGHT VEGAN PUDDING WAS A MYTH? THINK AGAIN. DR. OETKER ORGANICS HAS A LINE OF DRY PUDDING THAT IS SO GOOD YOU MIGHT FIND YOURSELF BUYING IT IN BULK. THERE ARE A VARIETY OF FLAVORS SUCH AS CHOCOLATE, VANILLA, BUTTERSCOTCH, COCONUT, AND BANANA. AVAILABLE AT WHOLE FOODS AND MANY HEALTH FOOD STORES, OR YOU CAN ORDER IT ONLINE AT WWW.VEGANESSENTIALS.COM.

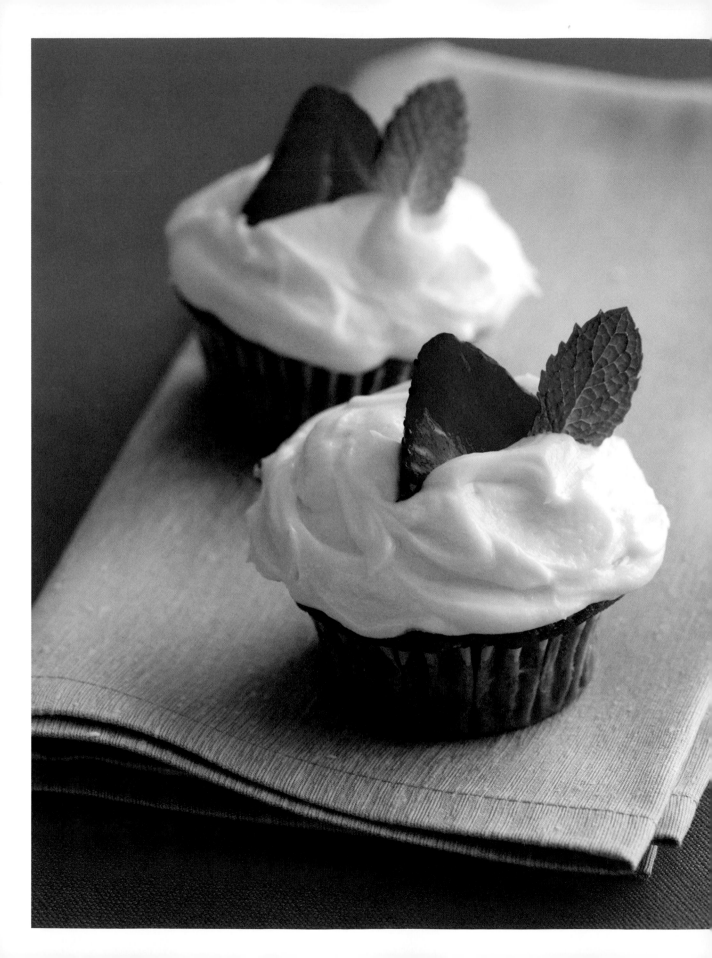

Strawberry Cupcakes

I have a confession to make. I am completely and utterly addicted to cupcakes. They are my Achilles heel. When I lived next door to my BFF Keesha in Florida we would put the kids to bed, and bake strawberry cupcakes as a mindless, temporary relief from the woes of raising infants. Oh the power of cupcakes!

MAKES 1 DOZEN CUPCAKES

2 cups (255 g) unbleached all-purpose flour
1 teaspoon baking powder
½ teaspoon baking soda
½ teaspoon salt
½ cup (120 ml) canola oil
½ cup (120 ml) almond milk
1 cup (200 g) evaporated cane sugar
2 teaspoons pure vanilla extract
1 teaspoon almond extract
⅓ cup (75 g) silken tofu
1¼ cups (200 g) chopped fresh or frozen
   strawberries

Preheat the oven to 325° F (165° C). Line a 12-cup muffin pan with crimped paper liners.

In a large bowl, sift in the flour. Add in the baking powder, baking soda, and salt; stir until combined. In a separate large bowl, whisk together the oil, milk, sugar, and extracts until well combined. In a food processor or blender, purée the tofu and strawberries until creamy. Add the strawberry mixture to the milk mixture and whisk until combined. Create a small well in the dry mixture and pour in the wet ingredients. Stir to combine but do not overmix. Pour the batter into prepared muffin pan, filling each liner about half to two-thirds full. Bake 20 to 25 minutes, or until a toothpick inserted in the center of the cupcakes comes out clean. Remove from the oven and place on a wire rack to cool completely. Top with Buttercream Frosting (see recipe on page 272).

Srv: 1 Cupcake | Cal: 210 | Fat: 10 g | Sat Fat: 0.5 g |
Col: 0 mg | Carb: 30 g | Fib: 1 g | Pro: 2 g

Chocolate Cupcakes

I know it's a basic, everyday cupcake flavor, but I feel it should be a staple in a cookbook, the go-to recipe for almost every occasion. This has a nice hint of orange that pairs well with the chocolate.

MAKES 12 CUPCAKES

2½ (320 g) cups unbleached all-purpose flour

¾ cup (70 g) unsweetened cocoa powder

½ teaspoon baking powder

¾ teaspoon baking soda

½ teaspoon salt

½ cup (120 ml) almond milk

1 teaspoon apple cider vinegar

½ cup (115 g) Earth Balance, at room temperature

1 cup (200 g) evaporated cane sugar

1 teaspoon vanilla extract

½ cup (120 ml) orange juice

1 teaspoon grated orange peel

Preheat the oven to 350° F (180° C). Line a 12-cup muffin pan with crimped paper liners.

In a large bowl, sift together the flour and the cocoa powder. Add the baking powder, baking soda, and salt. In a separate small bowl mix together the milk and apple cider vinegar and let sit until lightly curdled.

In a separate large bowl, beat together the Earth Balance and the sugar with an electric mixer until fluffy, about 2 minutes. Add the vanilla and beat an additional 30 seconds. Pour the flour and milk mixtures into the sugar mixture and stir until well combined. Add the orange juice and orange peel and stir together, but do not overmix. Pour the batter into the prepared muffin pan, filling each liner about two-thirds full. Bake about 15 minutes, or until a toothpick inserted in the center of the cupcakes comes out clean. Remove from the oven and set on a wire rack to cool completely. When cooled, top with your favorite frosting. I love these with the Peanut Butter Frosting (see recipe on page 273).

Srv: 1 Cupcake | Cal: 220 | Fat: 8 g | Sat Fat: 3.5 g | Col: 0 mg | Carb: 37 g | Fib: 3 g | Pro: 4 g

Soft Ginger Cookies

This is similar to a gingerbread cookie, so soft and moist. It deserves a warning sign: Addicting. You may need group therapy after one batch.

MAKES 24 COOKIES

2 cups (500 ml) unbleached all-purpose flour

½ teaspoon baking soda

1 teaspoon baking powder

1 teaspoon ground cinnamon

1 teaspoon ground nutmeg

1 cup (200 g) evaporated cane sugar

½ cup (115 g) Earth Balance, at room temperature

½ cup (120 ml) applesauce

2 tablespoons molasses

2 teaspoons ground ginger

1 teaspoon grated fresh ginger, or 1 tablespoon small pieces crystallized ginger

1 teaspoon vanilla extract

Preheat the oven to 350° F (180° C). Lightly grease a cookie sheet.

In a medium bowl, sift the flour. Add the baking soda, baking powder, cinnamon, and nutmeg.

In a separate large bowl, beat the sugar and the Earth Balance with an electric mixer until fluffy, about 2 minutes. Add the applesauce, molasses, ground and fresh ginger, and the vanilla. Beat for 1 minute. Add the flour mixture to the wet ingredients and slowly stir together, being careful to avoid overmixing. Place in the refrigerator to chill for 1 hour and then roll the dough into small balls and place on the prepared cookie sheet. Lightly press on the dough with your fingers to flatten a little, but make sure they aren't too thin. Bake about 8 minutes. Let the cookies cool on the baking sheet 5 minutes, then transfer to a wire rack to cool completely.

Srv: 1 Cookie (28 g) | Cal: 90 | Fat: 3 g | Sat Fat: 1 g | Col: 0 mg | Carb: 16 g | Fib: 0 g | Pro: 1g

Jenny & Heather's Mini Lemon Cheesecake Bites with a Strawberry Sauce

MAKES 24 MINI CHEESECAKES

¼ cup (30 g) toasted walnuts

¼ cup (30 g) toasted pecans

1 tablespoon safflower oil

½ cup (40 g) rolled oats

¼ cup (50 g) evaporated cane sugar plus 2 tablespoons

6 tablespoons (90 ml) maple syrup, divided

½ teaspoon ground cinnamon plus ¼ teaspoon

1 teaspoon vanilla extract, divided

½ teaspoon almond extract

3 pinches salt

1 (8-ounce/225 g) container vegan cream cheese

2 tablespoons freshly squeezed lemon juice plus 1 teaspoon

1 tablespoon unbleached all-purpose flour

4 to 5 fresh strawberries

Preheat the oven to 350° F (180° C).

Place the walnuts, pecans, oil, oats, 2 tablespoons of the sugar, 2 tablespoons of the maple syrup, ½ teaspoon of the cinnamon, ½ teaspoon of the vanilla, the almond extract, and a pinch of salt in a food processor and pulse until well combined. The mixture should smell like cookie dough and should stick together after pulsed approximately 20 times.

Lightly coat a mini cupcake pan with oil and place 1 tablespoon of the crust inside each section. Press the crust into the pan using the bottom of a shot glass and damp hands. Bake 7 minutes. Let cool on rack.

Meanwhile, clean the food processor and add the cream cheese, 2 tablespoons of the maple syrup, the remaining sugar, 2 tablespoons of the lemon juice, the flour, ¼ teaspoon of the cinnamon, a pinch of salt, and the remaining ½ teaspoon vanilla extract. Pulse until the mixture looks uniform and creamy. Top the cooled crusts with 1 tablespoon filling per section. Bake 20 to 25 minutes, or until the cheesecakes look browned. Let cool, then chill at least 30 minutes or up to 2 hours for the best consistency. Slide a small knife or toothpick around each cheesecake to remove from the pan.

To make the strawberry sauce, place the strawberries, the remaining maple syrup, the remaining lemon juice, and a pinch of salt in a blender. Purée until the mixture is uniform. Strain through a fine strainer.

Drizzle the strawberry sauce over the cheesecakes when serving.

Srv: 1 Mini Cheesecake (26 g) | Cal: 60 | Fat: 3.5 g | Sat Fat: 0 g | Col: 0 mg | Carb: 7 g | Fib: 0 g | Pro: 2 g

THE SPORK SISTERS: JENNY & HEATHER GOLDBERG

Some bitches were born to save the world. Sisters and BFFs Jenny and Heather Goldberg might have sprung from the womb in Superwoman aprons.

At an age when most college kids are making out in dorm rooms and eating crap in the school cafeteria, these sisters made the connection between the health of the planet and the destructive influence of the meat and dairy industries, and fiercely got to work. They thought the best way to stick it to the man was to be vegan, and make vegan food kick-ass. The rest, as they say, is written in the recipes.

The sisters have caused ripples in Los Angeles and beyond as they have led an army of carnivores to vegan salvation with their company, Spork Foods. A gourmet vegan food company based in Los Angeles, Spork Foods offers cooking classes, healthy-eating consultations, and small-scale catering. These crusading sisses are making healthy food delicious, while teaching people about the benefits of organic, seasonal, and local ingredients for their bods and the planet.

My love for the Spork sisters goes much further than their legendary vegan cashew cheese. I have a soft spot in my heart for these girls because they open their home to anyone. Men, women, kids, vegans, vegetarians, or meat eaters—they don't judge. Whether it's a mother-daughter duo looking to fit more plant-based foods into their weekly routine, or a boyfriend looking to cook more for his veggie girlfriend, Spork Foods' goal is to show the sexier side of the vegan diet. Learn more about Spork Foods and the dynamic duo at www.sporkfoods.com.

Nielsen-Massey Pure Vanilla Extracts

Imitation isn't always so flattering. It may look like the real thing on the outside, but on the inside, it's still a wannabe with some serious jealousy issues.

Take vanilla, for instance—the pure and imitation. On the surface, both forms are flavor activators for foods like chocolate, fruit, and nuts. But, on the inside, only one is really delivering. Scientists have found more than two hundred fifty natural flavor and aroma enhancers in real vanilla.

Though the flavor doesn't lie, pure vanilla extract wasn't always an easy find. The years and intense labor it requires to grow, ship, and convert to extract historically has made the good stuff a rare commodity.

Well, not anymore. My hands-down, all-time favorite brand for pure baking extracts, Nielsen-Massey Vanillas, has been catering to bakers with a distinguished taste since 1907. Located in Illinois, the family-owned and managed business has one game plan: to ensure you get the most from your frostings, puddings, and creamy confections.

In my household, we live, eat, and breathe their signature extract, Madagascar Bourbon Pure Vanilla. But the baking savior also purveys exotic premium blends like Tahitian Pure Vanilla and Mexican Pure Vanilla, and more versatile products like pure vanilla sugar, pastes, and whole beans.

Aside from pure vanilla, Nielsen-Massey boasts an arsenal of aromatic extracts, including coffee, chocolate, almond, lemon, orange, peppermint, orange blossom, and rose water.

All extracts are gluten-free and made from natural botanical oils in an alcohol base. Expect to pay a little more for pure extract, but if you follow the rules and use a teaspoon or two sparingly, it will prove its worth.

Nielsen-Massey pure extracts can be found at Whole Foods, specialty health food stores, and some major grocery retailers. Or purchase online at www.nielsenmassey.com

Peach Crisp

During the summer, my favorite fruits at the farmers' market are peaches. They have so many amazing health benefits, too. Peaches are a solid source of antioxidants, they are high in water and fiber to assist in the digestive process, and they boast carotenoids, which protect the eyes. Hmmm . . . should I keep going?

MAKES 6 SERVINGS

4 cups (615 g) peeled, cored, and sliced fresh peaches (about 5 to 6 peaches)

1 cup (85 g) rolled oats

1 cup (110 g) granola, homemade or store-bought

½ teaspoon salt

2 tablespoons lemon zest

1 teaspoon ground cinnamon

½ teaspoon ground nutmeg

½ cup (120 ml) brown rice syrup

⅓ cup (75 ml) coconut oil

3 tablespoons water

Preheat the oven to 350° F (180° C). Spread the peaches in a 13 x 9-inch (33 x 23 cm) baking dish.

In a large mixing bowl, combine the oats, granola, salt, lemon zest, cinnamon, and nutmeg, mixing until well combined. In a separate medium bowl, whisk together the brown rice syrup, coconut oil, and water. Stir the wet ingredients into the dry ingredients. Spoon the mixture evenly over the peaches. Bake 30 minutes, or until the top of the granola mixture is golden.

Srv: 184 g | Cal: 360 | Fat: 15 g | Sat Fat: 11 g | Col: 0 mg | Carb: 55 g | Fib: 5 g | Pro: 6 g

Amaretto Macerated Cherry and Coconut Cream Napoleons

....

When I was a little girl, I was obsessed with maraschino cherries, but needless to say, they weren't the healthiest sweet in the fridge. Good thing I found a new healthy dessert obsession. This will require some extra energy and patience to make, but you will feel like you're a prime candidate for the Food Network once you're through. Better start scouting for an agent.

MAKES 4 SERVINGS

2 (14-ounce/400 g) cans light coconut milk, refrigerated for at least 4 hours

3 tablespoons agar agar (preferably powdered)

¾ cup evaporated cane sugar plus 1 tablespoon

2 cups (560 g) frozen Bing cherries (or pitted fresh)

¼ cup (60 ml) amaretto

1 teaspoon almond extract

¼ cup (55 g) Earth Balance, melted

1 (16-ounce/455 g) box phyllo dough

½ teaspoon coconut extract

½ cup (50 g) shredded coconut, toasted

½ cup (55 g) sliced almonds, toasted

Open the refrigerated cans of coconut milk and remove the cream from the top. Spoon the cream into a small bowl and set aside. In a small saucepan, heat the remaining coconut milk and the agar agar. Whisk constantly over medium-high heat, until boiling. Once boiling, reduce the heat to medium heat and continue to whisk until the agar agar is dissolved, about 8 minutes. The agar agar may not dissolve completely, especially if you used the agar agar flakes instead of the powder, but it should be softened. Remove from the heat and transfer to a large metal bowl. Put in the freezer 10 to 15 minutes to cool. Remove the bowl from the freezer and add the reserved coconut cream coconut extract and ½ cup (65 g) of the sugar. Using an electric mixer, beat the cream mixture until it thickens. Pour the blended mixture into a fine mesh sieve or strainer, positioned over a bowl larger than the strainer. Using a spatula, press the mixture through the sieve so that the gelatin pieces remain in the sieve and the smooth coconut cream gets pushed through into the bowl. Put the bowl in the refrigerator and chill until it is thick enough to hold its shape.

Preheat the oven to 400° F (200° C). In a small saucepan, heat the cherries, the remaining ⅓ cup of the sugar, and the amaretto over medium heat, about 20 minutes. Remove from the heat and transfer to a small bowl. Stir in the almond extract. Chill in the refrigerator for 4 hours.

Using a pastry brush or a paper towel, coat the bottom and sides of a half-size cookie sheet with sides with 1 teaspoon of the melted Earth Balance. Unroll the phyllo dough and trim the stack to fit the pan. Place one sheet of the dough in the pan. Brush with a small amount of the Earth Balance. Sprinkle with a pinch of the remaining 2 tablespoons of sugar. Repeat until you have a stack of 8 layered sheets. Using a sharp knife, cut the stacked dough into four large squares, making sure to cut all the way to the bottom of the pan. Bake 15 to 20 minutes, or until golden and crisp. Remove from the oven. Maintain oven temperature.

Spread the shredded coconut on an ungreased shallow baking pan and place in the oven 5 minutes, or until just lightly toasted. Remove from the oven to cool. Spread the almonds in one layer on an ungreased shallow baking pan and toast in the oven until they are fragrant and just lightly toasted, about 10 minutes. Remove from the oven to cool. Place one piece of the sugared phyllo on a plate. Top with about 2 tablespoons of the thickened chilled pastry cream. Top with a few of the macerated cherries. Top with another phyllo square, pastry cream, and cherries. Add one more phyllo square on top. Top with a couple of the cherries. Drizzle some of the cherry juice around the plate. Sprinkle the almonds and coconut, for garnish. Repeat for the other three portions.

Srv: 379 g | Cal: 520 | Fat: 22 g | Sat Fat: 8 g | Col: 0 mg | Carb: 79 g | Fib: 4 g | Pro: 5 g

Coconut Panna Cotta

I never thought it would be possible to have such a creamy and rich vegan dessert, but here it is. A brilliant and determined chef friend of mine gave me some of her trade secrets to pull this one off. You have to refrigerate the custards for a couple hours to set, so it's a good one to make on the weekend.

MAKES 6 SERVINGS

¾ cup (180 ml) cream of coconut (like Coco Lopez)

¾ cup (180 ml) light coconut milk

¼ teaspoon coconut extract

½ packet of vegan gelatin mix, unsweetened and unflavored

2 tablespoons cold water

⅓ cup (50 g) frozen mixed berries

½ cup (120 ml) hot water (or more)

½ cup (100 g) evaporated cane sugar

1 teaspoon almond extract

5 fresh strawberries, minced, for garnish

¼ cup (25 g) toasted coconut, for garnish

> **BITCHWORTHY: VEGAN GELATIN**
> FINDING A VEGAN GELATIN TO MAKE A CUSTARD-LIKE DESSERT WAS A VERY HAPPY DAY FOR ME. LIEBER'S UNFLAVORED JEL IS AVAILABLE AT WHOLE FOODS, AND MANY NATURAL FOOD STORES, AND YOU CAN ORDER IT ONLINE AT WWW.VEGAESSENTIALS.COM

In a medium saucepan, heat the cream of coconut, coconut milk, and coconut extract to a simmer over medium-high heat. In a medium bowl, mix the gelatin and cold water together until the gelatin dissolves completely. Add the gelatin mixture to the coconut mixture and whisk, until well dissolved. Continue to simmer 3 more minutes. Pour the coconut mixture into six small ramekins and cover with plastic wrap. Refrigerate for 2 to 3 hours to set.

In a separate medium saucepan, heat the berries with the hot water over medium heat. When they are defrosted and starting to break down, add the sugar and stir until it forms a sauce. Add more hot water if necessary, one tablespoon at a time. The sauce should be slightly thick. Remove from the heat and stir in the almond extract. Strain the berry sauce to extract the seeds. Drizzle a little of the berry sauce on each serving plate. Remove the panna cotta custards from the refrigerator and run a knife or toothpick along the sides of the ramekins to loosen. Carefully turn each ramekin upside down onto a plate. Remove the ramekin and garnish with strawberries and coconut.

Srv: 1 Ramekin (155 g) | Cal: 250 | Fat: 14 g | Sat Fat: 13 g | Col: 0 mg | Carb: 33 g | Fib: 2 g | Pro: 2g

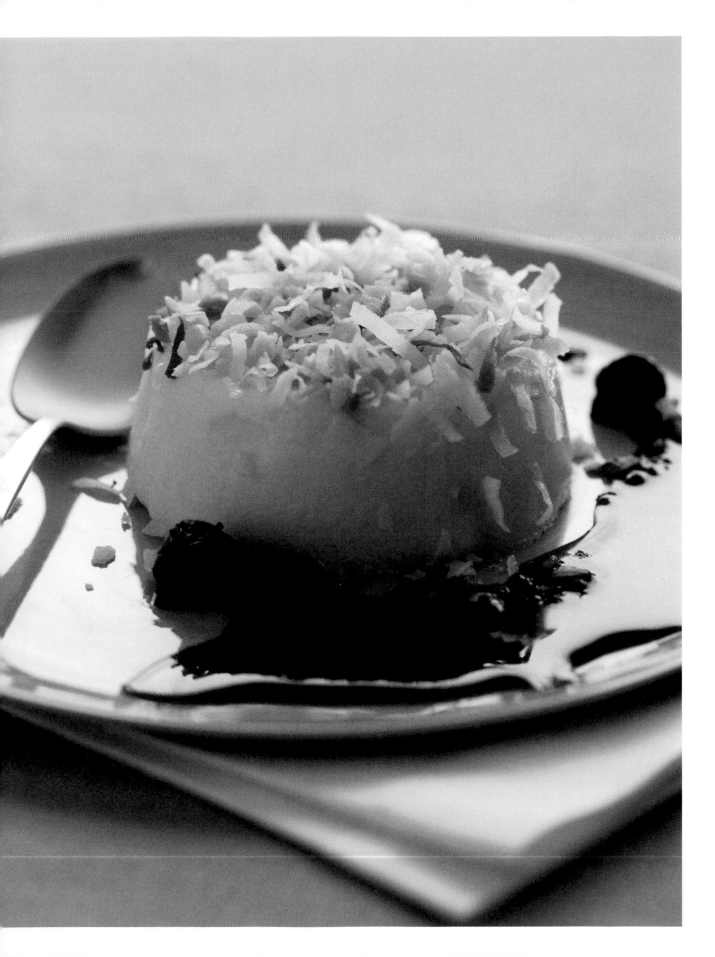

Mixed Berry Cobbler

Every summer my mom stocks the freezer in the garage with fresh berries that she has picked herself. She uses them for pies, muffins, and pancakes. Every time I make a berry cobbler it brings me back to my mom's kitchen.

MAKES 6 SERVINGS

4 cups (600 g) frozen mixed berries (raspberries, blueberries and blackberries)

½ cup (120 ml) hot water

1½ cups (300 g) evaporated cane sugar

2 cups (300 g) fresh blueberries

½ cup (65 g) vegan white or yellow cake mix

2 tablespoons dark brown sugar

1 cup (115 g) chopped pecans, toasted

6 tablespoons (55 g) Earth Balance, very cold

BITCHWORTHY: BAKE A BITCH A CAKE

LOOKING FOR A VEGAN CAKE MIX? CHECK OUT CHERRYBROOK KITCHEN FOR A SWEET TOOTH'S PARADISE OF VEGAN CAKE, COOKIE, AND BROWNIE MIXES. ALL-NATURAL CAKE MIXES ARE PEANUT, DAIRY, NUT, AND EGG-FREE. THEY EVEN CARRY FROSTINGS, WHEAT-FREE OPTIONS, AND PANCAKE MIXES. HOLD THE PHONE. PANCAKES?! WHERE'S MY DAMN CREDIT CARD. VISIT WWW.CHERRYBROOKKITCHEN.COM TO PURCHASE.

Preheat the oven to 375° F (190° C).

In a large saucepan, combine the mixed berries, water, and sugar and cook over medium heat. When the berries are defrosted and just starting to break down, add the fresh blueberries and stir until heated through. Add more water if necessary, 1 tablespoon at a time. The berries should remain whole and the sauce should be slightly thick. With a slotted spoon, divide the berries into six ramekins. Add 1 tablespoon of the sugar juice to each ramekin.

In a separate bowl, combine the cake mix and the brown sugar. Top the ramekins with ¼-inch (6 mm) layer of the cake and brown sugar mixture. Sprinkle a layer of the pecans over the cake mix. Place 1 tablespoon of the Earth Balance on top of the pecans on each ramekin. Place the ramekins on a cookie sheet and put in oven. Bake about 20 minutes, or until the topping turns golden brown and bubbly but the pecans are not burned. Remove from the heat. Serve warm with vanilla soy or coconut milk ice cream.

Srv: 1 Ramekin 196 g | Cal: 330 | Fat: 15 g | Sat Fat: 3.5 g | Col: 0 mg | Carb: 58 g | Fib: 5 g | Pro: 2 g

Lavender Shortbread Cookies

The lavender extract makes these cookies so unique. Plus, they are so easy to make. These are perfect for your fancy tea parties when you dig out your grandma's collection of expensive china teacups.

MAKES 2 DOZEN COOKIES

1 cup (225 g) Earth Balance, at room temperature
½ cup (100 g) evaporated cane sugar
2 cups (255 g) unbleached all-purpose flour
¼ teaspoon salt
1 teaspoon lavender extract

LAVENDER EXTRACT
YOU CAN FIND LAVENDER EXTRACT AT SPECIALTY KITCHEN STORES, OR ORDER IT ONLINE AT WWW.STARKAYWHITE.COM.

Using an electric mixer, beat the Earth Balance and sugar in a large bowl until fluffy, about 2 to 3 minutes. Sift in the flour, and add the salt, and lavender extract. Mix together until well combined. Place the dough onto a floured surface and roll the dough into 2 separate logs. Wrap each log in plastic wrap and chill in the refrigerator about 30 minutes.

Preheat the oven to 350° F (175° C). Remove the dough from the refrigerator, slice into ½-inch (12 mm) pieces, and transfer to a large cookie sheet. Bake 8 to 10 minutes. Remove from the oven and let cool on the cookie sheet 5 minutes. Transfer to a wire rack to cool completely.

Srv: 1 Cookie (21 g) | Cal: 110 | Fat: 7 g | Sat Fat: 3 g | Col: 0 mg | Carb: 11 g | Fib: 0 g | Pro: 1 g

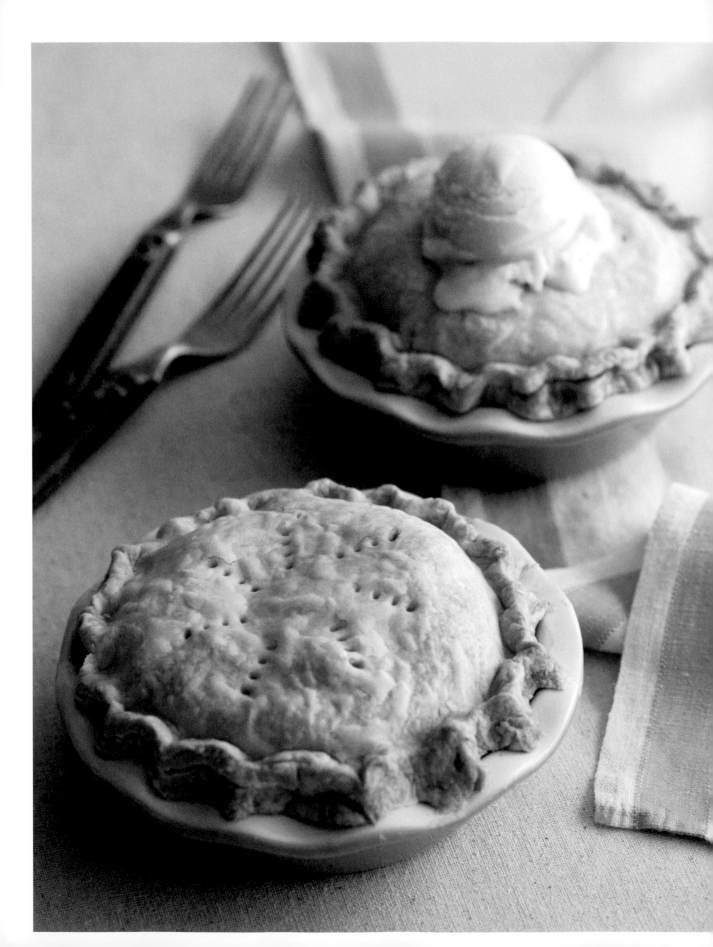

Jack's Grandma's Apple Pie

This is my favorite recipe in the entire cookbook—my mom's famous apple pie. She has been baking it for at least forty years, and can easily make it with her eyes closed.

VEGAN PIE DOUGH RECIPE

MAKES 1 PIE SHELL

You can also use this recipe to make Veggie Pot Pies (see page 211).

2 cups (255 g) unbleached all-purpose flour

1 teaspoon salt

¼ cup (60 ml) cold water, plus 7 tablespoons ice water

¾ cup (170 g) Spectrum vegetable shortening

In a large bowl, mix together the flour and salt. In a measuring cup, add ¼ cup (60 ml) of the cold water, then add the vegetable shortening to equal 1 cup (240 ml) of water and shortening combined. Lightly pack the shortening to remove air bubbles. Scoop out the shortening from the measuring cup with a spoon and add to the flour mixture, discarding the water. Using a pastry cutter, cut the shortening into the flour mixture until small flaky dough balls start to form. Add the 7 tablespoons of ice water, one tablespoon at a time, and continue mixing. You can add another tablespoon of water if your dough seems too hard. If it's too soft, chill the dough in the refrigerator for 30 minutes.

THE SKINNY: WHY DOES THE RECIPE CALL FOR ICE WATER?

ICE WATER KEEPS THE FAT CHILLED WHEN YOU'RE MAKING A PASTRY. IF THE FAT IS WARM, IT RELEASES WATER AND MOISTENS THE FLOUR MAKING YOUR PASTRY HARD AS NAILS.

PIE RECIPE

MAKES 8 SERVINGS

2 Vegan Pie Doughs (double recipe to make 2 balls of dough)

5 Granny Smith appl3es, peeled, cored, and cute into 1/4 –inch (6 mm) slices

2 Fuji apples, peeled, cored, and cut into ¼-inch (6 mm) slices

¾ cup (150 g) evaporated cane sugar

½ teaspoon ground cinnamon

½ teaspoon ground nutmeg

4 teaspoons Earth Balance

Preheat oven to 350° F (180° C)

In a large bowl, combine the apple slices, sugar, cinnamon, and nutmeg. Mix well to coat the apples. Set aside. Lightly flour a flat, clean surface and roll out one of the balls with a rolling pin. Place in a round glass pie pan. Press the dough along the edges of the pie pan. Add the apple filling, along with any juice in the bottom of the bowl. Place each teaspoon of the Earth Balance separately on top of the apples. Roll out the second ball of dough and place on top of the pie. Pinch around the edges of the pie to cover the apples and cute off any remaining long pieces of dough. Make about six ½-inch (12 mm) cuts in the top crust to release the steam during baking. Bake about 1 hour, or until the pie is bubbling. Remove from the oven. Serve warm with vanilla soy or coconut milk ice cream.

Srv: 1 Slice (208 g) | Cal: 390 | Fat: 20 g | Sat Fat: 5 g | Col: 0 mg | Carb: 53 g | Fib: 3 g | Pro: 4 g

Edible Florals

Add Some Color, Texture, and Flavor to Your Desserts

Flowers aren't just for show. Put them in your mouth, girl! Flowers can be a pretty decoration and an edible garnish for a sweet dish. As long as you are buying organic florals, a few petals or buds of some different varieties will add texture and zest for a picture-perfect dish.

LAVENDER: Therapeutic on the mind and tongue, lavender carries a sweet, floral taste with citrus notes. Lavender complements a handful of dishes ranging from stews to sorbets to chocolate cake. Add to a glass of Champagne with a pinch of fresh petals for a low-calorie, delicious treat.

DANDELION: The buds of dandelions have an almost savory, honey-like fragrance and flavor. The leaves can be steamed, sautéed, or tossed in salads, and the petals add some character to any dish. These guys are sweetest when picked young and eaten quickly, since the mature ones are bitter.

CARNATION: Usually available year-round, carnations have long been a finishing touch for wedding cakes and premium liqueur. The petals add soft, floral flavor to desserts.

ROSE: All varieties are edible with a stronger punch in the darker roses. Depending on the type, color, and the soil conditions of where they were grown, roses have a subtle taste reminiscent of green apples or strawberries and can range from fruity to minty to spicy. Ideal for syrups, jams, ice cream, salads, and beverages. *Note: Remove the bitter white portion of the petals.*

PEONY: Add peony petals to a summer salad, water, lemonades, iced or hot tea, and punches for a bit of freshness. In China, the petals are a delicacy for tea time.

SIP ON THIS: FREEZE SOME PETALS WITH WATER IN AN ICE CUBE TRAY TO GIVE BEVERAGES A FRESH, FLORAL KICK. PERFECT FOR THOSE HOT SUMMER DAYS BY THE POOL.

■ Follow a few dos and don'ts when it comes to snacking on flowers.

Not all florals are edible. Some can actually make you very sick. Do your research before you start feasting on the flower garden.

Remove the pistils and stamens and wash thoroughly before adding to your plate.

Make sure there were no pesticides used in the growth process.

Introduce into your diet in small quantities to make sure you have no allergies and your digestive system approves.

Coconut Macaroons

Macaroons have always felt like a heavy snack, but these Coconut Macaroons are so light and fluffy. These are great as housewarming gifts or for welcoming new neighbors. A little brownnosing never hurt anyone.

MAKES 3 DOZEN COOKIES

⅓ cup (75 g) Earth Balance
¾ cup (150 g) evaporated cane sugar
2 tablespoons EnerG-Egg Replacer
3 tablespoons warm water
1 cup (95 g) sweetened coconut flakes
4 ounces (115 g) chopped bittersweet chocolate

BITCHIONARY: DOUBLE-BOILER
A NIFTY PIECE OF KITCHEN EQUIPMENT THAT CONSISTS OF TWO FITTED SAUCEPANS. THE LARGER SAUCEPAN IS PARTIALLY FILLED WITH WATER BROUGHT TO A SIMMER OR BOIL, WHILE THE INNER SAUCEPAN USES THE HEAT TO MELT CHOCOLATE, AND COOK CUSTARDS OR SAUCES. IMPROVISING TRICK: CREATE YOUR OWN "DOUBLE-BOILER" BY USING A LARGE SAUCEPAN AND A METAL BOWL.

In a medium saucepan, add the Earth Balance and the sugar and cook over medium heat, stirring constantly, until the butter is melted. Remove from the heat and transfer to a medium-size bowl and set aside.

In a small bowl, whisk together the egg replacer and water until fluffy. Add to the Earth Balance mixture and beat with an electric mixer until all of the ingredients are fluffy, about 2 minutes. Stir in the coconut flakes. Place the batter in the freezer and allow to chill for 15 minutes.

Preheat the oven to 400° F (200° C). Remove the batter from the freezer and roll into small mounds. Lightly oil a cookie sheet and place the small mounds on the cookie sheet. Bake 10 to 12 minutes, or until the coconut starts to become light brown on the sides. Remove from the oven and allow to cool 5 minutes on a cookie sheet. Transfer to a wire rack to cool completely.

Melt the chopped chocolate in a double boiler. When the cookies are cooled, drizzle the melted chocolate over the tops or dip the bottoms into the melted chocolate.

Srv: 1 Cookie (19 g) | Cal: 90 | Fat: 6 g | Sat Fat: 3.5 g | Col: 0 mg | Carb: 10 g | Fib: 1 g | Pro: 1 g

Pistachio and Cardamom Cookies

....

Pistachio and cardamom are two ingredients that were destined for one other. Their flavors complement each other just right. Cardamom is one of those exotic spices that make you feel like you are a world traveler. Warning: These cookies may provide unexpected bouts of giddiness.

MAKES 3 DOZEN COOKIES

1 cup (225 g) Earth Balance, at room temperature

¾ cup (150 g) evaporated cane sugar

1 teaspoon vanilla extract

¼ cup (60 ml) almond milk

1 teaspoon lemon zest, finely grated

⅓ cup (40 g) chopped pistachio nuts

2⅔ (335 g) cups unbleached all-purpose flour

2 teaspoons ground cardamom

Using an electric mixer, beat the Earth Balance and the sugar in a large bowl until fluffy, about 2 to 3 minutes. Add the vanilla and beat until combined. Stir in the milk, lemon zest, and pistachios until combined. Sift in the flour and the cardamom. Mix with a wooden spoon to form a soft dough. Cover with plastic wrap and refrigerate 30 minutes.

Preheat the oven to 350° F (180° C). Remove the mixture from the refrigerator and make tablespoon-size dough balls. Place the dough balls on a cookie sheet 1½-inches (4 cm) apart. Flatten lightly with fingers and bake 13 to 15 minutes, or until lightly golden. Remove from the oven and let sit on the cookie sheet for 5 minutes. Transfer to a wire rack to cool completely.

....

Srv: 1 Cookie 30 g | Cal: 140 | Fat: 8g | Sat Fat: 3 g | Col: 0 mg | Carb: 16 g | Fib: 1 g | Pro: 2 g

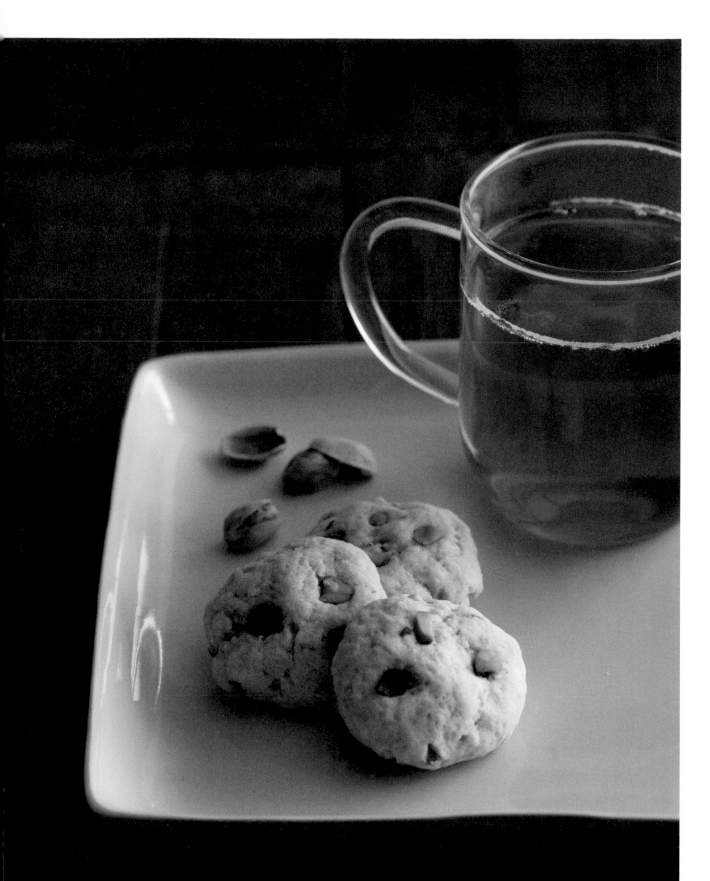

Buttercream Frosting

This is a great go-to frosting for cupcakes, cakes, and cookies. It's a vegan twist on my lovely grandmother's Christmas cookie frosting. I practically camped out at the mailbox as a kid waiting for her cookies to come in the mail. A thin layer of this frosting can be used for decorating sugar cookies, too.

MAKES 1½ CUPS

2 cups (200 g) confectioners' sugar
¼ cup (55 g) Earth Balance, at room temperature
1½ teaspoons vanilla extract
3 tablespoons almond milk

Using an electric mixer, beat the sugar and the Earth Balance in a medium bowl until fluffy, 3 to 4 minutes. Add the vanilla and the almond milk and beat for an additional 2 minutes.

Srv: 28 g | Cal: 110 | Fat: 3.5 g | Sat Fat: 1.5 g | Col: 0 mg | Carb: 20 g | Fib: 0 g | Pro: 0 g

Variation: Lemon Buttercream Frosting

MAKES 1½ CUPS

2 cups (200 g) confectioners' sugar
¼ cup (55 g) Earth Balance, at room temperature
3 tablespoons freshly squeezed lemon juice
1 teaspoon finely grated lemon peel

Using an electric mixer, beat the sugar and the Earth Balance in a medium bowl until fluffy, 3 to 4 minutes. Add the lemon juice and lemon peel, and beat an additional 2 minutes.

Srv: 28 g | Cal: 110 | Fat: 3.5 g | Sat Fat: 1.5 g | Col: 0 mg | Carb: 20 g | Fib: 0 g | Pro: 0 g

Peanut Butter Frosting

When paired with anything chocolate, this is divine!

MAKES 1½ CUPS

2 cups (200 g) confectioners' sugar
¼ cup (65 g) organic creamy peanut butter
1 teaspoon vanilla extract
¼ cup (60 ml) almond milk

Using an electric mixer, beat together the confectioners' sugar and the peanut butter in a medium bowl until creamy. Add the vanilla and almond milk, and beat an additional 2 minutes.

Srv: 30 g | Cal: 110 | Fat: 3 g | Sat Fat: 0 g | Col: 0 mg | Carb: 21 g | Fib: 0 g | Pro: 1 g

ALMOND MILK: AGE DEIFIER
VITAMINS A AND E IN ALMOND MILK HELP LUBRICATE, TONE, AND SOFTEN THE SKIN TO FIGHT OFF DRYNESS AND THE EFFECTS OF AGING. ITS HIGH CONCENTRATION OF ESSENTIAL FATTY ACIDS ALSO HELPS TO REGULATE OIL TO WARD OFF ACNE AND BLACKHEADS.[129]

DRINKS

Basic Smoothie-On-the-Go

Fruitastic. **There is a melting pot of berries and fruits in this yummy smoothie. Plus, the raved-about superfood, açai berry, has anti-aging abilities and helps with weight loss.**

MAKES 2 SERVINGS

⅔ cup (165 ml) chilled orange juice

1 (6-ounce/170 g) container vanilla soy yogurt

½ cup (70 g) frozen strawberries

1 banana, sliced

¼ teaspoon pure vanilla extract

1 tablespoon ground açai powder

Put all of the ingredients in a blender and blend until well combined. Serve immediately.

Srv: 263 g | Cal: 210 | Fat: 2 g | Sat Fat: 0 g | Col: 0 mg | Carb: 45 g | Fib: 2 g | Pro: 5 g

Jackie's Energy Booster

MAKES 2 SERVINGS

1 handful fresh spinach

1 cup (150 g) sliced bananas

1 scoop (1 ounce/30 g) soy protein powder

2 tablespoons flaxseed oil

¼ cup (60 ml) water

¼ cup (35 ml) ice cubes

Put all of the ingredients in a blender and blend until ice cubes are all crushed and the ingredients are well combined and creamy. Serve immediately.

Srv: 168 g | Cal: 220 | Fat: 14 g | Sat Fat: 1.5 g | Col: 0 mg | Carb: 18 g | Fib: 3 g | Pro: 9 g

BITCH I LOVE: JACKIE WARNER

Jackie Warner is the busiest bitch I know. Between running her Beverly Hills-based sports medicine and fitness club, and starring in her own reality TV series on Bravo, I have no idea how the woman even finds time to sleep. And that's just half her day. Tag on overseeing her own fitness apparel line, a workout DVD series, and a protein shake and energy-bar brand, and Jackie has somehow found a way to fit 72 hours into a 24-hour workday. And I thought I had my shit together.

But no matter how much you want to hate her, Jackie didn't just get lucky. Success didn't fall into her pretty little lap. She wasn't just on the right treadmill at the right time. No, ladies. This success story can be credited to good old-fashioned blood, sweat, and tears—the entrepreneur's American dream. A small-town Midwestern girl moves to Los Angeles to show the fitness industry that heavy lifting isn't just a job reserved for a man. Give her a tougher task.

On top of her crazy schedule, Jackie's also committed herself to creating new opportunity for those suffering from financial burdens and obesity. She has fought the system to get gym memberships and exercise therapy covered under traditional medical insurance plans. Additionally, Jackie has introduced SkyLab, a weeklong life camp where she coaches overweight clients on exercise, proper nutrition, and sustaining goals in the real world.

I don't know how Jackie does it. But she does. And in the thick of it, she even finds a way to look hot as hell in sweaty gym clothes. I'll say it now, and I'll say it again. I may be a one-man woman, but if I ever decide to bat for the other team, Jackie, I know just where to find you.

Learn more at www.jackiewarner.com.

HEALTHY, ALL-NATURAL
SODA POPS
THAT MAKE ME GO MMMM

Every once in a while, when I'm feeling crazy, I want to do something really daring. I'm talking something completely out of my norm. Something that would make my husband gasp and send the babysitter running home crying to her mother. Something that reminds me I'm a wild, wacky bitch, and the family minivan is just a cover.

Maybe . . . something with an aluminum tab.

Forget piercing my belly button or adding some hot pink color streaks to my hair. What better way to show people I'm bonkers than to drink a soda? Hold your horses. I'm not talking about a diet soda or iced tea in a can. What do I look like, a raging lunatic?

I'm talking about all-natural, artificial- and preservative-free sodas. They may be tough to find in this wild, wild world of ours, but honey, as long as I've had my eight glasses of water for the day, I'm up for anything. Get ready to live a little.

ZEVIA All-Natural Zero Calorie Soda: Zevia contains only pure ingredients, with no artificial sweeteners, flavors, or colors. It satisfies your thirst with zero calories, zero net carbs, and little to no sodium. Plus, it's sweetened with Stevia (doesn't contain aspartame). It comes in flavors like orange, cola, twist, root beer, and black cherry. Available at Whole Foods, specialty health food stores, and some major grocery retailers. www.zevia.com

DRY SODA: This soda option doesn't only call my name in an über-modern bottle, but it's all-natural and flavored with fruit, flower, and herb extracts. Each bottle contains only forty-five to seventy calories and is sweetened with a small dose of pure cane sugar. Available at Whole Foods and other health food stores. www.drysoda.com

IZZE SPARKLING JUICE: If it's the taste you're looking for, Izze contains pure fruit juice, no refined sugars, caffeine, or preservatives, and no artificial colors or flavors. It is low in calories and comes in delicious flavors like pomegranate, peach, apple, clementine, grapefruit, and blueberry. Available at major retailers like Whole Foods, Target, and Starbuck's Coffee. www.izze.com

GUS (GROWN-UP SODA): GuS is 100-percent all-natural, kosher, and made with real juices and extracts. No preservatives or caffeine. Sweetened with natural cane sugar and sealing the deal at only ninety to ninety-eight calories per bottle. www.drinkgus.com

HOT LIPS SODA: Real fruit soda pop filtered with pure cane sugar and organic lemon juice, Hot Lips contains no supplements, artificial flavors, concentrates, or corn syrup. Even the bottles are locally manufactured from 80 percent recycled glass. www.hotlipssoda.com

---

THE SKINNY: THE UGLY TRUTH ABOUT DIET SODA

How's this for a tall glass of shut the hell up? Diet soda is gross. It contains an artificial sweetener called aspartame, which is broken down into phenylalanine, aspartic acid, and methanol. (P.S. When ingested, methanol converts to formaldehyde in the body—an embalming fluid and dangerous neurotoxin. Yuck.) Aspartame has triggered class-action lawsuits and victim support groups, with states like New Mexico and Hawaii attempting to get it banned.[130] Put it down already . . . you're too pretty to hold that can.

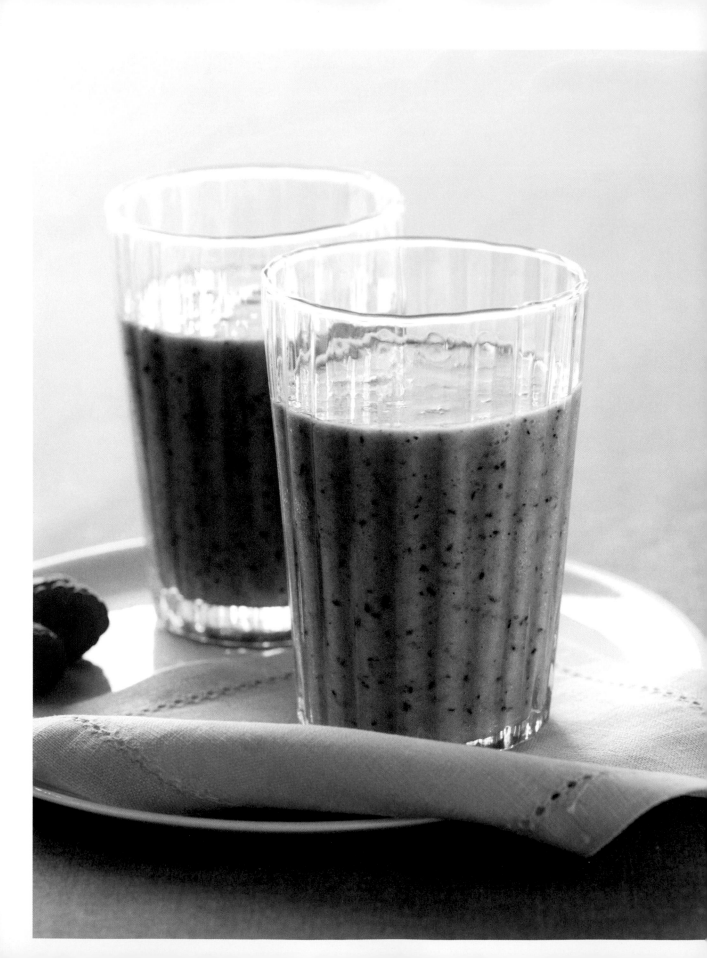

Wake-Up Smoothie

Skip the cup of coffee, and get your energy from a nutrient-rich morning shake. It's also a great snack after working out. Wheat germ packs a punch with folic acid, iron, and zinc, while the flaxseeds provide the omega-3 fatty acids.

MAKES 2 SERVINGS

1 (6-ounce/170 g) container vanilla soy yogurt
½ cup (120 ml) chilled orange juice
½ cup (80 g) frozen blueberries
1 banana, sliced
2 tablespoons wheat germ
1 tablespoon flaxseed oil or ground flaxseeds

Put all of the ingredients in a blender and blend until well combined. Serve immediately.

Srv: 256 g | Cal: 270 | Fat: 10 g | Sat Fat: 0.5 g | Col: 0 mg | Carb: 40 g | Fib: 5 g | Pro: 6 g

Nutty Monkey

The Nutty Monkey is similar to a breakfast sandwich I get at a little café in Venice Beach, but the world has enough breakfast sandwiches. I decided to make it into a smoothie! It's the adult version of a PB&J. Enjoy.

MAKES 2 SERVINGS

1 cup (240 ml) almond milk
1 frozen banana, cut into chunks
¼ cup (65 g) organic creamy peanut butter
2 tablespoons whole, raw almonds
1 teaspoon wheat germ
2 tablespoons all-natural strawberry jam

Put all of the ingredients in a blender and blend until well combined. Serve immediately.

Srv: 229 g | Cal: 350 | Fat: 22 g | Sat Fat: 4 g | Col: 0 mg | Carb: 32 g | Fib: 6 g | Pro: 11 g

Peach Delight

A light-hearted pick-me-up to make you feel just peachy.

MAKES 2 SERVINGS

¼ cup (55 g) silken tofu
½ cup (120 ml) chilled orange juice
¼ cup (60 ml) peach-coconut yogurt
2 peaches, peeled and sliced
1 tablespoon flaxseed oil
Ground nutmeg, to taste

Put all of the ingredients in a blender and blend until well combined. Serve immediately.

Srv: 301 g | Cal: 210 | Fat: 9 g | Sat Fat: 0.5g | Col: 0 mg | Carb: 31 g | Fib: 3 g | Pro: 4 g

Green Dream

This is the powerhouse of juices. If you have a juicer, you should treat yourself to this once a week to get a hefty dose of your essential nutrients. The apples and cherries soften the green veggies and the ginger brings the heat.

MAKES 2 SERVINGS

4 kale leaves
1 Fuji apple
½ cucumber
2 celery stalks
1 large lemon
Handful of cherries, pitted
1 teaspoon fresh ginger, sliced

Thoroughly rinse all of the ingredients. Juice all the ingredients in a juicer. Serve immediately.

Srv: 292 g | Cal: 90 | Fat: 0.5 g | Sat Fat: 0 g | Col: 0 mg | Carb: 22 g | Fib: 4 g | Pro: 2 g

Antioxidant Sangria

Toast, ladies. This refreshing red sangria is full of all the right stuff. Heart-healthy *resveratrol* in red wine, the one-two punch of açai and pomegranate in potent antioxidants, and plenty of vitamins and minerals from fresh, seasonal fruit. Okay, just one glass.

MAKES 2 SERVINGS

3 watermelon chunks
8 blueberries
½ ounce (15 ml) agave nectar
1 ounce (30 ml) VeeV Açaí Spirit (see page 291)
¾ ounce (20 ml) pomegranate juice, such as POM Wonderful
2 ounces (60 ml) red wine
Seasonal fruit, for garnish

Muddle the watermelon, blueberries, and agave nectar in the bottom of a bar glass. Add the VeeV, pomegranate juice, and red wine. Shake well with ice. Strain into 2 ice-filled rocks glasses and garnish with seasonal fresh fruit.

Srv: 178 g | Cal: 170 | Fat: 0 g | Sat Fat: 0 g | Col: 0 mg | Carb: 21 g | Fib: 1 g | Pro: 0 g

Minty Cantaloupe Surprise

The combination of the cantaloupe and fresh mint in this drink is definitely a surprise. Truly refreshing.

MAKES 2 SERVINGS

½ cantaloupe, seeded, peeled, and chopped into cubes
½ cup (120 ml) chilled orange juice
1 cup (155 g) fresh or frozen peaches
¼ cup (25 g) finely chopped fresh mint leaves

Place all of the ingredients in a blender and blend until well combined. Serve immediately.

Srv: 282 g | Cal: 140 | Fat: 0.5 g | Sat Fat: 0 g | Col: 0 mg | Carb: 30 g | Fib: 5 g | Pro: 4 g

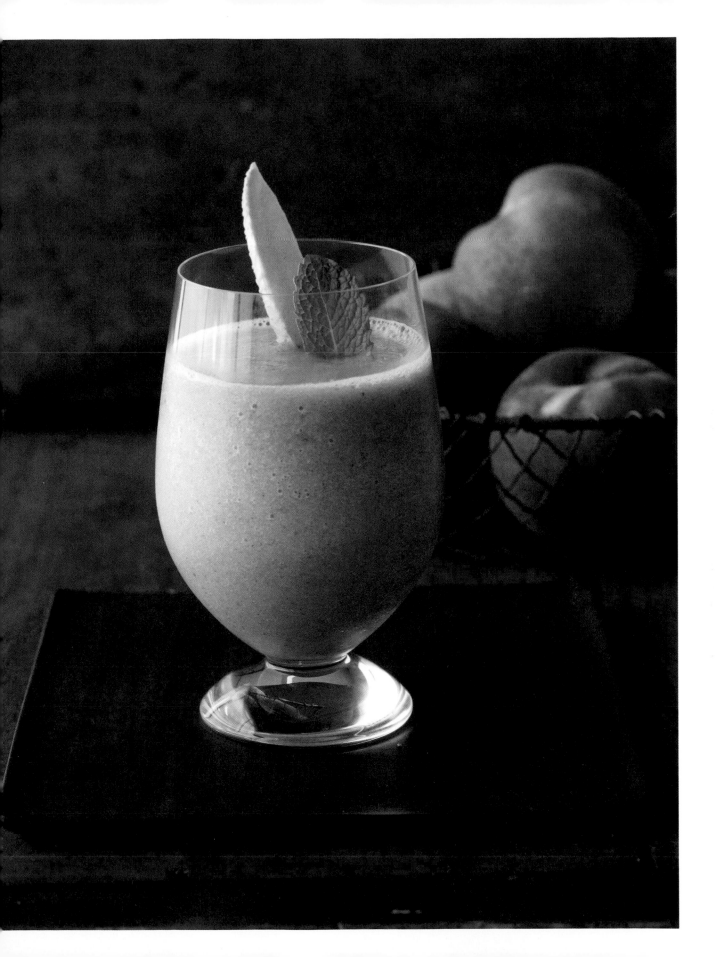

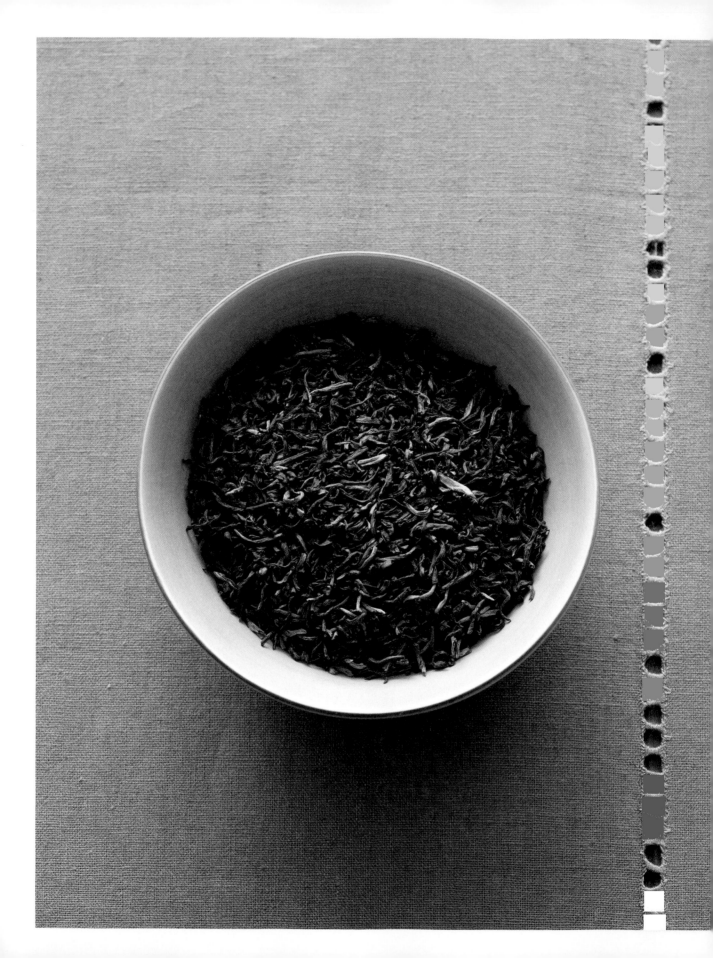

My Cup of Tea | The Healing Powers of Nature's Antioxidant Beverage

Real bitches drink tea. If you don't know your antioxidant count from your loose-leafs, well, I hate to pull the fine china out from under you, Ms. Thang. You ain't worth your crumpets in tea bags.

If you want to impress Mum at the next gathering, I suggest you push the term coffee break out of your high-brow vocabulary for a moment, and get acquainted with a handful of some of the healthiest teas in the pantry. Coffee was never your cup of tea, anyway.

GREEN TEA: Green tea is pulling plenty of antioxidants and high in a very powerful polyphenol called *catechin*. Catechins are thought to be responsible for green tea's cancer-fighting properties, which may protect against a slew of cancers, including those of the bladder, colon, esophagus, pancreas, rectum, and stomach. Green tea also helps to protect against cardiovascular disease, lowers LDL ("bad") cholesterol and blood sugar, and triggers the release of the "feel-good" chemical, dopamine. And for those who think the coffee diet is a smart way to shed that double chin, think again. Green tea helps burn some major calories.

BLACK TEA: Carrying similar anticancer properties to green tea, black tea helps reduce the production of total and LDL ("bad") cholesterol, and lowers triglycerides associated with cardiovascular disease. Black tea also cuts your risk of heart attack and stroke by improving blood vessel function.[132]

BITCHWORTHY: To get the amount of antioxidants found in two cups of black tea, you'd have to drink one glass of red wine, seven glasses of orange juice and twenty glasses of apple juice. Hope you're sitting close to the potty. [133]

CHAMOMILE TEA: A must-have in my household, chamomile tea is a great reliever for cramps, irritable bowel syndrome, insomnia, anxiety, and the stomach flu. Overworked and exhausted? Steep a chamomile tea bag in warm water for five minutes, let cool to room temperature, lay on your eyes, and relax.

WHITE TEA: Let me let you in on a little secret. White tea packs more antioxidants than any other tea. It is also the least processed of the crew and higher in polyphenols. White tea helps to strengthen bones; aids in detoxification; promotes healthy teeth, gums, and skin; and acts as an antibacterial.

MINT TEA: Mint tea is one of the best herbs for the digestive system. Sip a cup to calm belly aches, combat gas, relax stomach muscles, and keep your system free of bad bacteria. Mint tea also relaxes your nervous system to ward off stress and anxiety. If you feel a cold coming on, the mint herb is a pro at relieving flu symptoms.[134]

The Pink Fizzy

Yes, this *Skinny Bitch* is saying "Let's Drink Ladies"! Everyone has something to celebrate on occasion, and when you do, look no further. The juices blend so well with the sparkling wine, and you get a healthy dose of pomegranates.

MAKES 4 SERVINGS

Handful of pomegranate seeds
½ cup (120 ml) pomegranate juice
½ cup (120 ml) pink grapefruit juice
1 cup (240 ml) sparkling wine,
  such as Champagne

Divide the handful of pomegranate seeds among 4 Champagne flutes. In a large measuring cup, add the pomegranate and pink grapefruit juices and stir until mixed. Pour 2 ounces of the juice into each Champagne flute. Top each glass with 2 ounces of sparkling wine.

Srv: 1 Glass (4 oz) | Cal: 90 | Fat: 0 g | Sat Fat: 0 g | Col: 0 mg | Carb: 10 g | Fib: 1 g | Pro: 1 g

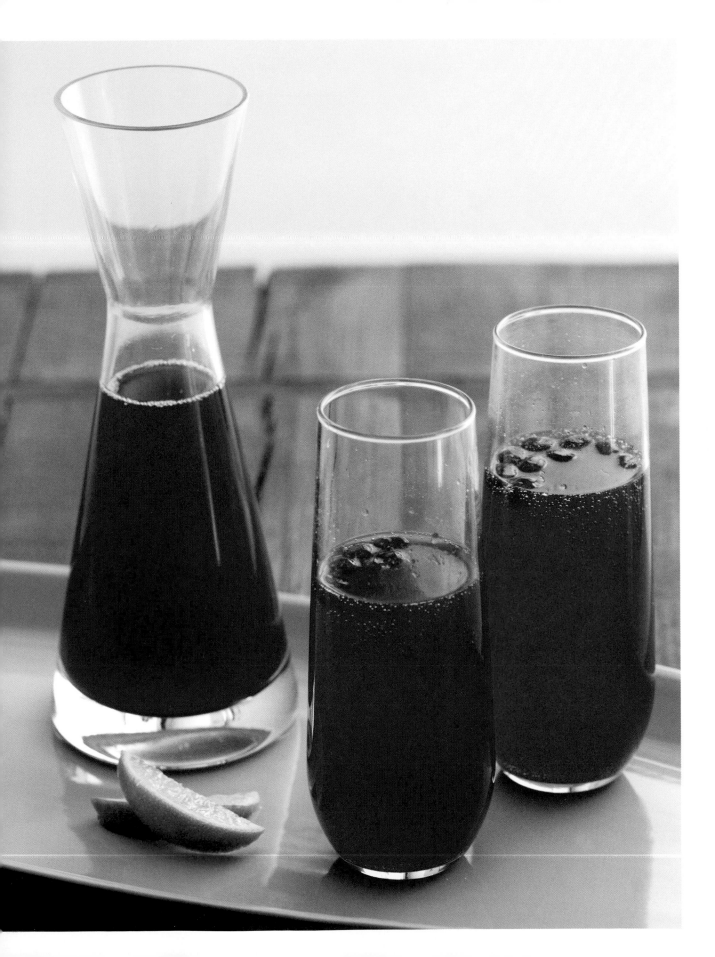

Skinny Lemonade

The Skinny Lemonade is perfect for lounging poolside with girlfriends. And since it comes in at just under 100 calories per serving, it looks like you may be able to show off that new bikini, too.

SERVES 2

1½ ounces (45 ml) VeeV Açaí Spirit
½ ounce (15 ml) agave nectar
2 lemon wedges
Club soda
Lemon wedges, for garnish

Combine the VeeV and agave nectar in a shaker filled with ice; squeeze in the juice from the lemon wedges and shake well. Strain into 2 ice-filled rocks glasses and top with club soda. Garnish with lemon wedges.

Srv: 85 g | Cal: 95 | Fat: 0 g | Sat Fat: 0 g | Col: 0 mg | Carb: 5 g | Fib: 0 g | Pro: 0 g

VEEV—THE WORLD'S FIRST AÇAI SPIRIT

Let's face it. We all need a cocktail every now and then. But, rather than convince yourself that the vodka and soda you're chugging has cancer-fightin' benefits (you've had seven for heaven's sake), why not pour yourself something that actually does support a healthy cause.

Introducing the world's first açai spirit, Veev. Made with the nutrition world's most buzzed-about superfood, Veev contains 100-percent all-natural ingredients like prickly pear and acerola cherry. The spirit prides itself on 57 percent more antioxidants than pomegranates, and thirty times more heart-healthy anthocyanins than red wine. Somebody grab me a coaster.

As an environmental front runner, Veev is a carbon-neutral company and the only distillery in the world to get their power through renewable wind energy. They have a good heart, too. One dollar of every bottle sold is given back to the Brazilian rainforest—right where the beautiful little açai berry comes from. The money benefits the Sustainable açai Project, which goes directly to the farming communities that harvest the acaí berries, and protects surrounding flora and biodiversity.

With hints of exotic berries, Veev tastes great on the rocks or with a low-calorie option like soda water. But I suggest you take advantage of the Antioxidant Sangria and The Skinny Lemonade, created for my favorite Skinny Bitches by the guys at Veev.

You can purchase Veev online at www.bevmo.com or www.southernwine.com.

SOURCES CONSULTED

"About Local Harvest." Aboutlocalharvest.org, accessed Nov. 2, 2009. http://www.localharvest.org/about.jsp

"Almonds, Soaked and Dehydrated." Shapeyou.com, accessed Dec. 5, 2009. http://www.shapeyou.com/award_products/display/almonds_soaked_dehydrated

"Anti Depression Foods." Myfit.ca, accessed Feb. 2, 2010. http://www.myfit.ca/anti-depression-foods.asp

"Aphrodisiac Foods." Gourmetsleuth.com, accessed Nov. 20, 2009. http://www.gourmetsleuth.com/Articles/Nutrition-Health-Food_Labeling-646/aphrodisiac-foods.aspx

"Aspartame: What is the negative side?." Medicinenet.com, accessed Oct. 2, 2009. http://www.medicinenet.com/artificial_sweeteners?page8.htm

Barley, Lisa "White Bread vs. Wheat Bread." Vegetariantimes.com, accessed Oct. 14, 2009. http://www.vegetariantimes.com/features/editors_picks/389

"Bell Peppers." Worldshealthiestfoods.com, accessed Jan. 4, 2010. http://www.whfoods.com/genpage.php?tname=foodspice&dbid=50

Bitten, Mark "Real Food Can Be Cheaper Than Junk Food." *The New York Times* on the Web, accessed Nov. 20, 2009 http://bitten.blogs.nytimes.com/2009/05/29/real-food-can-be-cheaper-than-junk-food/

"Black Tea or Green Tea—Which is Healthier?" About.com, accessed Dec. 4, 2009. http://chinesefood.about.com/library/weekly/aa021103a.htm

Blumenthl, Brett. "10 Worst Food Additives & Where They Lurk" Gaiam Life, accessed Dec. 2, 2009. http://life.gaiam.com/gaiam/p/10-Worst-Food-Additives-Where-They-Lurk.html

Bose, Debopriya. "Table Salt vs Sea Salt-Difference Between Sea Salt and Table Salt."

Bowden, Jonny Ph.D., C.N.S. *The 150 Healthiest Foods on Earth*. Massachusetts: Fair Winds Press, 2007.

Brodsky, Ruthan. "4 Food Additives to Avoid" Ezinearticles.com, Oct. 25, 2009. Accessed Jan. 20, 2010. http://ezinearticles.com/?4-Food-Additives-to-Avoid&id=3150881

Burke, Cindy. *To Buy or Not To Buy Organic*. New York: Marlowe & Company, 2007.

Buzzle.com, accessed Dec. 4, 2009. http://www.buzzle.com/articles/table-salt-vs-sea-salt-difference-between-sea-salt-and-table -salt.html

Campbell, T. Colin, and Thomas M. Campbell II, *The China Study*. Texas: BenBella Books, 2006.

"Carbon Footprint Calculator: What's My Carbon Footprint?" Nature.org, accessed Jan. 2, 2010. http://www.nature.org/initiatives/climatechange/calculator/

"Choosing the right cooking oil." Pccnaturalmarkets.com, accessed Nov. 8, 2009. http://pccnaturalmarkets.com/guides/tips_cooking_oils.html

Clark, Donna. "Evaporated Cane Juice. A Healthier Way to Sweeten Your Food" Brightbulb.com, Aug. 7, 2009. Accessed Dec. 11, 2009. http://www.brighthub.com/health/diet-nutrition/articles/45020.aspx

"Climate Change Mitigation" Sekala.net, accessed Jan. 22, 2010. http://www.sekala.net/guidance.php?cnt=International&lang=English&mlD=2&clD=33

Craven, Jackie. "What is Feng Shui? Architects and designers find inspiration in ancient Eastern ideas." About.com. Accessed Dec. 23, 2009. http://architecture.about.com/cs/fengshui/a/fengshui.htm

Dalelden, George. "1100 + Antioxidant-Rich Foods Studied and Ranked." Suite101.com, Oct. 8, 2009. Accessed Dec. 14, 2009. http://food-facts.suite101.com/article.cfm/a_ranking_of_antioxidanr_values_of_foods

Damato, Ph.D, Dr. Gregory. "GM-Soy Destroy the Earth and Humans for Profit." Naturalnews.com, May 27, 2009. Accessed Jan. 23, 2010. http://www.naturalnews.com/026334_soy_Roundup_GMO.html

"Dangerous food additives that should be avoided." Vitalearthminerals.com, accessed Jan. 3, 2010. http://www.vitalearthminerals.com/v/articles/dangerous_food_additives.html

"Definition of Free Radicals." Antioxidant-health-benefits.com http://www.antioxidants-health-benefits.com/definition-of-free-radicals.html

"Dictionary-Soy Sauce." Answers.com, accessed Oct. 20, 2009. http://www.answers.com/topic/soy-sauce

"Diet and Physical Activity: What's the Cancer Connection?" Cancer.org, Oct. 22, 2009. Accessed Jan. 5, 2010. http://www.cancer.org/docroot/PED/content/PED_3_1x_Link_Between_Lifestyle_and_CancerMarch03.asp

"Directory of Less Refined Sweeteners", Care2.com, accessed March 20. http://www.care2.com/channels/holidays/sweeteners.html

Earle, " Declining Ocean Biodiversity." Globalissues.org, Feb. 2009. Accessed Jan. 25, 2010. http://www.globalissues.org/article/171/loss-of-biodiversity-and-extinctions#DecliningOceanBiodiversity

"Fact Sheet: Climate Change and Intensive Livestock Production." Beyondfactoryfarming.org, accessed Nov. 30, 2009. http://www.beyondfactoryfarming.org/files/climatechange2.pdf

"Factory Farming." Farmforward.org, accessed Dec. 1, 2009. http://www.farmforward.com/farming-forward/factory-farming

"Facts about Pollution From Livestock Farms." National Resources Defense Council, accessed Dec. 20, 2009. http://www.nrdc.org/water/pollution/ffarms.asp

"FDA Should Ban Potassium Bromate and Bromated Flour" Nowpublic.com, April 29, 2009. Accessed Feb. 3, 2010. http://www.nowpublic.com/health/fda-should-ban-pitassium-bromate-and-bromated-flour

"Feed." Sustainabletable.org, accessed Nov. 20, 2009.
http://www.sustainabletable.org/issues/feed/

"Feng Shui Kitchen Made Easy." Crystalsbay.net, accessed Feb. 8, 2010.
http://www.crystalsbay.net/feng-shui-kitchen.html

"Fight Climate Change with Diet Change." Goveg.com, accessed Dec. 2, 2009.
http://www.goveg.com/environment-globalWarming.asp

"Fight Global Warming with Food." Environmental Defense Fund, July 28, 2009. Accessed Feb. 2, 2010,
http://www.edf.org/article.cfm?contentid=6604

"5 Ways Your Breakfast Affects Your Mood." Stanford-wellsphere.com, Sept. 7, 2009. Accessed Jan. 9, 2010.
http://stanford.wellsphere.com/general-medicine-article/5-ways-your-breakfast-affects-your-mood/790946

Foer, Jonathan Safran. *Eating Animals*, New York: Little, Brown and Company, 2009.

"Frequently Asked Questions." soyfoods.org
http://www.soyfoods.org/health/faq

"From Field To Feedlot To Fork: The Impacts of Meat and Dairy on Global Warming." Coolfoodscampaign.org, accessed Dec. 20, 2009.
http://coolfoodscampaign.org/your-tools/global-warming-and-your-food/from-field-to-feedlot-to-fork/

Geagan, Kate. *Go Green, Get Lean*. New York: Rodale Books, 2009.

"Global Warming." Global-warming-truth.com, accessed Jan. 15, 2009.
http://www.global-warming-truth.com/global-warming/

"Green Tea." University of Maryland Medical Center, Umm.edu, accessed Jan. 28, 2010.
http://www.umm.edu/altmed/articles/green-tea-000255.htm

Goodland and Anhang, "Livestock and Climate Change: What if the key actors in Climate Change are. . .cows, pigs, and chickens?" Meatthefacts.org, Nov. 5, 2009. Accessed Feb. 10, 2010.
http://meatthefacts.org/wp/category/urgency/

"Global climatic change and environmental crisis and its solution." Psrast.org, accessed Nov. 25, 2009.
http://www.psrast.org/globecolcr.htm

Goodwin-Nguyen, Sarah. "Vegetarianism is Good for the Environment: How Reducing Meat, Fish, and Poultry Consumption Helps the Planet." Suite101.com, July 6 2009; accessed Jan. 29, 2010.
http://ecosystem-preservation.suite101.com/article.cfm?why_vegetarianism_is_good_for_the_environment

Group, Dr. Edward. "The Health Benefits of Olive Oil." Globalhealing-center.com, Dec. 29, 2008. Accessed Jan. 20, 2010.
http://www.globalhealingcenter.com/natural-health/benefits-of-olive-oil/

"Health Effects of Cut Flower Pesticides: What the Studies Show." Organicconsumers.org, Feb. 2006. Accessed Jan. 5, 2010.
http://www.organicconsumers.org/valentines/flower-studies.pdf

"Healthy Nutritious Super Foods for Perfect Health." Knol.google.com, accessed Jan. 5, 2010.
http://knol.google.com/k/yogesh-gupts/healthy-nutritious-super-foods-for/94kytesywpfk/24#

Heppard, Cheryl. "Foods for Brain Health. A Healthy Brain Depends on Healthy Eating." Suite101.com, Feb. 14, 2010. Accessed Feb. 20, 2010.
http://vitamins-minerals.suite101.com/article.cfm/build-your-brain-with-superfoods

"How do I know if something is organic?" Organic.org, accessed Nov. 1, 2009.
http://www.organic.org/home/faq

"How Healthful is Soy?" Thedailygreen.com, Sept. 21, 2008. Accessed Oct. 20, 2009.
http://www.thedailygreen.com/environmental-news/latest/soymilk-460908

"How To Choose Food for Brain Health for Your Child." Ehow.com, accessed Jan. 2, 2010.
http://www.ehow.com/how_4542278_choose-food-brain-health-child.html

"Huge Spill of Hog Waste Fuels an Old Debate with North Carolina." *The New York Times* on the Web, June 6, 1995; accessed Jan. 20, 2009.
http://www.nytimes.com/1995/06/25/us/huge-spill-of-hog-waste-fuels-an-old-debate-in-north-carolina.html?pagewanted=1

"Humane Eating and the Three Rs." Humane Society of the United States, accessed April 14, 2010.
http://www.hsus.org/farm/humaneeating/

"Interesting facts about Spinach." Stumblerz.com, Sept. 10, 2009. Accessed Jan. 7, 2010.
http://www.stumblerz.com/interesting-facts-about-spinach/

Irani, Sarah. "Orgasmic Organics: 20 Tasty Aphrodisiacs to Put Sizzle in Your Sex Life." Ecosalon.com, Jan. 7, 2009. Accessed Nov. 26, 2009.
http://www.ecosalon.com/orgasmic-organic-aphrodisiac-foods-for-great-healthy-sex/

Jegtvig, Sheneen. "Eating Healthy Food Aids Learning." About.com, Aug. 20, 2008. Accessed Dec. 7, 2009.
http://nutrition.about.com/od/nutritionforchildren/a/dietandlearning.htm

Jerome, Louie. "10 Health Benefits of Drinking Beer." Healthmad.com, Aug., 20 2007. Accessed Jan. 5, 2010.
http://healthmad.com/health/10-health-benefits-of-drinking-beer/

"Lactose Intolerance." National Digestive Diseases Information Clearing House, accessed April 10, 2010.
http://digestive.niddk.nih.gov/ddiseases/pubs/lactoseintolerance/

Lanier, Carolyn. "The benefits of almond milk." Helium.com, accessed Feb. 9, 2010.
http://www.helium.com/items/806258-the-benefits-of-almond-milk

Laskawy, Tom. "For first time, GM soybeans may be losing favor among farmers", Grist.org, Feb. 25, 2010. Accessed March 20.
http://www.grist.org/article/for-first-time-gm-soybeans-may-be-losing-favor-among-farmers/

"Least Contaminated: The Clean Fifteen." Foodnews.org, accessed Nov. 1, 2009.
http://www.foodnews.org/methodology.php

"Low Carbon Diet." Circleofresponsibility.com, accessed Dec. 5, 2009.
http://www.circleofresponsibility.com/page/321/low-carbon-diet.htm

McManis, Sam. "Get the lowdown on soy sauce and sodium." *The Miami Herald* on the Web, Aug. 4, 2009. Accessed Jan. 4, 2010.
http://www.miamiherald.com/2009/08/04/1169204/get-the-lowdown-on-soy-sauce-and.html

McMillan, Clinton "Why is White Bread So Bad for You? What "Mono" Taught Me about White Bread." Associatedcontent.com, Aug. 1, 2007. Accessed Jan. 22, 2010.
http://www.associatedcontent.com/article/328704/why_is_white_bread_so_bad_for_you.html?cat=5

Moll, Jennifer "What is the Amount of Cholesterol You Need to Consume Each Day?" About.com, Nov. 30, 2009. Accessed Jan. 5, 2010.
http://cholesterol.about.com/od/aboutcholesterol/a/howmuch.htm

"Most Contaminated: The Dirty Dozen." Foodnews.org, accessed Nov. 1, 2009.
http://www.foodnews.org/methodology.php

Murphy, Karen. "Ten Things You Should Know About Factory Farming" Causecast.org, accessed Nov. 5, 2009.
http://www.causecast.org/news_items/8581-ten-things-you-should-know-about-factory-farming

Napolitano, Wenona. "Harmful and Unnatural Floral Practices: Flower Power." Everything.com, accessed Nov. 20, 2009. http://www.everything.com/Flower-PowerHarmful-and-Unnatural-Floral-Practices/

"Nitrates May be Environmental Trigger For Alzheimer's, Diabetes And Parkinson's Disease." Sciencedaily.com, July 6, 2009. Accessed Nov. 20, 2009. www.sciencedaily.com/releases/2009/07/090705215239.htm

Oakland, Chun Suzanne Senator "Hawaii Senate Aspartame Resolution Requesting FDA to Resind Approval for United States Markets." prlog.org, March 12, 2008. Accessed Dec. 9, 2009. http://www.prlog.org/10056715

"Obesity and overweight." World Health Organization, accessed Nov. 7, 2009. http://www.who.int/dietphysicalactivity/publications/facts/obesity/en/

Olmstead, Carol M. "Feng Shui Weight Loss Tips." Bellaonline.com, accessed Nov. 24, 2009. http://www.bellaonline.com/articles/art381.asp

"Omega-3 fatty acids." Worldshealthiestfoods.com, accessed Jan. 5, 2010. http://whfoods.com/genpage.php?tname=foodspice&dbid=84

"Organic Labeling and Marketing Information" ams.usda.gov April 2008. www.ams.usda.gov/AMSv1.0/getfile?dDocName=STELDEV3004446

"Panna: Methyl Bromide Use in California." Pesticide Action Network, accessed Jan. 14, 2010. http://www.panna.org/files/mbUseInCA.dv.html

Peng, Chan Lee. "Beware! Something Unusual May Be in Your Food", Healthmad.com, June 10, 2009. Accessed Jan 10, 2010. http://healthmad.com/nutrition/beware-something-unusual-may-be-in-your-food/

Plank, Nina. "Is Organic Food Worth the Price?" Oprah.com, accessed Jan. 20, 2010. http://www.oprah.com/food/Food-Writer-Nina-Planck_Gives-O-the-Lowdown-on-Organic-Food/print/1

Poisso, Lisa. "Cheat Sheet: 20 worst food additives" Supereco.com, June 1, 2009. Accessed Jan. 10, 2009. http://www.supereco.com/news/2009/06/01/cheat-sheet-20-worst-food-additives/

"Propylene Glycol, Alcohol." Natural-health-information-center.com, accessed Jan. 30, 2010. www.natural-health-information-centre.com/propylene-glycol.html

"Propylene Glycol." Supereco.com, Nov. 19, 2008. Accessed Dec. 20, 2009. http://www.supereco.com/glossary/propylene-glycol/

Rastegar, "Food Print-Make Green Count." *Food Safety Magazine*, Jan 2010. Accessed Feb. 3, 2010. http://www.foodsafetymagazine.com/article.asp?id=3526&sub=sub2

Readers Digest. *Food Cures: Fight Disease with Your Fork!*. New York: Reader's Digest Association, 2007.

"References." Animalfreeshopper.com, accessed Jan. 22, 2010. www.animalfreeshopper.com/References/Environment/Land.aspx

Reilly, Christopher T. "Top 20 Foods High in Antioxidants." Suite101.com, July 18, 2008. Accessed Jan. 5, 2010. http://vitamins-minerals.suite101.com/article.cfm/top_20_foods_high_in_antioxidants

Richard, Wendy "Making Sense of Food Labels." Gaiam Life, accessed Jan. 10, 2010. http://life.gaiam.com/gaiam/p/Making-Sense-of-Food-Labels.html

Roan, Shari. "Soy doesn't harm, and may even help breast cancer survivors, study finds." *Los Angeles Times* Article Collections, on the Web, Dec. 9, 2009. Accessed Jan. 5, 2010.

http://www.latimes.com/news/nationworld/nation/la-sci-soy9-2009dec09,0,6546847.story

Robbins, John "What About Soy." Foodrevolution.org, accessed Nov.2, 2009. http://www.foodrevolution.org/what_about_soy.htm

Roggio, Doran. "Go Nuts with Nuts." Health.learninginfo.org, accessed Dec. 4, 2009. http://health.learninginfo.org/health-benefits-nuts.htm

Sandborg, Alyx. "What is seitan? Nutritional facts and instructions on making a protein-rich meat substitute." Essortment.com, accessed Jan 20, 2010. http://www.essortment.com/all/whatisseitan_rkgb.htm

Sanela, "The Top 10 Aphrodisiac Foods." Alternet.org, March 23, 2009. Accessed Nov. 20, 2009. http://www.alternet.org/health/132846

Sheridan, Kate. "Free Feng Shui Tips: Kitchen Arrangement Advice." Essortment.com, accessed Nov. 24, 2009. http://www.essortment.com/home/freefengshuit_sloj.htm

Simonis, Daric. "Is Olestra Safe?" Technical Communication-University of Wisconsin, accessed Nov. 3, 2009. http://tc.engr.wisc.edu/UER/uer96/author6/index.html

"Sodium (Salt or Sodium Chloride)." Americanheart.org, accessed Feb. 4, 2010. http://www.americanheart.org/presenter.jhtml?identifier=4708

"Soymilk." Soyfoods Association of America, accessed April 10, 2010. http://www.soyfoods.org/products/soy-fact-sheets/soymilk-fact-sheet

"Soy Sauce." Foodreference.com, accessed Dec. 23, 2009. http://www.foodreference.com/html/fsoysauce.html

Stec, Laura, and Cordero, Eugene Ph.D. *Cool Cuisine: Taking the Bite Out of Global Warming.* Salt Lake City: Gibbs Smith, 2008

Stevens, Melissa, MS, RD, LD. "The Whole Truth and Nutting But the Truth", Clevelandclinic.org, accessed April 12, 2010. http://my.clevelandclinic.org/heart/prevention/nutrition/nuts.aspx

"Sustainable Dictionary." Sustainabletable.org, accessed Jan 3. 2010. http://www.sustainabletable.org/intro/dictionary/

"Sugar's effect on your health" Healingdaily.com, accessed Dec. 16, 2009. http://www.healingdaily.com/detoxification-diet/sugar.htm

"Swiss Chard" Worldshealthiestfoods.com, accessed Jan. 30, 2010. http://www.whfoods.com/genpage.php?tname=foodspice&dbid=16

Tateishi, Dr. Kazu. "Natural Remedy: Five-Element Vegetable Broth & Brown Rice Tea." Ancientpathweb.com, accessed Feb. 20, 2010. http://ancientpathweb.com/VegeBroth.aspx

"TED Case Studies: Basmati." American University, accessed Feb. 20, 2010. http://www1.american.edu/ted/basmati.htm

"The Advantages of Red Wine." Ehow.com, accessed Jan. 6, 2010. http://www.ehow.com/about_5156940_advantages-red-wine.html

"The Anti-Cancer Diet: 12 Dietary Changes That Will Lower Your Cancer Risk." Askdrsears.com, accessed Jan. 2, 2009. http://www.askdrsears.com/html/4/t040300.asp

"The Cause of a Weak Immune System." Immunesystemremedies.com, accessed Dec. 20, 2009. http://www.immunesystemremedies.com/weak-immune-system.html

"The dangers of food colorings." hubpages.com, accessed Jan. 10, 2010. http://hubpages.com/hub/The-dangers-of-food-colorings

"The Health Benefits of Eggplant." Elements4health.com, accessed Feb. 20, 2010. http://www.elements4health.com/eggplant.html

"12 Dangerous Food Additives: The Dirty Dozen Food Additives You

Really Need to be Aware of." Sixwise.com, April 5, 2006. Accessed
Dec. 20, 2009.
http://www.sixwise.com/newsletters/06/04/05/12-dangerous-food-
additives-the-dirty-dozen-food-additives-you-really-need-to-be-
aware-of.htm

V, Cat. "Fun Facts About Tea." Theteadrinker.com, Feb. 3, 2009.
Accessed Nov. 27, 2009.
http://theteadrinker.blogspot.com/2009/02/fun-facts-about-
tea.html

Vaughn, Dondra. "The Truth About Processed Foods." Farmers
Almanac, March 16 2009. Accessed Feb. 3, 2010.
www.farmersalmanac.com/recipes/a/the-truth-about-processed-foods

"Vitamin D" Mayoclinic.com, accessed Nov. 7, 2009.
www.mayoclinic.com/health/vitamin-d/NS_patient-vitamind

Voropay, Elena. "Color Therapy for Yoga." Wordpress.com, Aug. 9,
2007. Accessed Dec. 28, 2009.
http://powerofnature.wordpress.com/2007/08/09/colour-therapy-for-yoga/

Walser, Maggie L. "Carbon Footprint." Eoearth.org, Aug. 23, 2008.
Accessed Nov. 20, 2009.
http://www.eoearth.org/article/Carbon_footprint

Weiss, Jean. "12 Food Additives to Avoid" Health.msn.com, accessed
Jan. 3, 2010.
http://health.msn.com/nutrition/slideshow.aspx?cp-
documentid=100204508&imageindex=12

"What are the health benefits of tempeh?", Tempeh.info, accessed Feb
20, 2010.
http://www.tempeh.info/health/tempehhealth.php

"What is Broccolini?" Wisegeek.com, accessed Dec. 5, 2009,
http://www.wisegeek.com/what-is-broccolini.htm

Wolpe, Rabbi David. "Eating Animals: Jonathan Safran Foer's New
Book Asks Why Don't We Eat Pets?", *Huffingtonpost,* Oct 29, 2009.
Accessed April 12, 2010.
http://www.huffingtonpost.com/rabbi-david-wolpe/eating-animals-
jonathan_b_337578.html

"Worst Food Additives." Vitalearth.net, accessed Jan. 5, 2010.
http://www.vitalearth.net/dangerous_food_additives.html

"Worst Food Additives" Vitalearthminerals.com, accessed Dec. 3, 2009.
http://www.vitalearthminerals.com/v/articles/dangerous_food_
additives.html

Wuerthner, George. "Factory Farming's Long Reach." All-creatures.org,
accessed Jan. 10, 2009.
http://www.all-creatures.org/articles/env-factory.html

Walton, Geri. "Artificial Colors and Bugs" Newrinkles.com, Jan. 6,
2009. Accessed Dec. 15, 2009.
http://www.newrinkles.com/index.php/nutrition/
artificial-colors-and-bugs

Zeratsky, Katherine, R.D., L.D. "Is sea salt better for our health than
table salt." Aug. 27, 2007:accessed Jan. 20, 2010.
http://www.mayoclinic.com/health/sea-salt/AN01142

Zeratsky, Katherine R.D., L.D. "Nutrition and healthy eating"
Mayoclinic.com, Jan. 9, 2010. Accessed Feb. 5, 2010.
http://www.mayoclinic.com/health/monosodium-
glutamate/AN01251

ENDNOTES

[1] "The Anti-Cancer Diet: 12 Dietary Changes That Will Lower Your Cancer Risk." Askdrsears.com.

[2] "Obesity and overweight." Who.int.

[3] Bitten, "Real Food Can Be Cheaper Than Junk Food." *The New York Times*, Bitten.blogs.nytimes.com.

[4] Foer, *Eating Animals*, 43.

[5] Ibid., 58.

[6] "Fight Climate Change with Diet Change." Goveg.com.

[7] "Low Carbon Diet." Circleofresponsibility.com.

[8] Foer, 174.

[9] "Fact Sheet: Climate Change and Intensive Livestock Production." Beyondfactoryfarming.org.

[10] "Eating Animals: Jonathan Safran Foer's New Book Asks Why Don't We Eat Pets?." *The Huffington Post*, Huffingtonpost.com.

[11] "Fact Sheet: Climate Change and Intensive Livestock Production." Beyondfactoryfarming.org.

[12] "Facts about Pollution From Livestock Farms." Nrdc.org.

[13] "Sustainable Dictionary." Sustainabletable.org.

[14] "Huge Spill of Hog Waste Fuels an Old Debate with North Carolina," *The New York Times,* Nytimes.com.

[15] "Global Warming." Globalwarmingtruth.com.

[16] "Feed." Sustainabletable.org.

[17] "Climate Change Mitigation." Sekala.net.

[18] Goodland and Anhang, "Livestock and Climate Change: What if the key actors in Climate Change are. . .cows, pigs, and chickens?." Meatthefacts.org.

[19] Goodwin-Nguyen, "Vegetarianism is Good for the Environment: How Reducing Meat, Fish, and Poultry Consumption Helps the Planet." Suite101.com.

[20] Rastegar, "Food Print-Make Green Count." Foodsafetymagazine.org.

[21] Wuerthner, "Factory Farming's Long Reach." All-creatures.org.

[22] Ibid.

[23] "Human Eating and the Three Rs." The Humane Society, hsus.org.

[24] Earle, "Declining Ocean Biodiversity," Globalissues.org.

[25] "Global climatic change and environmental crisis and its solution." Psrast.org.

[26] "Factory Farming." Farmforward.org.

[27] "From Field To Feedlot To Fork: The Impacts of Meat and Dairy on Global Warming." Coolfoodscampaign.org.

[28] "Fight Global Warming with Food." Edf.org.

[29] Walser, "Carbon Footprint." Eoearth.org.

[30] "Carbon Footprint Calculator: What's My Carbon Footprint?." Nature.org.

[31] Geagan, *Go Green, Get Lean,* 4.

[32] Stec, and Cordero, *Cool Cuisine: Taking the Bite Out of Global Warming,* 6.

[33] "References." Animalfreeshopper.com.

[34] Stec, and Cordero, 5.

[35] Vaughn, "The Truth About Processed Foods." Farmersalmanac.com.

[36] "Diet and Physical Activity: What's the Cancer Connection?." Cancer.org.

[37] Burke, *To Buy or Not To Buy Organic,* 13.

[38] "Nitrates May be Environmental Trigger For Alzheimer's, Diabetes And Parkinson's Disease." Sciencedaily.com.

[39] Moll, "What is the Amount of Cholesterol You Need to Consume Each Day?." Cholesterol.about.com.

[40] "Sodium (Salt or Sodium Chloride)." Americanheart.org.

[41] Richard, "Making Sense of Food Labels." Life.gaiam.com.

[42] "How do I know if something is organic?." Organic.org.

[43] "Organic Labeling and Marketing Information." Agricultural Marketing Service, U.S Department of Agriculture, Ams.usda.gov.

[44] Plank, "Is Organic Food Worth the Price?." Oprah.com.

[45] Murphy, "Ten Things You Should Know About Factory Farming." Causecast.org.

[46] "About Local Harvest." Aboutlocalharvest.org.

[47] "Panna: Methyl Bromide Use in California." Panna.org.

[48] "Most Contaminated: The Dirty Dozen" Foodnews.org.

[49] "Least Contaminated: The Clean Fifteen." Foodnews.org.

[50] Poisso, "Cheat Sheet: 20 worst food additives." Supereco.com.

[51] Walton, "Artificial Colors and Bugs." Newrinkles.com.

[52] "The dangers of food colorings." Hubpages.com.

[53] "Aspartame: What is the negative side?." Medicinenet.com.

[54] Blumenthl, "10 Worst Food Additives & Where They Lurk." Life.gaiam.com.

[55] "Worst Food Additives." Vitalearthminerals.com.

[56] "FDA Should Ban Potassium Bromate and Bromated Flour." Now-public.com.

[57] "Dangerous food additives that should be avoided." Vitalearthminerals.com.

[58] "Propylene Glycol, Alcohol." Natural-health-information-center.com.

[59] "Propylene Glycol." Supereco.com.

[60] Weiss, "12 Food Additives to Avoid." Msn.com.

[61] "Worst Food Additives." Vitalearth.net.

[62] Zeratsky, "Nutrition and healthy eating." Mayoclinic.com.

[63] "12 Dangerous Food Additives: The Dirty Dozen Food Additives You Really Need to be Aware of." Sixwise.com.

64 Brodsky, "4 Food Additives to Avoid." Ezinearticles.com.

65 Simonis, "Is Olestra Safe?" Technical Communications: University of Wisconsin.

66 "12 Dangerous Food Additives: The Dirty Dozen Food Additives You Really Need to be Aware of." Sixwise.com.

67 Blumenthal, "10 Worst Food Additives & Where They Lurk." Life.gaiam.com.

68 "Sugar's effect on your health." Healingdaily.com.

69 Clark, "Evaporated Cane Juice: A Healthier Way to Sweeten Your Food." Brighthub.com.

70 "Directory of Less Refined Sweeteners." Care2.com.

71 "What are the health benefits of tempeh?." Tempeh.info.

72 "What exactly is Seitan? Nutritional facts and instructions on making a protein-rich meat substitute." Essortment.com.

73 "Beware! Something Unusual May Be in Your Food." Healthmad.com.

74 "Frequently Asked Questions." Soyfoods.org.

75 Roan, "Soy doesn't harm, and may even help breast cancer survivors, study finds." *Los Angeles Times*, latimes.com.

76 Damato, "GM-Soy Destroy the Earth and Humans for Profit" Naturalnews.com.

77 Robbins, "What About Soy." Foodrevolution.org.

78 "Lactose Intolerance." National Digestive Diseases Information Clearinghouse, digestive.niddk.gov.

79 "Soymilk." Soyfoods.org.

80 "Vitamin D," Mayoclinic.com.

81 Campbell and Campbell, *The China Study*, 6.

82 Group, "The Benefits of Organic Hemp Milk." Hemp.org.

83 "How Healthful is Soy?." Thedailygreen.com.

84 McMillen, "Why is White Bread So Bad for You? What "Mono" Taught Me about White Bread." Associatedcontent.com.

85 Barley, "White Bread vs. Wheat Bread." Vegetariantimes.com.

86 "Dangerous Food Additives." Vitalearthminerals.com.

87 "Choosing the right cooking oil." Pccnaturalmarkets.com.

88 *Readers Digest: Food Cures: Fight Disease with Your Fork!*, 14-25.

89 "The Whole Truth and Nutting But the Truth." Clevelandclinic.org.

90 "Almonds, Soaked and Dehydrated." Shapeyou.com.

91 Jegtvig, "Eating Healthy Food Aids Learning." About.com.

92 "5 Ways Your Breakfast Affects Your Mood." Wellsphere.com.

93 "How To Choose Food for Brain Health for Your Child." Ehow.com.

94 Heppard, "Foods for Brain Health. A Healthy Brain depends on Healthy Eating." Suite101.com.

95 "Interesting facts about Spinach." Stumblerz.com.

96 Montala, "Health Benefits of Lemon Grass." Buzzle.com.

97 "Aphrodisiac Foods." Gourmetsleuth.com.

98 Irani, "Orgasmic Organics: 20 Tasty Aphrodiacs to Put Sizzle in Your Sex Life." Ecosalon.com.

99 Sanela, "The Top 10 Aphrodisiac Foods." Alternet.org.

100 "Aphrodisiac Foods." Gourmetsleuth.com.

101 Craven, "What is Feng Shui? Architects and designers find inspiration in ancient Eastern ideas." About.com.

102 Sheridan, "Free Feng Shui Tips: Kitchen Arrangement Advice." Essortment.com.

103 "Feng Shui Kitchen Made Easy." Crystalsbay.net.

104 Voropay, "Color Therapy for Yoga," Powerofnature.wordpress.com.

105 Olmstead, "Feng Shui Weight Loss Tips." Bellaonline.com.

106 "The Cause of a Weal Immune System." Immunesystemremedies.com.

107 Food Cures, 104 108.

108 Ibid.,198.

109 "TED Case Studies: Basmati." *American University*, American.edu.

110 Group, "The Health Benefits of Olive Oil." Globalhealingcenter.com.

111 "What is Broccolini?." Wisegeek.com.

112 "Definition of Free Radicals." Antioxidant-health-benefits.com.

113 Dalelden, "1100 + Antioxidant-Rich Food's Studied and Ranked." Suite101.com.

114 Food Cures, 39.

115 Reilly, "Top 20 Foods High in Antioxidants." Suite101.com.

116 Roggio, "Go Nuts with Nuts." Health.learninginfo.org.

117 "Green Tea." Umm.edu.

118 "The Advantages of Red Wine." Ehow.com.

119 "Swiss Chard." Whfoods.com.

120 Tateishi, "Natural Remedy: Five-Element Vegetable Broth & Brown Rice Tea." Ancientpathweb.com.

121 "Dictionary-Soy Sauce." Answers.com.

122 McManis, "Get the lowdown on soy sauce and sodium." *The Miami Herald*, Miamiherald.com.

123 "For first time, GM soybeans may be losing favor among farmers." Grist.org.

124 "Soy Sauce." Foodreference.com.

125 "Bell Peppers." Whfoods.com.

126 Jerome, "10 Health Benefits of Drinking Beer." Healthmad.com.

127 "The Health Benefits of Eggplant." Elements4health.com.

128 Zeratsky, "Is sea salt better for our health than table salt." Mayoclinic.com.

129 Lanier, "The benefits of almond milk." Helium.com.

130 Oakland, "Hawaii Senate Asoartame Resolution Requesting FDA to Rescind Approval for United States Markets." Prlog.org.

131 "Healthy Nutritious Super Foods for Perfect Health." knoll.google.com

132 "Black Tea or Green Tea—Which is Healthier?." About.com.

133 V, "Fun Facts About Tea." Theteadrinkerblogspot.com.

134 Coleman, "Health benefits of mint tea." Examiner.com.

ACKNOWLEDGMENTS

Thank you to my amazing team at Running Press for all of your support, enthusiasm, and dedication: Jennifer Kasius, Seta Zink, Craig Herman, Chris Navratil, Josh McDonnell, and Peter Costanzo. I will always be in debt to you for helping shape my career. To my agent, Laura Dail, thank you for always looking out for me, and for exuding the right mix of kindness, compassion, and business savvy to help me discover what I was meant to do.

To Denise Vivaldo and your super-talented team at Food Fanatics, the amount of time, energy and passion you put into your everyday work has never failed to shine through the end result. To say you are a joy to be around would be a mere understatement. To food photographer, Matt Armendariz, and his assistant, Teri Lyn Fisher, thank you for bringing such beauty and life to my book. It was exactly what I wanted. My dear friend Candice Kumai, I am so grateful for your friendship, and I am forever inspired by your passion for food and life. To Noriyuki Sugie, Amy Jurist, and Christy Morgan, you are brilliant chefs and cooks. It is people like you that encourage me to not be afraid to try new things in the kitchen, for you have perfected the art. To my interns, Lisa Hayim and Elise Mische, thank you for all the hours and weekends you put into research and fact checking for this cookbook. I'm counting on you hardworking women to help educate a new generation on eating healthier and treating animals with the love and respect they deserve.

Stephanie Macy-Hanses, you gave me something that was debatably the most important to creating this cookbook. You gave me *time*. Knowing that my little one was safe and happy in your hands gave me minimal working mother guilt.

Sarah Rosenhaus, god bless your amazing design talent, and thank you for being such a good "mommy friend." You help keep me sane.

Julie C. May, thank you for your friendship, hard work, and uplifting spirit. Healthy Bitch Daily would be nothing if it weren't for you and your love for starting new things.

Carly Harrill, you have helped me in so many ways. Thank you for your creativity, attention to detail, late-night slumber parties in my office, and for helping me bring something so big to life. I'm grateful to have you as a friend, as well.

To my good friends, Jesse Sarr and Ali Benden, I completely dropped off the face of the earth while working on this book, but know that I am grateful for your unconditional friendship, encouragement, and support.

Erin Mathis, you are truly one of a kind. Thank you for your benevolence, and for your generous heart.

Kay Warren, you inspire me to be a better person and I thank you from the bottom of my heart for all of your kindness and for walking with me in the beginning of my new journey.

Keesha Whitehurst Fredricksen, thank you isn't enough for all that you bring to my life. I cherish your support, guidance, humor, and love. Let's do this, sister.

To my parents Rob and Linda, thank you for being so amazing and allowing me to find my own path in life. It might just be safe to say I found it. To my sisters, Jeri and Chrissy, my nieces Amanda, Melissa, and Alex, and my nephew Elliot, all my love.

To my husband Stephane, the words *thank you* will never quite be enough. I am blessed for your patience while I worked non-stop on this book, and for reminding me what is important when things get overwhelming. Your brilliance as a chef is what helped me realize that I had a love for it, too. You are my cheerleader. You are my rock. You are my love. *Je T'Aime*.

Jack, I didn't know it was humanly possible to love someone as much as I love you. Thank you for choosing me as your mommy. You have brought an eternity of joy into my soul, and I promise to do my best to inspire you to follow your heart. I hope one day you will understand that this was all for you.

Last but certainly not least, I want to send all my love and everlasting gratitude to the fans around the world that have made *Skinny Bitch* such a success. You inspire me every day to get my ass to work, and help women empower themselves to get healthy. Watching strong, independent women make a difference in this world is what gave me the strength to move forward with an idea that some thought would never catch on. You are my role models.

CHEF CONTRIBUTORS

DENISE VIVALDO

Denise Vivaldo is a jack of all cooking trades. An author, spokesperson, educator, culinary producer, and product consultant, Denise has been a professionally trained chef for 25 years. Catering more than 10,000 parties in her lifetime, Denise has cooked for such prominent personalities as Ronald Reagan, Prince Charles, Bette Midler, Cher, Arnold Schwarzenneger, and Maria Shriver. Her company, Food Fanatics, specializes in food styling, recipe development, and support for cookbooks. www.foodfanatics.net

NORIYUKI SUGIE

Chef Noriyuki Sugie has traveled the globe to perfect his unique signature style that melds traditional Japanese cuisine with classic French technique. His resume includes stints working with renowned chefs like Yutaka Ishinabe in Japan, Michel Trama in France, and Tetsuya Wakuda in Australia, before embarking on his culinary odyssey in America at prestigious restaurants like Charlie Trotter's in Chicago and Asiate at the Mandarin Oriental Hotel in New York. Under his new umbrella, IRONNORI, Chef Nori now works as an international consultant to create concepts and menus for gourmet restaurants and bistros. www.ironnori.com

CHRISTY MORGAN

Christy Morgan, "The Blissful Chef," is a vegan macrobiotic chef residing in Los Angeles, California. She has helped foodies transition to a healthier, happier lifestyle with her personal chef services and cooking classes. Her blog includes recipes, cooking videos, health information, and more on ways you can live a blissful life with delicious food and optimal health. www.theblissfulchef.com

AMY JURIST

A personal chef and in-demand caterer, Amy Jurist is the owner and founder of Amy's Culinary Adventures. She began her culinary education abroad in France and Switzerland attending classes through CIA-Hyde Park, before returning to Hollywood to formalize her training at the professional program at the Westlake Culinary Institute. Aside from her catering business, Chef Amy has mastered creativity behind the stove with a series of the most sought-after underground "bootleg" dinners (aka "food raves") in Southern California. www.amysculinaryadventures.com

INDEX